Yearbook of Pediatric Endocrinology 2007

Endorsed by the European Society for Paediatric Endocrinology

Editors

Jean-Claude Carel
Ze'ev Hochberg

Associate Editors

John C. Achermann
Gary Butler
Francesco Chiarelli
Mehul Dattani
Heiko Krude
Claire Levy-Marchal
Mohamad Maghnie
Ken Ong
Lars Sävendahl
Olle Söder
Martin Wabitsch
Stefan A. Wudy

KARGER

Sponsored by a grant from Pfizer Endocrine Care

© Copyright 2007 by S. Karger AG, P.O. Box, CH–4009 Basel (Switzerland)
www.karger.com
Printed in Switzerland on acid-free paper by Reinhardt Druck, Basel
ISBN 978–3–8055–8324–4

Claire Levy-Marchal

Unité 690 INSERM, Hôpital Robert Debré
FR–75935 Paris Cedex 19, France
E-Mail Claire.Levy-Marchal@rdebre.inserm.fr

Mohamad Maghnie

Department of Pediatrics, IRCCS Giannina Gaslini
University of Genova
Largo G. Gaslini, IT–16147 Genova, Italy
Tel. +39 0105636574; Fax +39 0105538265; E-Mail mohamadmaghnie@ospedale-gaslini.ge.it

Ken Ong

Medical Research Council Epidemiology Unit
Institute of Metabolic Science, Addenbrooke's Hospital, Box 285
Cambridge CB2 0QQ, UK
Tel. +44 (0)1223 330315; Fax +44 (0)1223 330316; E-Mail ken.ong@mrc-epidcam.ac.uk

Lars Sävendahl

Pediatric Endocrinology Unit; Q2:08
Karolinska Institutet, Department of Woman and Child Health
Karolinska University Hospital, Solna, SE–17176 Stockholm, Sweden
Tel. +46 8 517 72369; Fax +46 8 517 75128; E-Mail lars.savendahl@ki.se

Olle Söder

Pediatric Endocrinology Unit, Q2:08
Karolinska Institutet, Department of Woman and Child Health
Karolinska University Hospital, Solna, SE–17176 Stockholm, Sweden
Tel. +46 8 517 75124; Fax +46 8 517 75128; E-Mail olle.soder@kbh.ki.se

Martin Wabitsch

Pediatric Endocrinology, Diabetes and Obesity Unit, Department of Pediatrics and Adolescent Medicine
University of Ulm, Eythstrasse 24
DE–89075 Ulm, Germany
Tel. +49 731 5002 6714; +49 731 5002 7789; E-Mail martin.wabitsch@uniklinik-ulm.de

Stefan A. Wudy

Pediatric Endocrinology and Diabetology
Steroid Research and Mass Spectrometry Unit, Center of Child and Adolescent Medicine
Justus Liebig University, Giessen
Feulgenstrasse 12
DE–35392 Giessen, Germany
Tel. +49 641 994 3410; Fax +49 641 994 3419; E-Mail stefan.wudy@paediat.med.uni-giessen.de

Table of Contents

Preface

Dozens of supporting experiments, hundreds of sustaining observations, and even the successful engineering of ingenious machines that are based on a theory, do not make a scientific theory eternal. The temporary nature of scientific theories is one of science's most remarkable features. This apparent weakness of science is also one of its main strengths. It is a common error to assume that scientific theories are certain and forever true. Theories hold true only for the experimental conditions that supports them, and they do not seize an all-inclusive truth about a subject. This temporary nature of science is the foundation of our *Yearbook of Pediatric Endocrinology*.

The 2007 *Yearbook of Pediatric Endocrinology* brings you abstracts of articles that reported the year's breakthrough developments in the basic sciences and evidence-based new knowledge in clinical research and clinical practice that are relevant to the field.

Increasingly, we now cite articles from the Public Library of Science (PLoS) journals, which has revolutionized the journals arena. PLoS provides open access to works of exceptional significance in all areas of biological science, but has also developed tools and materials to engage the interest and imagination of the public, and help non-scientists to understand and enjoy scientific discoveries and the scientific process.

This is the fourth volume of the *Yearbook of Pediatric Endocrinology*, and traditionally the Associate Editors will present their chapters at the 2007 European Society for Paediatric Endocrinology (ESPE) annual meeting in Helsinki. Our twelve Associate Editors and their coauthors have done an enormous work to discover this year's advances, and provide their chapters in a timely fashion.

We wish to also acknowledge for the fourth year in a row the generous support by Pfizer that makes the Yearbook project possible.

Readers of all four volumes of the Yearbook might have wondered whether the cover color has a meaning, and what it represents. It is known as IKB 79 [International (Ives) Klein Blue], a distinctive ultramarine which Ives Klein registered as a trademark color in 1957. He considered that this color had a quality close to pure space and he associated it with immaterial values beyond what can be seen or touched. In his words, 'Blue has no dimensions, it is beyond dimensions. At first there is nothing, then there is profound nothing, after that a blue profundity. Other colors bring associations to concrete, material and tangible ideas, while blue recalls at most the sky and the sea, but also Western spirituality and Eastern mysticism, the symbol of eternity and … what is most abstract in tangible and visible nature'. We invite the reader to contemplation in line with our cover's Blue.

Ze'ev Hochberg (Haifa)
Jean-Claude Carel (Paris)

Pituitary

Mohamad Maghnie[a], Andrea Secco[a] and Sandro Loche[b]

[a]Department of Pediatrics, Istituto di Ricovero e Cura a Carattere Scientifico, Giannina Gaslini, University of Genova, Italy
[b]Ospedale Regionale per le Microcitemie, Cagliari, Italy

Mechanism of the year

A new progeroid syndrome reveals that genotoxic stress suppresses the somatotroph axis

Niedernhofer LJ, Garinis GA, Raams A, Lalai AS, Robinson AR, Appeldoorn E, Odijk H, Oostendorp R, Ahmad A, van Leeuwen W, Theil AF, Vermeulen W, van der Horst GT, Meinecke P, Kleijer WJ, Vijg J, Jaspers NG, Hoeijmakers JH

Center for Biomedical Genetics, Medical Genetic Center, Department of Cell Biology and Genetics, Erasmus Medical Center, Rotterdam, The Netherlands

Nature 2006;444:1038–1043

Background: Experimental evidence reconciling the apparently disparate mechanisms of progeroid syndrome and natural ageing is lacking. Patients with xeroderma pigmentosum (XPF) carrying a mutation and severe progeroid symptoms, along with mice-generated models, may serve to understand mechanisms related to ageing.

Methods: Cell lines were established from skin biopsies of patients or from mouse embryos. Nucleotide excision repair was measured by a clonogenic survival assay after exposure of cells to UV irradiation. Transcription-coupled nucleotide excisin repair and XPF-ERCC1, an endonuclease required for repair of helix-distorting DNA lesions, were measured. XPF cDNA were sequenced and Ercc1$^{-/-}$ mice were generated. IGF-1 and insulin concentrations were determined.

Results: Ercc1$^{-/-}$ mice showed mild retardation and growth arrest in the second week followed by death at 4 weeks. There was a striking similarity between the symptoms of patients and mice as well as between their final outcomes. Expression data from XPF–ERCC1-deficient mice indicated increased cell death and antioxidant defenses, a shift towards anabolism, and reduced GH/IGF-1 signalling.

Conclusion: DNA damage triggers a highly conserved metabolic response, either directly or by interfering with transcription or replication through the GH/IGF-1/insulin pathway, responsible for resources shifting from growth to somatic preservation and life extension.

Several progeroid syndromes are caused by defects in cellular response to DNA damage, including Cockayne syndrome, Werner syndrome, ataxia telangiectasia and trichothiodystrophy, suggesting a close relationship between ageing and genome maintenance. On the other hand, the mitogenic GH/IGF-1 pathway is a determinant of lifespan as shown by the fact that prolonged dampening of the axis genetically or by caloric restriction promotes longevity, whereas persistent upregulation shortens life. Nucleotide excision repair is a multistep 'cut-and-patch' mechanism that removes distorting lesions affecting one strand of DNA, such as those resulting from ultraviolet radiation damage. Two subpathways exist: (1) transcription-coupled nucleotide excision repair – its defect causes Cockayne syndrome and trichothiodystrophy – which removes lesions that block RNA polymerases and rescues transcription and prevents cell death, and (2) global genome nucleotide excision repair – its defect causes XPF – which operates genome-wide preventing mutations. In this study, the authors describe a 15-year-old boy with severe XPF mutation and a combination of progeroid symptoms and sunburn. In addition, the Ercc1$^{-/-}$ mice model exhibits a similar phenotype and pattern of senescence of the patient with the XPF defect. In these mice, circulating insulin and IGF-1 levels were reduced without any evidence of hypothalamic-pituitary defect, suggesting a possible suppression of the GH axis as an adaptive response to DNA damage. Diverse metabolic changes and increased apoptotic cells in the Ercc1$^{-/-}$ mice were similarly altered in aged mice. This model is in favor of the hypothesis that ageing is genetically regulated but is also the consequence of the accumulation of stochastic damage which in turn is responsible for functional decline.

The human growth hormone gene contains a silencer embedded within an Alu repeat in the 3'-flanking region

Trujillo MA, Sakagashira M, Eberhardt NL
Department of Medicine, Mayo Clinic/Mayo Foundation, Rochester, Minn., USA
Mol Endocrinol 2006;20:2559–2575

Background: Alu family sequences consist of middle, repetitive short interspersed elements spread throughout vertebrate genomes. Although most Alu repeats are transcriptionally silent, they might have a functional role and may even contribute to genetic diseases. The 3'-flanking region of human growth hormone (hGH)-1 and hGH-2 genes contains an Sx Alu repeat, whose close proximity to the hGH coding region makes it an ideal candidate for studying the potential transcription role of these sequences. *Methods:* Plasmid construction, deletion of the sequences 3' containing the 3' Alu element, and functional analysis of the hGH-1 3'-flanking region sequences were carried out. *Results:* hGH expression in transfected rat anterior pituitary tumor cell (GC) cells was increased in the reporter constructs in which the Sx Alu sequences were deleted. This result is consistent with the hypothesis of the presence of a repressor element within this region, mapping between nts 2158 and 2572 (the region comprising the Sx Alu repeat). Functional analysis and gene sequences lead to the identification of four discrete entities that are essential for silencer function: a core repressor domain, an anti-silencer domain (comprising mediators of the orientation-independent silencer activity), and two domains flanking the core repressor domain/anti-silencer domain that regulate silencer activity in a core repressor domain-dependent manner. The hGH-1 silencer was found to be active in human placental syncytiotrophoblast, supporting the hypothesis that the hGH 3'-flanking region silencer is a tissue-specific element and promoter-dependent. The silencer was able to inhibit transcription by a mechanism involving histone deacetylation, resulting in a significant decrease of RNA polymerase II recruitment to the promoter. *Conclusion:* This study provides a comprehensive functional analysis of the hGH 3'-flanking region sequences and found that a silencer/anti-silencer cassette resides in the proximal 3'-flanking region of the hGH gene.

As they are the most effectively transposed primate-specific short interspersed elements, Alu elements are present in more than 1 million copies in the human genome and include most recently transposed subsets of AluY elements that are polymorphic in humans. Although Alu elements are commonly thought to play an essential role in the shaping and functioning of primate genomes, the understanding of the impact of recent Alu insertions on human gene expression is far from being comprehensive. Mobilization of Alu elements is thought to occur through an RNA polymerase III-derived transcript by means of a retroposition process. The effect does not depend on sequences of Alu elements and their orientation, but is likely to be cell type specific [1]. Although Alu sequences accumulate preferentially in gene-rich regions, the probability that the insertion event occurs within or in a coding region is extremely low; consequently, Alu insertions would contribute to only 0.1% of genetic diseases, and their consequences at the molecular level have only been studied in a few cases. Alu-containing exons may also be skipped through an Alu-mediated rearrangement, as in Hunter disease, or as in Apert syndrome, through disruption of a *FGFR2* splice site. Skipping of an Alu-containing exon has also been described in the *BRCA2* gene for breast cancer, as well as in *HESX1* transcript carrying a deletion of exon 3, leading to pituitary aplasia and coloboma. Although Alu sequences have been associated with silencing activity in many genes, the data presented in this study represent the most detailed dissection of the specific Alu sequences that mediate silencing activity. Further studies will be required to establish whether the domains in the hGH-1 3'Alu element are related to those that mediate repression in other gene systems or whether the hGH-associated 3'Alu members have evolved specialized regulatory features, including those domains that lie outside the Alu repeat which are involved in modulating silencer function.

Mohamad Maghnie/Andrea Secco/Sandro Loche

Identification of novel peptide hormones in the human proteome by hidden Markov model screening

Mirabeau O, Perlas E, Severini C, Audero E, Gascuel O, Possenti R, Birney E, Rosenthal N, Gross C
Mouse Biology Unit, EMBL, Monterotondo, Italy
Genome Res 2007;17:320–327

Background: Several methods have been used to identify new peptide hormones, including biochemical purification coupled with functional assays. The advent of genomic sequence and bioinformatics search strategies has contributed to the development of more powerful systematic bioinformatics methods.

Methods: A bioinformatics search tool based on the hidden Markov model formalism that uses several peptide hormone sequence features to estimate the likelihood that a protein contains a processed and secreted peptide of this class was employed.

Results: This method allows for the identification of two novel peptide hormones named spexin and augurin. Biochemical investigations revealed their presence in secretory granules in a transfected pancreatic cell line. Spexin was expressed in the submucosal layer of the mouse esophagus and stomach. Augurin was found to be expressed in mouse endocrine tissues, such as pituitary and adrenal tissue, as well as in the choroids plexus and atrioventricular node of the heart.

Conclusion: This study proposes the use of a bioinformatics tool to identify novel peptide hormones that might be actively involved in endocrine homeostasis.

The study of peptide hormones has received considerable attention because of their role in modulating a wide range of physiological functions. In fact a large group of peptide hormones serves as both hormones and neurotransmitters as they are secreted into the bloodstream by endocrine cells and released into the synapse by neurons. Peptide hormones are short peptides (<100 amino acids) produced by the proteolytic cleavage of pre-pro-hormone precursors. Following signal peptide removal by the signal peptidase complex, the pro-hormone undergoes cleavage at specific sites by pro-hormone convertases. In many cases, processed peptides undergo post-translational modification, with <50% of peptide hormones becoming amidated at their C-terminus. Mature peptides pass through the secretory pathway and are released into extracellular space, where they can bind to specific cell surface receptors and modulate cellular functions. Several methods have been used to identify new peptide hormones including biochemical purification and functional assays. This study used a sequence-based approach to identify two candidate novel peptide hormones called spexin and augurin, both co-localized with insulin in the secretory pathway; they were processed and secreted following transfection in endocrine cells. This is an additional example that shows that such peptide hormone symbiosis is likely to exist, i.e. obestatin and salusin, produced by the ghrelin and Torsin2A genes, respectively. These findings confirm that peptide hormones in the human proteome can be identified using a bioinformatics approach and that this method could be useful for the systematic screening of proteomes for biologically active peptides.

Important for clinical practice

HESX1 mutations are an uncommon cause of septo-optic dysplasia and hypopituitarism

McNay DE, Turton JP, Kelberman D, Woods KS, Brauner R, Papadimitriou A, Keller E, Keller A, Haufs N, Krude H, Shalet SM, Dattani MT
Biochemistry, Endocrinology, and Metabolism Unit, Institute of Child Health, London, UK
m.dattani@ich.ucl.ac.uk
J Clin Endocrinol Metab 2007;92:691–697

Background: Mutations in the transcription factor HESX1 were described in patients with septo-optic dysplasia and hypopituitarism.

Methods: Patients with either septo-optic dysplasia or isolated pituitary dysfunction, optic nerve hypoplasia, or midline neurological abnormalities were screened for mutations in the HESX1 gene. Molecular analysis was performed by heteroduplex detection for mutations in the coding and regulatory regions of the gene.

Results: A novel functionally significant heterozygous mutation (E149K) was found in a patient with isolated GH deficiency and digital abnormalities. The overall incidence of coding region mutations was <1%.

Conclusions: Mutations of HESX1 gene are a rare cause of septo-optic dysplasia and hypopituitarism.

Hormonal, pituitary magnetic resonance, LHX4 and HESX1 evaluation in patients with hypopituitarism and ectopic posterior pituitary lobe

Melo ME, Marui S, Carvalho LR, Arnhold IJ, Leite CC, Mendonca BB, Knoepfelmacher M
Unidade de Endocrinologia do Desenvolvimento, Laboratorio de Hormonios e Genetica Molecular LIM 42, Disciplina de Endocrinologia, HCFMUSP, Brazil
medna@usp.br
Clin Endocrinol (Oxf) 2007;66:95–102

Background: LHX4 and HESX1 are transcription factors which play a crucial role in early stages of pituitary development. Mutations in the genes encoding for these proteins cause hypopituitarism which can be associated with ectopic posterior lobe. This study analyzed LHX4 and HESX1 genes and characterized pituitary hormone profiles and their relationships with magnetic resonance imaging (MRI) findings.

Methods: 62 patients with hypopituitarism and ectopic posterior lobe were evaluated. Molecular analysis of LHX4 and HESX1 genes was performed by PCR and automatic sequencing.

Results: In 42 patients, the pituitary stalk was not visualized at MRI whereas in 20 the pituitary stalk was visible. Most patients (95%) with non-visible stalk had combined pituitary hormone deficiency with ACTH deficiency in 85%. In patients with visible pituitary stalk, combined pituitary hormone deficiency was found in 50% of the cohort while ACTH deficiency occurred in 20%. The frequency of ectopic posterior lobe was found to be similar whether the stalk was visible or not. No mutations of the two genes were identified. Three new polymorphisms of the LHX4 gene were found.

Conclusions: Mutations of LHX4 and HESX1 genes are rare causes of hypopituitarism.

Genetic screening of combined pituitary hormone deficiency: experience in 195 patients

Reynaud R, Gueydan M, Saveanu A, Vallette-Kasic S, Enjalbert A, Brue T, Barlier A
Laboratoire de Biochimie et Biologie Moléculaire, Hôpital de la Conception, Marseille, France
J Clin Endocrinol Metab 2006;91:3329–3336

Background: Combined pituitary hormone deficiency can be caused by mutations in transcription factor genes. This study screened a large number of patients with combined pituitary hormone deficiency for mutations known to cause hypopituitarism.

Methods: 195 patients with CPHD from the international GENHYPOPIT network were studied for mutations in POU1F1, PROP1, LHX3, LHX4, and HESX1 genes.

Results: Total prevalence of mutations was 13.3 and 52.4% in 20 patients with familial combined pituitary hormone deficiency. No mutations in HESX1 gene were found in 16 patients with septo-optic dysplasia. A mutation of the LHX4 gene was found in one familial case of combined pituitary hormone deficiency. No mutations in LHX3 gene were found in 109 patients with no extrapituitary abnormalities; 20 had a PROP1 mutation. A mutation in Pit1 gene was found in 1 patient with GH and TSH deficiency.

Conclusions: Mutations in PROP1 gene are the most frequent type in patients with combined pituitary hormone deficiency.

The pathophysiology of combined pituitary hormone deficiency is just beginning to be elucidated, with mutations in genes encoding transcription factors expressed at different stages of pituitary development. Several transcription factors are involved in pituitary development and in the regulation of the transcription of specific pituitary genes. Among them, two closely related genes, LHX3 and LHX4, are believed to share redundant biological properties. LHX3 and LHX4 are members of the LIM homeodomain family of transcription factors and are essential for normal pituitary development. Mutations in the LHX3 gene cause combined pituitary hormone deficiency with rigid cervical spine. More recently, mutations of the LHX3 gene have also been found associated with milder

Table 1. Summary of current gene/MRI correlations in congenital hypopituitarism

Gene	Prevalence	Prevalence among familial cases	Hormone deficiencies	MRI findings					
				Ectopic posterior pituitary	Small anterior pituitary	Skull base abnormalities	Pituitary stalk abnormalities	Optic nerve abnormalities	Extra-pituitary abnormalities
HESX1	<1% of cases labeled as SOD		•	•	•	•	•	•	•
LHX4	2.5%[1]	increased	•	•	•	•	•		•
PROP1	≈20% of cases with PP in place	50%	•		•[2]				
POU1F1	1/17 (5.8%)		•		•[3]				

Data are collected from: McNay et al., J Clin Endocrinol Metab 2007; Melo et al., Clin Endocrinol (Oxf) 2007; Reynaud et al., J Clin Endocrinol Metab 2006, and from previous publications on the topic cited herein.

[1]Based on 1/39 reported by Reynaud et al.: JCEM 2006. The case has been already described by Machinis K et al., Am J Hum Genet 2001;69:961–968 (two families were described).

[2]PROP1: anterior pituitary gland can be small, normal or large.

[3]POU1F1: anterior pituitary gland can be normal with evolution to small pituitary.

hypopituitary phenotypes including isolated GH deficiency. Mutations in the HESX1 gene have been described in association with septo-optic dysplasia, with pituitary aplasia as well with isolated defects of the hypothalamic-pituitary axis. Human PROP-1 gene mutations induce combined pituitary hormone deficiency that includes GH, PRL, TSH, gonadotrope and sometimes late ACTH deficiency. Mutations in POU1F1, also known as PITt-1, are associated with GH, TSH, and prolactin deficiency. These three studies show that mutations in LHX3, LHX4 and HESX1 genes are a rare cause of hypopituitarism and septo-optic dysplasia. Mutations of PROP1 gene are the most frequent and therefore remain the first to be looked for. Mutations in PIT-1 gene should be looked for in patients with GH and TSH deficiency. Establishing endocrine and MRI phenotypes is extremely helpful in the selection and management of patients with hypopituitarism, both in terms of possible genetic counselling and for early diagnosis of evolving anterior pituitary hormone deficiencies (table 1).

Adult height in patients with permanent growth hormone deficiency with and without multiple pituitary hormone deficiencies

Maghnie M, Ambrosini L, Cappa M, Pozzobon G, Ghizzoni L, Ubertini MG, di Iorgi N, Tinelli C, Pilia S, Chiumello G, Lorini R, Loche S
Department of Pediatrics, Istituto di Ricovero e Cura a Carattere Scientifico Giannina Gaslini, University of Genoa, Genoa, Italy
mohamadmaghnie@ospedale-gaslini.ge.it
J Clin Endocrinol Metab 2006;91:2900–2905

Background: Adult height in childhood-onset growth hormone deficiency (GHD) has been reported as being greater in patients with multiple pituitary hormone deficiencies than in patients with isolated GHD. These data, however, have not been based on the re-evaluation of GH status after adult height achievement and in addition the outcome of patients with permanent isolated GHD has not been adequately evaluated.

Methods: This was a retrospective multicenter study conducted in university research hospitals and a tertiary referral endocrine unit. 39 patients with IGHD (26 males, 13 females) and 49 with multiple pituitary hormone deficiencies (31 males, 18 females) were re-valuated for GH secretion after adult height achievement. GHD was based on peak GH levels <3 µg/l after an insulin tolerance test or peak GH <5 µg/l after two other tests. Magnetic resonance imaging (MRI) showed congenital hypothalamic-pituitary abnormalities in 73 patients, while no relevant MRI alterations were seen in 15 subjects. Height SD score (SDS) was analyzed at GHD diagnosis, at the onset of puberty (either spontaneous or pharmacological), and at the time of GH withdrawal.

Results: Median height SDS at diagnosis was not significantly different between isolated GHD and multiple pituitary hormone deficiencies patients. Those with isolated GHD entered puberty at a median age of 12.6 years in girls and 13.4 years in boys. In multiple pituitary hormone deficiencies, puberty was induced at a median age of 13.5 years in girls and 14.0 years in boys. Median height SDS at Tanner stage II was similar in both isolated GHD and multiple pituitary hormone-deficient patients. No significant differences in median height SDS were seen at the beginning of puberty between IGHD and MPHD subjects, or in total pubertal height gain and in median adult height (males 168.5 vs. 170.3 cm, females 160.0 vs. 157.3 cm). A positive correlation was found between adult height SDS of the IGHD subjects, height at the time of diagnosis and total pubertal height gain. Differently, adult height SDS of the multiple pituitary hormone-deficient subjects showed a positive correlation with both the duration of GH treatment and height SDS at the time of GHD diagnosis.

Conclusion: No significant differences exist in adult height between patients with permanent isolated GHD with spontaneous puberty and multiple pituitary hormone deficiencies with induced puberty.

In this study, patients with multiple pituitary hormone deficiencies and those with isolated GHD reached similar adult heights, regardless of the timing of puberty, a finding that directly contradicts most earlier studies in the literature. Indeed, the current body of literature suggests that patients with multiple pituitary hormone deficiencies reach a taller adult height than patients with isolated GHD. However, these studies may be biased because no distinction between patients with permanent GHD and transitory GHD within the isolated GHD group was considered. Thus, when GHD is permanent (a diagnosis that should be confirmed in adulthood), GH therapy results in an adult height that is comparable to that of isolated GHD and multiple pituitary hormone-deficient subjects. In fact, this study suggests that the delaying puberty does not increase adult height gain.

Clinical characterization of familial isolated pituitary adenomas

Daly AF, Jaffrain-Rea ML, Ciccarelli A, Valdes-Socin H, Rohmer V, Tamburrano G, Borson-Chazot C, Estour B, Ciccarelli E, Brue T, Ferolla P, Emy P, Colao A, De Menis E, Lecomte P, Penfornis F, Delemer B, Bertherat J, Wemeau JL, De Herder W, Archambeaud F, Stevenaert A, Calender A, Murat A, Cavagnini F, Beckers A
Department of Endocrinology, Centre Hospitalier Universitaire de Liège, Domaine Universitaire du Sart Tilman, Liège, Belgium
J Clin Endocrinol Metab 2006;91:3316–3323

Background: Familial pituitary adenomas usually occur in the context of multiple endocrine neoplasia type 1 (MEN1) or Carney Complex (CNC). This article presents an international, multicenter, retrospective study to identify non-MEN1/CNC families with isolated pituitary adenomas. The characteristics of families with isolated pituitary adenomas and their phenotypic presentation were analyzed and compared with a matched population of patients with sporadic pituitary tumors.

Methods: Families with isolated pituitary adenomas are defined as families containing two or more members with anterior pituitary tumors and no evidence of MEN1 or CNC. Molecular genetic analysis of the MEN1 and PRKAR1A genes was performed to exclude MEN1 or CNC. The study analyzed patients between 1970 and 2004 and was performed in 22 centers in Belgium, France, Italy and The Netherlands. The control group comprised 2,600 patients with sporadic pituitary adenoma. Immunohistochemistry for LH, FSH, TSH, GH, prolactin, ACTH and α-subunit was carried out in the tumor tissue of 74 patients who underwent surgery.

Results: A total of 64 families with isolated pituitary tumors were identified, which included 138 affected individuals (52 males, 86 females). 55 were prolactinomas, 47 somatotropinomas, 28 non-secreting adenomas, and 8 ACTH-secreting tumors. A single tumor phenotype occurred in 30 families, and heterogeneous phenotype in 34. Patients with FIPA were younger at diagnosis than sporadic cases. Macroadenomas

were more frequent in heterogeneous than in homogeneous FIPA families. Prolactinomas from heterogeneous families were larger and had more frequent suprasellar extension than sporadic cases. Isolated familial somatotropinoma cases were younger at diagnosis than sporadic cases. Familial non-secreting adenomas were younger at diagnosis and had more frequent invasive tumors than the sporadic cases.
Conclusions: This study shows that familial isolated pituitary adenomas and sporadic adenomas have differing clinical characteristics and may represent a novel endocrine neoplasia that requires further genetic characterization.

This multicenter international study succeeded in collecting a high number of patients with a condition as rare as familial pituitary adenoma. Careful scrutiny of their clinical history revealed that they differ clinically from patients with sporadic pituitary adenoma. Interestingly, germline mutations in the aryl hydrocarbon receptor-interacting protein gene has been identified in subjects pituitary adenoma (for details, see *New gene* section) indicating that it is possible to identify the causative genetic defects in the low-penetrance conditions even in the absence of a strong family history. Unravelling the genetic basis of this rare condition would be of great help in elucidating the pathogenesis of pituitary adenomas.

Pituitary autoantibodies in autoimmune polyendocrine syndrome type 1

Bensing S, Fetissov SO, Mulder J, Perheentupa J, Gustafsson J, Husebye ES, Oscarson M, Ekwall O, Crock PA, Hokfelt T, Hulting AL, Kampe O
Department of Molecular Medicine and Surgery, Karolinska Institutet, Karolinska University Hospital, Stockholm, Sweden
sophie.bensing@ki.se
Proc Natl Acad Sci USA 2007;104:949–954

Background: Mutations in the autoimmune regulator (AIRE) are responsible for autoimmune polyendocrine syndrome type 1 (APS1), a rare autosomal recessive disease. Diagnosis of APS1 and prediction of disease manifestations are based on a finding of high titer autoantibodies (Aabs) toward intracellular enzymes. The aim of this study was to identify pituitary autoantigens in subjects affected by APS1.
Methods: Screening of a pituitary cDNA expression library with APS1 sera.
Results: A Tudor domain containing protein 6 (TDRD6) cDNA clone was identified. Incubation of in vitro translated TDRD6 fragments with APS1 sera generated positive immunoreactivity in 42 out of 86 patients (49%), but not with sera from patients affected by other autoimmune diseases or from healthy subjects. Sera from 3/6 APS1 patients affected by growth hormone (GH) deficiency showed, by means of immunohistochemistry, a reaction with a small number of guinea pig anterior pituitary cells that was not seen with the sera from healthy controls. Only 40–50% of these cells were GH-positive, while other APS1 Aab-positive cells were probably a novel subpopulation of anterior pituitary cells. Furthermore, 4 of 6 patient's sera stained a fiber plexus in the pituitary intermediate lobe, recognizing monoamine- and GABA-synthesizing enzymes.
Conclusion: This study identified TDRD6 as a major autoantigen recognized by APS1 patients' sera and demonstrates recognition of specific pituitary cell populations or specific nervous tissues by sera from some GH-deficient patients.

The autoimmune polyendocrine syndrome type I (APSI) is a rare autosomal recessive disease with a complex picture drawn by decades of clinical observation and research. Autoantibody screening along with mutational analysis of the disease gene AIRE are important diagnostic tools for this life-threatening syndrome. The initial manifestation appeared within the age range of 0.2–18 years, with an occurrence of mucocutaneous candidiasis in 60% of patients, hypoparathyroidism in 32%, and adrenocortical failure in 5%. 23% of the patients had one to six other manifestations including hepatitis, keratoconjunctivitis, chronic diarrhea and periodic rash with fever [2]. By immunoscreening of a human pituitary cDNA library, the authors of this study have identified TDRD6 (the function of which is still not completely understood) as a major autoantigen in APS1. TDRD6 is known to be mainly expressed in the testis and only at very low levels in other endocrine tissues like the pituitary, adrenal gland, and pancreas. The identification of autoantibodies against guinea pig anterior pituitary cells in sera from half of the GH-deficient APS1 patients may represent an additional marker for autoimmune forms of GH deficiency.

Pegvisomant for the treatment of gsp-mediated growth hormone excess in patients with McCune-Albright syndrome

Akintoye SO, Kelly MH, Brillante B, Cherman N, Turner S, Butman JA, Robey PG, Collins MT
Department of Oral Medicine, School of Dental Medicine, University of Pennsylvania, Philadelphia, Pa., USA
akintoye@dental.upenn.edu
J Clin Endocrinol Metab 2006;91:2960–2966

Background: Approximately 20% of the patients affected by McCune-Albright syndrome (MAS) suffer from GH excess. MAS is due to sporadic, post-zygotic, activating mutations of Gsα, the cAMP-regulating protein encoded by the GNAS gene (gsp oncogene). Approximately one third of the sporadic cases of acromegaly are associated with the same genetic disorder. The aim of this study was to evaluate the effects of pegvisomant, a GH receptor antagonist, on gsp oncogene-related GH hypersecretion and the skeletal disease (fibrous dysplasia of the bone) associated with MAS.
Methods: A randomized, double-blind, placebo-controlled crossover clinical trial was conducted at the National Institutes of Health. Five patients with GH excess-related MAS were treated with Pegvisomant for 12 weeks (20 mg/day s.c. injection). Primary outcome was IGF-1 normalization; secondary outcomes were attainment of lower serum IGF binding protein-3 (IGFBP-3) concentration, reduction of fatigue and sweating, improvement of markers of bone metabolism and bone pain.
Results: Mean reduction of serum IGF-1 was -236.4 ng/ml (53%, $p < 0.005$) at 6 weeks and -329.8 ng/ml (62%, $p < 0.001$) at 12 weeks, while IGFBP-3 levels were lower by 0.8 mg/l (24%, $p < 0.01$) and 2.9 mg/l (37%, $p < 0.005$) respectively. No significant variations were found in signs and symptoms of acromegaly, in markers of bone metabolism, in bone pain, or in pituitary size. Retrospective analysis, performed to evaluate the efficacy of pegvisomant in comparison with other medications (long-acting octreotide ± dopamine agonist) in the same group, showed no significant differences between the two regimens.
Conclusion: IGF-1 and IGFBP-3 levels benefit from pegvisomant treatment in patients affected by gsp-mediated GH excess without improvement of fibrous dysplasia.

McCune-Albright syndrome and acromegaly: effects of hypothalamopituitary radiotherapy and/or pegvisomant in somatostatin analog-resistant patients

Galland F, Kamenicky P, Affres H, Reznik Y, Pontvert D, Le Bouc Y, Young J, Chanson P
Service d'Endocrinologie et des Maladies de la Reproduction, Hôpital de Bicêtre, Kremlin-Bicêtre, France
J Clin Endocrinol Metab 2006;91:4957–4961

Background: Acromegaly may be associated with McCune-Albright syndrome and often cannot be surgically treated mainly due to technical complications related to dysplasia of the skull base bone. While partial recovery after somatostatin analogs has been reported, a secondary bone sarcomatous transformation makes the use of radiotherapy controversial.
Methods: Retrospective analysis of efficacy and tolerability of various therapeutic options in 6 patients affected by acromegaly secondary to McCune-Albright syndrome was reported. Treatment with fractionated radiotherapy (45–55 Gy) was performed in 5 of the 6 patients (not eligible for surgery and not responsive to somatostatin analogs) who failed to normalize GH/IGF-1 concentrations. Three patients (2 previously irradiated) were also treated with pegvisomant.
Results: A decrease of GH and IGF-1 concentrations (median follow-up 5 years, range 0.5–9) and a parallel improvement of acromegalic symptoms were documented after radiotherapy. Bone sarcomatous transformation occurred in 1 patient at the mandibular site/outside the radiation field. No evidence of normalization of GH/IGF-1 concentrations was observed in the 5 patients receiving radiotherapy alone and/or in combination with somatostatin analogs; a rapid (5–9 months) normalization of IGF-1 levels was observed in the 6 patients treated with pegvisomant (10–20 mg/day).
Conclusion: Radiotherapy may be taken into consideration for the treatment of acromegaly in patients with McCune-Albright syndrome who are not eligible for surgery and not responsive to somatostatin analogs. The risk of bone sarcomatous transformation remains uncertain. This small series of patients affected by severe GH excess confirms the efficacy of pegvisomant in the reduction of IGF-1 levels.

About 20% of adult patients with McCune-Albright syndrome have GH excess and conventional treatments of GH excess include (1) surgery, (2) radiotherapy, which is usually avoided because of potential sarcomatous transformation of bone fibrous dysplasia, and (3) medications such as short- and long-acting analogs of somatostatin, dopamine receptor agonists and more recently the GH receptor antagonist, pegvisomant. Pegvisomant is a pegylated GH analog with eight amino acid sub- stitutions in GH-binding site 1 and the substitution of glycine for alanine at position 120, resulting in both enhanced affinity for the growth hormone receptor and prevention of functional growth hormone-receptor signalling. Pegvisomant blocks the growth hormone-mediated generation of IGF-1 in approximately 90% of patients. During therapy with this agent, growth hormone levels reportedly increase by as much as 76% over baseline levels, an event probably attributable to a loss of negative feedback by lowering IGF-1 levels. Accordingly, IGF-1 measurement is the biomarker for monitoring the success of treatment [3]. Pegvisomant at well-tolerated s.c. doses was considerably more effica- cious than octreotide in suppressing the GH axis, resulting in substantial and sustained inhibition of circulating IGF-1, IGF-2, and IGFBP-3 concentrations [4]. The results of these two studies on the short- term treatment of McCune-Albright syndrome and GH excess provide evidence in favor of further testing of the hypothesis that pegvisomant, through blocking the GH receptor-mediated signal trans- duction pathways, could be effective in treating IGF-1-related diseases. In other words, even in the absence of positive treatment effects on bone in these studies, the reduction of IGF-1 and IGFBP-3 may help avoid direct structural and functional tissue damage, as well as impeding the development of secondary systemic illnesses due to prolonged exposure to elevated endogenous levels of GH/IGF-1. Additional studies in a large cohort with pegvisomant, alone or in combination with somatostatin analogs, may be promising for the treatment of this challenging disorder.

New Mechanisms

Regulation of pituitary cell function by adiponectin

Rodriguez-Pacheco F, Martinez-Fuentes AJ, Tovar S, Pinilla L, Tena-Sempere M, Dieguez C, Castano JP, Malagon MM
Department of Cell Biology, Physiology and Immunology, University of Cordoba, Cordoba, Spain
Endocrinology 2007;148:401–410

Background: Adiponectin is a 30-kDa belonging to the family of adipokines produced by adipose tissue. Adipokines play important roles in the regulation of food intake and energy balance. Adiponectin acts on two specific membrane receptors whose expression has been demonstrated in a wide variety of tis- sues. Likewise, adiponectin mRNA also shows a widespread distribution. Adipokine is also abundantly expressed in the chicken anterior pituitary. Interestingly, GH has been shown to regulate adiponectin secretion and adiponectin receptor expression in human and mouse adipocytes. This study investigated the effect of adiponectin on pituitary cell function.
Methods: Dispersed isolated cells from rat anterior pituitary were used for in vitro experiments. Pituitary hormones were measured by RIA in culture media. PCR analysis was used to assess the expression of adiponectin and its two receptors, and real-time quantitative PRC was performed to evaluate changes in gene expression in rat pituitary cell cultures exposed to adiponectin.
Results: Adiponectin inhibited GH and LH release as well as both ghrelin-induced GH release and GnRH-stimulated LH secretion in short term (4 h) treated cell cultures. Adiponectin increased GHRH-R and GHS-R mRNA content and decreased that of GnRH-R. The pituitary expressed both adiponectin and its receptors.
Conclusions: The findings of this study indicate that adiponectin may play a neuroendocrine role in the control of pituitary function.

Pituitary function is primarily under the regulation of hypothalamic releasing and inhibiting hor- mones as well as under the regulation of the feedback action of target products. A number of peripheral hormones and metabolic substrates may also influence pituitary function, acting either directly on pituitary cells or via the central nervous system. This study showed that adiponectin, an adipocyte-derived cytokine, modulates pituitary function in vitro. These findings establish another relationship between peripheral metabolism and pituitary function and suggest that adiponectin may be a link factor in the regulation of metabolism, growth and reproduction.

Cell proliferation and vascularization in mouse models of pituitary hormone deficiency

Ward RD, Stone BM, Raetzman LT, Camper SA
Graduate Program in Cellular and Molecular Biology, University of Michigan, Ann Arbor, Mich., USA
Mol Endocrinol 2006;20:1378–1390

Background: Mutations in the transcription factors Pit1 and Prop1 are causes of pituitary hormone deficiency and hypopituitarism in mice and humans. The aim of this study was to provide additional information on the vascular system of the pituitary gland in these conditions, associated with pituitary dysfunction and abnormal pituitary morphology.

Methods: Experiments were conducted in Ames and Snell dwarf mice carrying mutations on Pit1 and Prop1 genes. Histological examination of pituitary cells was performed at various stages of fetal and postnatal life. The pituitary vascular system was studied from embryonic day 14.5 and throughout development.

Results: The main recognized feature of Pit1-deficient mice was pituitary hypoplasia after birth, due in the first instance to low cell proliferation rate, although a minor role was shown to be played by apoptosis. No significant alterations in Pit1 pituitary vascularization were found during pituitary development. In contrast, vascularization was significantly reduced in the Prop1-deficient mouse, where apoptosis seems to play a key role. In normal mice, caspase-3 is activated at postnatal day 11 in an apoptosis-independent manner in thyrotropes and somatotropes; this activation does not occur in mutant mice, suggesting that caspase-3 expression needs a normal Prop1 and/or Pit1 function.

Conclusion: These studies provide further insight into the mechanisms for the pituitary growth defect in both the Pit1 and Prop1 mouse models.

The great majority of genetic conditions associated with multiple pituitary hormone deficiency are linked to mutations in the transcription factors expressed at different stages of pituitary development and mainly to mutations in PIT1 (POU1F1) associated with GH, TSH, and prolactin deficiency, as well as in PROP1. Prop1 is one of the transcription factors involved in pituitary development through a progressive reduction of Hesx1 repressor activity. Its expression appears early in embryonic development and is crucial for the differentiation and function of somatotropes, thyrotropes, gonadotropes and lactotropes. While a small anterior pituitary is the most frequently observed pituitary feature in both mice and humans carrying PIT1 mutations, the mouse and human PROP1-deficient pituitary phenotype are different. Indeed, enlarged anterior pituitary with progression from a large and full sella turcica to suprasellar extention of a pituitary mass, followed by areas of cystic change and eventual regression to a large empty sella, has been described in subjects with PROP1 mutations. Several hypotheses have been posited in order to explain the phenomenon of pituitary hyperplasia followed by shrinkage of the pituitary gland including apoplexy. One study provides information about the role of Prop1 in pituitary gland growth, suggesting that pituitary hyperplasia could be due to trapped progenitor cells, while subsequent degeneration could be due to the apoptosis of undifferentiated cells. The same group's research enhances our understanding of the mechanism of PIT1 and PROP1 action by demonstrating that the vascular network of the pituitary gland is affected in Prop1-deficient mice. Inadequate pituitary vascularization in Prop1 may contribute to hypoxia-induced apoptosis whereas an apoptosis-independent caspase-3 activation occurs in normal thyrotropes and somatotropes, suggesting that these transcription factors are necessary for caspase-3 expression.

Mohamad Maghnie/Andrea Secco/Sandro Loche

Pituitary adenoma predisposition caused by germline mutations in the AIP gene

Vierimaa O, Georgitsi M, Lehtonen R, Vahteristo P, Kokko A, Raitila A, Tuppurainen K, Ebeling TM, Salmela PI, Paschke R, Gundogdu S, De Menis E, Makinen MJ, Launonen V, Karhu A, Aaltonen LA
Department of Clinical Genetics, Oulu University Hospital, Oulu, Finland
Science 2006;312:1228–1230

Background: Pituitary adenomas are common benign tumors accounting for approximately 15% of intracranial tumors. Understanding their molecular basis is of great interest. Given the incidence of the disease in Northern Finland, the authors hypothesized the existence of a form of low-penetrance pituitary adenoma predisposition. Low penetrance is defined as hereditary predisposition that relatively rarely leads to disease but which may have more influence on population level compared to high-penetrance disease susceptibility.

Methods: Three clusters of familial pituitary adenoma in Northern Finland were detected. Two clusters appeared to be linked by genealogy while the third appeared separate. A total of 14 patients in the two families were identified. Six had somatotropinoma, 4 had prolactinoma, and 4 had mixed pituitary adenoma. A population-based cohort of patients with somatotropinoma had previously been characterized. To identify the pituitary adenoma predisposition locus, whole-genomic single-nucleotide polymorphism genotyping was performed. Two analyses were performed, one on individuals with somatotropinoma/mixed adenoma (high stringency), and the other on all affected subjects (low stringency).

Results: Linkage analysis using high-stringency criteria provided evidence for linkage in chromosome 11q12-11q13, a region previously implicated in isolated familial somatotropinoma. Expression profiles were obtained in pituitary adenoma predisposed patients and carriers yielding 172 probe sets that mapped in the linked region. The two lowest p values were obtained for the two separate probe sets representing AIP (aryl hydrocarbon receptor interacting protein) gene. Another gene, galectin-12 (LGALS12), was also chosen on the basis of decreased expression. Out of 45 patients from the population-based cohort, a nonsense mutation (Q14X) and a G>A transversion were identified in 16% of patients diagnosed with somatotropinomas and in 40% of a subset of patients who were diagnosed when they were younger than 35 years of age. The possible role of AIP in pituitary adenoma predisposition in other populations was studied in three families with 2 affected individuals. No mutations were found in a German or a Turkish family, whereas a nonsense mutation R304X was detected in an Italian family. Loss of heterozygosity analysis indicated that AIP is likely to act as a tumor suppressor.

Conclusions: These data strongly associate loss of function mutations of AIP to PAP. AIP is an example of a low-penetrance tumor susceptibility gene.

Prevention and early identification of disease are cornerstones of modern medicine. In particular, early diagnosis of tumors is of special importance in order to establish adequate treatment and prevent morbidity. By applying sophisticated genetic analysis, the authors were able to show that mutations in the AIP gene accounted for 16% of all patients with pituitary somatotropinomas and for 40% of the subset who were diagnosed when they were younger than 35 years of age. AIP (aryl hydrocarbon receptor interacting protein) forms a complex with the aryl hydrocarbon receptor, a ligand-activated transcription factor which participates in the cellular signalling pathway. AIP likely acts as a tumor suppressor. Patients with untreated pituitary adenomas typically show slow development of potentially severe symptoms. Patients with pituitary adenomas usually come to our attention due to local compressive effects (visual defects, headache) or for symptoms related to oversecretion of pituitary hormones. Although genetic predisposition to tumors is suggested by epidemiological studies, dissecting the molecular basis of this susceptibility remains a difficult task. This study elegantly presents an example of low-penetrance tumor susceptibility genes, and shows that it is possible to make identification of predisposed individuals. Awareness of pre-existing risk may spare predisposed subjects from late diagnoses and associated morbidity. It is expected that genetic technology will enable us in the future to identify tumor susceptibility in other neoplasms as well.

Sustained Notch signaling in progenitors is required for sequential emergence of distinct cell lineages during organogenesis

Zhu X, Zhang J, Tollkuhn J, Ohsawa R, Bresnick EH, Guillemot F, Kageyama R, Rosenfeld MG
Howard Hughes Medical Institute, Department and School of Medicine, University of California at San Diego, La Jolla, Calif., USA
Genes Dev 2006;20:2739–2753

Background: Organogenesis in mammals is the result of the concerted actions of signalling pathways in progenitor cells that induce a hierarchy of transcription factors involved in organ and cell type differentiation. Sustained Notch activity is needed in order to ensure the persistence of the proliferating ability of some progenitor cells, which can give rise to specific late-arising cell types during pituitary organogenesis.
Methods: In situ hybridization was carried out to examine the expression pattern of the known mammalian Notch ligands and receptors, as well as the direct downstream targets of Notch signalling.
Results: Conditional deletion of Rbp-J, which encodes the major mediator of the Notch pathway, leads to premature differentiation of progenitor cells caused by loss of the expression of the basic helix-loop-helix (bHLH) factor Hes1 and conversion of the late (Pit1) lineage into the early (corticotrope) lineage. Notch signal activity is necessary to ensure expression of the tissue-specific paired-like homeodomain transcription factor, Prop1, required for generation of the Pit1 lineage. Terminal differentiation in postmitotic Pit1$^+$ cells requires reduction of Notch signalling, while Math3, the Notch-repressed Pit1 target gene, is essential to differentiation of GH-secreting cells.
Conclusion: Sustained Notch activity in progenitor cells prevents transformation of late-arising cell lineages to early-born cell lineages, ensuring differentiation of various cell types. This mechanism is probably common in mammalian organogenesis.

Recently, there has been the discovery in the adult anterior pituitary of a subset of cells with side population phenotype, enriched for expression of stem/progenitor cell-associated factors like Sca1, and of Notch1 and Hes (hairy and enhancer of split) 1, components of the classical developmental Notch pathway. The present study showed that Notch activity operates in a precise temporal window during pituitary development. The expression patterns reveal that both the ligands and the receptors of the Notch pathway are expressed in early stages of pituitary development, and that subsequent downregulation of expression correlates well with the onset of the pituitary gland maturation. In particular, Notch activation controls the formation of Pit1 precursors while downregulation at a later stage is necessary for terminal differentiation. Whereas in early developmental stages, Notch signalling plays a crucial role in the control of the lineage commitment of Pit1$^+$ precursors, in large part by directly regulating the expression of Prop1, its activity is considerably attenuated in Pit1$^+$ cells through the expression of other regulator factors. More specifically, one of these factors, Math3, a downstream transcription target of Pit1, is crucial for maturation and expansion of somatotropes through regulation of GHRHR expression. The role of these factors in the cell cycle and in differentiation remains open for further exploration.

Mutations within Sox2/SOX2 are associated with abnormalities in the hypothalamo-pituitary-gonadal axis in mice and humans

Kelberman D, Rizzoti K, Avilion A, Bitner-Glindzicz M, Cianfarani S, Collins J, Chong WK, Kirk JM, Achermann JC, Ross R, Carmignac D, Lovell-Badge R, Robinson IC, Dattani MT
London Centre for Paediatric Endocrinology, Biochemistry, Endocrinology, Institute of Child Health, University College London, London, UK
J Clin Invest 2006;116:2442–2455

Background: SOX2 is a member of the sex-determining region of the Y chromosome-related high mobility group box family of transcription factors. It is expressed in the developing central nervous system and placodes, where it plays critical roles in embryogenesis. Heterozygous Sox2 mice show a reduction in size and male infertility. Heterozygous mutations in SOX2 in humans have been found associated with bilateral anophthalmia/microphthalmia, developmental delay, short stature, and male genital tract abnormalities. This study investigated both the role of Sox2 in murine pituitary development and function and the presence of mutations in humans.

Mohamad Maghnie/Andrea Secco/Sandro Loche

Methods: The pituitaries of embryo and adult mice bearing the Sox2$^{\beta geo}$ mutation were studied by in situ hybridization. Mutation analysis of SOX2 was performed by PCR and direct sequencing. Wild-type and mutant proteins were generated and subcloned into an expression vector for transient transfection and cell localization experiments on CHO cell cultures. Wild-type and mutant SOX proteins were generated using the TNT quick-coupled transcription/translation system (Promega). Following transfection, cells were harvested and assayed for luciferase activity. 235 patients with congenital hypothalamopituitary disorders (142 males and 92 females) were screened for mutations within SOX2. 197 patients had congenital hypopituitarism without any other abnormality, 126 had septo-optic dysplasia, and 12 patients had anophthalmia or microphthalmia.

Results: Mice heterozygous for a targeted disruption of Sox2 did not manifest eye defects, but showed abnormal anterior pituitary development with reduced levels of growth hormone, luteinizing hormone and thyroid-stimulating hormone. Eight patients were identified with heterozygous sequence variations in SOX2. Six were de novo mutations that exhibited partial or complete loss of function. In addition to bilateral eye defects, these mutations were associated with anterior pituitary hypoplasia and hypogonadotropic hypogonadism, variable defects affecting the corpus callosum and mesial temporal structures, hypothalamic amartoma, sensorineural hearing loss, and esophageal atresia.

Conclusions: SOX2 plays a critical role in the normal development and function of the hypothalamic-pituitary and reproductive axes in both mice and humans.

Pituitary development, differentiation and function is under the regulation of a complex network of transcription factors and, ultimately, affects the secretion and function of hypothalamic releasing and inhibiting hormones. A number of transcription factors are expressed at different times in embryogenesis and affect the development of multiple cell lineages. Thus, mutations in these transcription factors not only can cause variable degrees of hypopituitarism, but endocrine dysfunction can be associated with extraendocrine abnormalities. The transcription factor SOX2, expressed from the earliest stages of development, plays an important role in the normal development of the brain and the pituitary, as well as to that of the eyes and inner ear. All patients with SOX2 mutations had marked gonadotropin deficiency and 2 had evidence of GH deficiency. TSH, ACTH, and prolactin secretion were normal. It is conceivable that dysregulation of hypothalamic secretion associated with SOX2 mutations could lead to hypoplasia of the anterior pituitary. A direct effect of Sox2 deficiency in germ cells, where the gene is known to be expressed, could also contribute to hypogonadism. It is also possible that SOX2 participates directly in the regulation of genes such as Hesx1, Prop1, and Aes, all of which show a similar phenotype when mutated. This study shows that mutations in the transcription factor SOX2 cause pituitary hypoplasia associated with a number of extraendocrine abnormalities. Careful clinical characterization of patients with congenital hypopituitarism is thus a crucial step for screening for mutations of candidate genes. Indeed, as in *HESX1* and *LHX4* mutations, both of which are associated with a variable MRI scan including ectopic posterior pituitary (EPP), patients with SOX2 mutations display normal anterior pituitary gland or structural hypothalamic-pituitary abnormalities such as anterior pituitary hypoplasia, EPP and absent infundibulum at MRI examination.

FOXL2 in the pituitary: molecular, genetic, and developmental analysis

Ellsworth BS, Egashira N, Haller JL, Butts DL, Cocquet J, Clay CM, Osamura RY, Camper SA
University of Michigan Medical School, Ann Arbor, Mich., USA
Mol Endocrinol 2006;20:2796–2805

Background: FOXL2 is a forkhead transcription factor expressed in the eye, ovary, and pituitary gland. Loss-of-function mutations of FOXL2 cause blepharophimosis, ptosis, and epicanthus inversus syndrome, a dominant disorder characterized by eyelid malformations. Since FOXL2 is implicated in the regulation of follicular growth and development, mutations can cause premature ovarian failure in some women, revealed as either primary or secondary amenorrhea. FOXL2 is expressed in the developing pituitary gland at embryonic days 10.5 and 12.5. Patients who are heterozygous for mutations in the FOXL2 gene do not have an obvious pituitary phenotype, whereas FOXL2 knockout mice are smaller than wild-type animals and have reduced IGF-1 levels, suggesting GH insufficiency. Thus, FOXL2 may play a role in pituitary development which is, however, not evidenced in heterozygotes if the pituitary is less sensitive than other affected tissues to reduction in FOXL2 levels. This study reports a comprehensive analysis of the developmental regulation and cell-specific expression of FOXL2 in the pituitary.

Methods: Mouse embryos were obtained from mating wild-type animals or from an intercross of heterozygous mice with mutations in *Prop1*, *PITX2*, *Lhx3*, or *Lhx4*. Immunohistochemistry and in situ hybridization were used to visualize FOXL2 in the pituitary at various embryonic ages. Ovarian tissue was also obtained. Culture cells were transfected to generate a FOXL2-VP16 fusion protein.

Results: FOXL2 protein is present in quiescent cells of the anterior pituitary from embryonic day 11.5 through adulthood, and is co-localized with non-proliferating differentiating cells. FOXL2 regulates αGSU gene (Cga) expression in a dose-dependent manner in culture cells. Transgenic mice that overexpress FOXL2 exhibit primarily appropriate expression in the anterior lobe with some ectopic expression in nearby tissue. αGSU is expressed in all areas that express the FOXL2 transgene including ectopic regions. Normal FOXL2 expression requires the transcription factor Lhx3 and Lhx4 but not of Prop1. Thus, FOXL2 is downstream of Lhx3 and Lhx4 in the genetic hierarchy of the control of pituitary development.

Conclusions: This study shows that FOXL2 is involved in the control of pituitary development and suggests a role for it in the regulation of αGSU gene expression.

In recent years, studies of animal models and humans affected by multiple pituitary hormone deficiencies have contributed to elucidating a complex cascade of transcription factors which participate in the control of pituitary development and function. So far, a number of genes have been characterized whose loss of function causes multiple pituitary hormone deficiencies, either associated or not with extraendocrine abnormalities. Among these are the LIM family genes, HESX1, Prop1 and Pit1, and the precise developmental expression of these genes has been elucidated. FOXL2 belongs to a class of transcription factors called forkhead factors that are important in a number of developmental processes. Deficiencies in individual forkhead genes have revealed their roles in speech and language disorders, diabetes, immunodeficiency, cleft palate, and eye development. Loss of function mutations of FOXL2 cause blepharophimosis, ptosis, and epicanthus inversus syndrome, a dominant disorder characterized by eyelid malformations. Since FOXL2 is implicated in the regulation of follicular growth and development, mutations can cause premature ovarian failure in some women, revealed as either primary or secondary amenorrhea. This important study shows that FOXL2 is expressed in the pituitary preceding that of most thyrotrope and gonadotrope markers and regulates αGSU gene expression. Most patients with congenital MPHD do not have a recognizable cause of their defect. Elucidating the complex hierarchy of transcription factors which participate in the control of pituitary development as well as their reciprocal interaction will help us to unravel the genetic basis of many undiagnosed cases.

Review

Craniopharyngiomas

Karavitaki N, Cudlip S, Adams CB, Wass JA
Department of Endocrinology, Oxford Centre for Diabetes, Endocrinology and Metabolism, Churchill Hospital, Headington, Oxford, UK
Endocr Rev 2006;27:371–397

Craniopharyngiomas are rare epithelial tumors arising along the path of the carniopharygeal duct. Two major histological subtypes have been described (adamantinomatous and papillary) with unknown pathogenesis. Despite their benign histological appearance, their frequent tendency to infiltrate into critical parasellar structures and their aggressive behavior may result in significant morbidity and mortality. Their optimal management is controversial and remains a subject of debate. The lack of prospective randomized studies (unlikely to be carried out) makes the therapy of craniopharyngiomas controversial. The goals for the primary or recurrent disease treatment should focus not only on long-term tumor control and survival, but also on the reduction of the disease and treatment-related morbidity and the preservation of quality of life.

A very useful review on a difficult topic. Craniopharyngiomas are the most common tumor affecting the hypothalamic-pituitary region and account for approximately 10% of all childhood intracranial tumors. Differential diagnosis between craniopharyngioma, Rathke's cleft cyst and other masses can often prove difficult. The information from this review provides a comprehensive and updated contribution to a better understanding and management of this locally devastating tumor. It highlights: (1) epidemiology, (2) pathogenesis, (3) clinical manifestations, (4) imaging features, (5) treatment options, (6) risk factors for recurrence, and (7) long-term outcome.

References
1. Lebedev YB, Amosova AL, Mamedov IZ, Fisunov GY, Sverdlov ED: Most recent AluY insertions in human gene introns reduce the content of the primary transcripts in a cell type specific manner. Gene 2007;390:122–129.
2. Perheentupa J: Autoimmune polyendocrinopathy-candidiasis-ectodermal dystrophy. J Clin Endocrinol Metab 2006;91: 2843–2850.
3. Melmed S: Medical progress: acromegaly. N Engl J Med 2006;355:2558–2573.
4. Yin D, Vreeland F, Schaaf LJ, Millham R, Duncan BA, Sharma A: Clinical pharmacodynamic effects of the growth hormone receptor antagonist pegvisomant: implications for cancer therapy. Clin Cancer Res 2007;13:1000–1009.

Thyroid

Heiko Krude

Institute of Pediatric Endocrinology, Charité University Medicine Berlin, Berlin, Germany

Again in the last 12 months a number of more than 3,000 references were published under the search heading 'thyroid'. Most of the papers are related to thyroid malignancies, a topic which has not seen a relevant pediatric contribution this year. The two papers with the highest impact factors and relevance to pediatric endocrinology deal with iodine and with interrelation of thyroid function and regulation of metabolism. Iodine got its share from a publication in the New England Journal of Medicine showing the possibly harmful effect of iodine overdose resulting in a pro-immunogenic effect. The *Cell* paper on metabolism and thyroid function was provided by the NURSA consortium which went out to analyze the expression of the known 49 nuclear receptors. As part of this 'mega-project', the researchers identified that most of the nuclear receptors are expressed in a coordinated and timely synchronized fashion referred to as 'megagenic entity' influencing metabolism. The thyroid hormone receptors α and β are members of this entity and are expressed in several tissues with daytime rhythmicity. These data may explain daily differences in thyroid hormone function despite the fact that circulating thyroid hormone remains constant around the clock.

Thyroid function around the clock: rhythmicity in the thyroid axis

Nuclear receptor expression links the circadian clock to metabolism
Yang X, Downes M, Yu RT, Bookout AL, He W, Straume M, Mangelsdorf DJ, Evans RM
Gene Expression Laboratory, The Salk Institute, La Jolla, Calif., USA
Cell 2006;126:801–810

Background: As sensors for fat-soluble hormones and dietary lipids, oscillations in nuclear receptor expression in key metabolic tissues may contribute to circadian entrainment of nutrient and energy metabolism.
Methods: Survey of the diurnal expression profiles of all 49 mouse nuclear receptors in white and brown adipose tissue, liver, and skeletal muscle.
Result: Of the 45 nuclear receptors expressed, 25 are in a rhythmic cycle and 3 exhibit a single transient pulse of expression 4 h into the light cycle. While thyroid hormones are generally constant, they found that TRα and TRβ dramatically cycle, suggesting that fundamental concepts such as 'basal metabolism' may need to be revisited.
Conclusion: The dynamic but coordinated changes in nuclear receptor expression, along with their key target genes, offer a logical explanation for the known cyclic behavior of lipid and glucose metabolism and suggest novel roles for endocrine and orphan receptors in coupling the peripheral circadian clock to divergent metabolic outputs.

Day-cycle rhythmicity of physiological functions is rendered by a sophisticated molecular clockwork which has a pendulum, so to say, of transcription factor activation and inactivation with a 24-hour phase (fig. 1). This molecular clock, which was discovered in *Drosophila* mutants and was shown to equally function in mice, is synchronized in the suprachiasmatic nucleus via light sensed in specialized melanopsin-positive ganglion cells of the retina. However, how the synchronized suprachiasmatic nucleus clock signals its day cycle to the several clocks of the different organs and tissues is still unknown. The cycling activation and inactivation of transcription factors lead to downstream target gene regulation dependent on the respective cell populations where the local clockworks tick. The present paper of Yang et al. describes for the first time the rhythmicity of the complete range of nuclear receptor genes in metabolic tissues of mice, e.g. white and brown adipose tissue, liver and muscle. All nuclear receptor genes which were identified as being expressed in a day-cycle-dependent way can be seen as targets of the molecular clockwork factors. Among them the authors found the

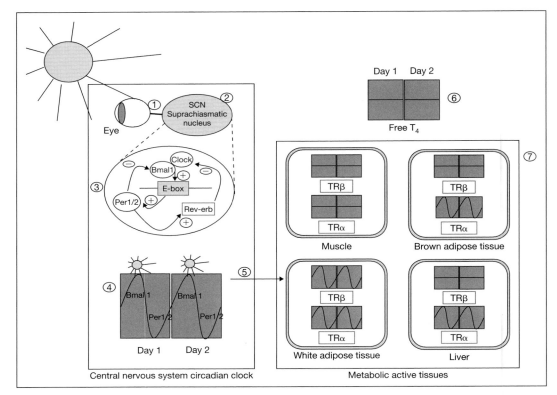

Fig. 1. Coordination of circadian timing of thyroid hormone receptor expression in metabolic tissues. Sunlight activation of melanopsin-positive retinal ganglion cells (1) which form a retinohypothalamic tract that projects to the suprachiasmatic nucleus (SCN) (2). Within SCN neurons a molecular clock mechanism of positive and negative feedback loops (3) leads to a rhythmic expression of KEY transcription factors like the clock-gene, bmal1 gene and perl1/2 gene products with a 24-hour cycle. Sunlight synchronizes the cycle with the day-night cycle via the retinohypothalamic tract (4). The information of the synchronized central clock mechanism is transferred to peripheral tissue with an unknown mechanism with the consequence of day-night cycle synchronized expression of target genes. By that mechanism, thyroid hormone receptors α and β are tissue-specific differentially expressed (6). The non-rhythmic secreted free T_4 exerts its effect on the metabolic tissues in a rhythmic function via the partially rhythmic expression of the two different thyroid hormone receptors (7).

thyroid hormone receptors α and β; both were rhythmic in white adipose tissue, α rhythmic in brown adipose tissue and liver while none of them are rhythmic in muscle. Since it has been shown that the free thyroid hormone is constantly present in serum all over a day cycle without fluctuation – most likely due to the long half-life of thyroid hormones – it was so far puzzling how thyroid effects are day-cycle-dependent, especially metabolic activity. The study of Yang et al. now explains this daytime-specific effect of thyroid hormone by the rhythmic expression of the receptors. However, one might argue that the long biological half-life of thyroid hormones for even several days as initiated via the classical nuclear signal transduction of thyroid hormone receptors is not compatible with a 24-hour rhythmicity. This well-taken argument is losing strength since the following paper published in *PNAS* this year further underlines the non-classical, non-nuclear receptor and rapid responses of thyroid hormone receptors.

Rapid signaling at the plasma membrane by a nuclear receptor for thyroid hormone

Storey NM, Gentile S, Ullah H, Russo A, Muessel M, Erxleben C, Armstrong DL
Membrane Signaling Group, Laboratory of Neurobiology, National Institute of Environmental Health Sciences,
National Institutes of Health, Department of Health and Human Services, Research Triangle Park, N.C., USA
Proc Natl Acad Sci USA 2006;103:5197–5201

Background: Many nuclear hormones have physiological effects that are too rapid to be explained by changes in gene expression and are often attributed to unidentified or novel G-protein-coupled receptors. Thyroid hormone is essential for normal human brain development, but the molecular mechanisms responsible for its effects remain to be identified.
Result: The authors present direct molecular evidence for potassium channel stimulation in a rat pituitary cell line (GH_4C_1) by a nuclear receptor for thyroid hormone, TRβ, acting rapidly at the plasma membrane through phosphatidylinositol 3-kinase (PI_3K) to slow the deactivation of $KCNH_2$ channels already in the membrane. Signaling was disrupted by heterologous expression of TRβ receptors with mutations in the ligand-binding domain that are associated with neurological disorders in humans, but not by mutations that disrupt DNA binding. More importantly, PI_3K-dependent signaling was reconstituted in cell-free patches of membrane from CHO cells by heterologous expression of human $KCNH_2$ channels and TRβ, but not TRα, receptors.
Conclusion: TRβ signaling through PI_3K provides a molecular explanation for the essential role of thyroid hormone in human brain development and adult lipid metabolism.

As mentioned above, this paper resolves the enigma of the rapid and transient effects of thyroid hormones on their receptors and of the need for a rhythmic expression of the thyroid hormone nuclear receptors. Because the biological half-life of the gene regulation function of the TRs is so long, it would make no sense that the TRs are expressed in a day-cycle-specific rhythm. But the rapid function via the cell membrane rather than via the nucleus creates a perfectly fitting picture of cycling thyroid hormone function: while the thyroid hormone levels themselves are constant (see next paper), the receptors are cycling and the rapid signal transduction pathways of the TRs at least give short-lasting cycling biological responses on metabolic functions.

Effects of evening versus morning thyroxine ingestion on serum thyroid hormone profiles in hypothyroid patients

Bolk N, Visser TJ, Kalsbeek A, van Domburg RT, Berghout A
Department of Internal Medicine, Erasmus Medical Centre, Rotterdam, The Netherlands
Clin Endocrinol (Oxf) 2007;66:43–48

Background: Standard drug information resources recommend that L-thyroxine be taken half an hour before breakfast on an empty stomach, to prevent interference of its intestinal uptake by food or medication. Cases were observed in which TSH levels improved markedly after changing the administration time of L-thyroxine to the late evening. Therefore, 12 female patients were studied on two occasions: on a stable regimen of morning thyroxine administration and 2 months after switching to night-time thyroxine using the same dose. On each occasion, patients were admitted for 24 h and serial blood samples were obtained.
Result: A significant difference in TSH and thyroid hormones was found after switching to bedtime administration of L-thyroxine. 24-hour average serum values amounted to (mean ± SD, morning vs. bedtime ingestion): TSH, 5.1 ± 0.9 vs. 1.2 ± 0.3 mU/l ($p < 0.01$); FT_4, 16.7 ± 1.0 vs. 19.3 ± 0.7 pmol/l ($p < 0.01$); T_3, 1.5 ± 0.05 vs. 1.6 ± 0.1 nmol/l ($p < 0.01$). There was no significant change in T_4, rT_3, albumin and TBG serum levels, nor in the T_3/rT_3 ratio. The relative amplitude and time of the nocturnal TSH surge remained intact.
Conclusion: L-Thyroxine taken at bedtime by patients with primary hypothyroidism is associated with higher thyroid hormone concentrations and lower TSH concentrations compared to the same L-thyroxine dose taken in the morning. At the same time, the circadian TSH rhythm stays intact. The findings are best explained by a better gastrointestinal uptake of L-thyroxine during the night.

While searching for a better treatment in patients with unsatisfying TSH levels despite high LT_4 doses, the authors tested the hypothesis that resorption of ingested LT_4 at night-time might be better than at day-time. And surprisingly they could show that taking LT_4 at night increases FT_4 and decreases TSH. Including several other LT_4 kinetic parameters they could show that the differences in 24-hour total T_4 levels are secondary to changes in the binding proteins TBG and albumin and that FT_4 remains impressively stable over 24 h. This paper has important practical implications for millions of patients worldwide who are told to take their thyroid hormone half an hour before breakfast and who may – if the data are confirmed – sleep half an hour longer and take their tablets in the evening. In addition, these data nicely show the daily rhythmicity of TSH, T_4 and FT_4. While TSH levels increase at night-time without change in FT_4 – most likely due to a lower biological activity of night-time TSH hypoglycosylation – total T_4 decreases over night parallel to the lower binding proteins TBG and albumin at night-time. The authors explain the lower night-time protein concentrations by postural changes with lower levels in supine positions. However, the changes in TSH bioactivity cannot be easily explained and might represent the effect of the molecular 24-hour clockwork within pituitary thyrotropic cells.

Linking eating and heating: new complex interrelations of the thyroid axis and metabolism

A central thermogenic-like mechanism in feeding regulation: an interplay between arcuate nucleus T₃ and UCP2

Coppola A, Liu ZW, Andrews ZB, Paradis E, Roy MC, Friedman JM, Ricquier D, Richard D, Horvath TL, Gao XB, Diano S
Department of Obstetrics, Gynecology & Reproductive Sciences, Yale University School of Medicine, New Haven, Conn., USA
Cell Metab 2007;5:21–33

Background: The active thyroid hormone, triiodothyronine (T_3), regulates mitochondrial uncoupling protein activity and related thermogenesis in peripheral tissues. Type 2 deiodinase (DII), an enzyme that catalyzes active thyroid hormone production, and mitochondrial uncoupling protein-2 (UCP2) are also present in the hypothalamic arcuate nucleus, where their interaction and physiological significance have not been explored.

Result: The authors report that DII-producing glial cells are in direct apposition to neurons coexpressing neuropeptide Y (NPY), agouti-related protein (AgRP), and UCP2. Fasting increased DII activity and local thyroid hormone production in the arcuate nucleus in parallel with increased GDP-regulated UCP2-dependent mitochondrial uncoupling. Fasting-induced T_3-mediated UCP2 activation resulted in mitochondrial proliferation in NPY/AgRP neurons, an event that was critical for increased excitability of these orexigenic neurons and consequent rebound feeding following food deprivation.

Conclusion: These results reveal a physiological role for a thyroid-hormone-regulated mitochondrial uncoupling in hypothalamic neuronal networks.

In the periphery, thyroid hormone exerts its influence on increased metabolic rate by an increase of the mitochondrial uncoupling protein activity, which leads to increased thermogenesis. This pathway of T_3-UCP2-mitochondria activation was surprisingly found also within the hypothalamus (fig. 2). Within arcuate nucleus glial cells, serum T_4 is transformed into the receptor-active T_3 by deiodinase 2. T_3 is subsequently transferred to the neighboring neuronal cells expressing NPY where UCP2-dependent mitochondrial activation leads to increased neuronal activity of the orexigenic, weight-increasing NPY cells. It seems that nature likes winning teams and the same efficient T_3 signal pathway known in the periphery is surprisingly used in the central nervous system too, however with an opposing effect. While the T_3-UCP2-mitochondria pathway in the periphery increases caloric use by increasing thermogenesis, the central T_3-UCP2-mitochondria pathway leads to stimulation of the NPY orexigenic pathway with the consequence of an increase of caloric intake. Maybe the simultaneous activation of burning calories and increasing calories by peripheral and central T_3 function respectively represent a wise counterbalancing system to avoid a too strong oscillation and to maintain energy homeostasis.

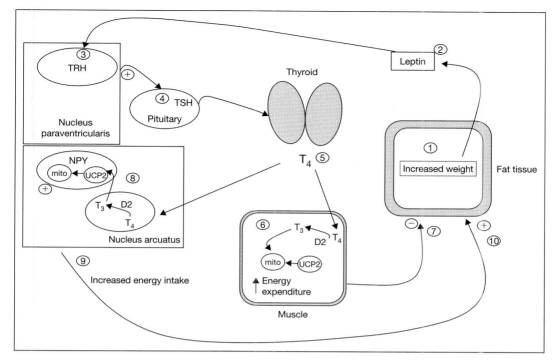

Fig. 2. Reciprocal activation of UCP2-mitochondrial activation by T_4. Increased fat tissue leads to increased leptin levels (1, 2). As recently shown, leptin activates the thyroid axis via TRH neurons in the nucleus paraventricularis (3, 4). Increased thyroid function (5) leads to stimulation of energy expenditure via UCP2 in muscle tissue (6) with the result of counteracting decrease of fat tissue (7). At the same time, increased T_4 activates in the hypothalamus the new pathway of UCP2-related activation of NPY neurons (8) which in turn leads to more food intake (9) and as a subsequent response increased fat tissue (10).

The role of intracerebroventricular administration of leptin in the stimulation of prothyrotropin releasing hormone neurons in the hypothalamic paraventricular nucleus

Perello M, Stuart RC, Nillni EA
Division of Endocrinology, Department of Medicine, Brown Medical School/Rhode Island Hospital, Providence, R.I., USA
Endocrinology 2006;147:3296–3306

Background: The authors have previously shown that leptin regulates proTRH in the paraventricular nucleus (PVN) of the hypothalamus through two pathways. The first one acts directly on proTRH neurons, and the second one (indirectly) acts through the melanocortin system (arcuate nucleus). However, it is unknown whether the direct or the indirect pathways of leptin action on proTRH neurons occurs on separated or on the same subsets of neurons within the PVN region.

Result: In this study they used immunostaining for the phosphorylated signal transducer and activator of transcription-3 to localize direct leptin signaling, and the phosphorylated cAMP response element binding protein to localize indirect signaling on proTRH neurons in animals intracerebroventricularly injected with leptin. They were able to identify two subsets of neuronal populations responsive to leptin, which are distributed in different regions within the PVN. proTRH neurons directly responsive to leptin were located mainly in the medial and posterior part of the PVN, and they were not primarily related to the hypothalamic pituitary thyroid axis. Whereas proTRH neurons indirectly responsive (through α-MSH) to leptin were located mainly in the anterior, medial, and periventricular part of the PVN, and related to the hypothalamic pituitary thyroid axis. In addition, α-MSH showed to affect the processing of proTRH and upregulated the prohormone convertase 1/3.

Conclusion: Together they show evidence supporting the hypothesis that in the PVN there are subpopulations of proTRH neurons responding to leptin, which is dependent upon the way leptin reaches its primary target(s) in the hypothalamus. These findings are critical to a better understanding of leptin-mediated actions on energy expenditure.

In contrast to the last paper that describes an effect of T_3 on metabolism, this paper confirms and describes in more detail the reciprocal effect of leptin itself on the thyroid axis. In leptin deficiency a mild form of central hypothyroidism has been described and in subsequent studies a direct stimulatory effect of leptin on the thyroid axis by activating the TRH gene was discovered. The leptin-stimulated proTRH gene expression leads to increased TSH and thyroid hormone levels. This central activation of thyroid function in times of increased leptin seems to represent one orexigenic counteractivity of the neuroendocrine feedback loop to maintain a set point of body weight. Interestingly, the authors could now show that two different neuron populations of the PVN are activated by leptin – one via the arcuate nucleus and α-MSH leading to activation of proTRH and prohormone convertase 1/3 – and the second by direct binding of leptin to the PVN. It remains unsolved which neuronal responses are targeted by this direct leptin binding to the PVN. However, these robust experimental data are in agreement with the observations described in the following paper in obese children who tend to have mildly elevated TSH and T_3 levels. These changes in the thyroid axis are more likely the consequence of a normal regulatory response than the indication of hypothyroidism causing obesity as discussed in the next paper.

Hyperthyrotropinemia in obese children is reversible after weight loss and is not related to lipids

Reinehr T, de Sousa G, Andler W
Vestische Kinder- und Jugendklinik, University of Witten/Herdecke, Datteln, Germany
T.Reinehr@kinderklinik-datteln.de
J Clin Endocrinol Metab 2006;91:3088–3091

Background: The objective of this study was to examine whether hyperthyrotropinemia is a cause or a consequence of obesity. The study was designed as a cross-sectional comparison between obese and lean children and includes a 1-year follow-up study. The study was set in a primary care facility. There were 246 obese and 71 lean children. A 1-year intervention program was based on exercise, behavior therapy, and nutrition education. The main outcome measures were TSH, free T_3 (FT_3), free T_4 (FT_4), high-density lipoprotein, low-density lipoprotein, and total cholesterol at baseline and 1 year later.
Results: TSH ($p = 0.009$) and FT_3 ($p = 0.003$) concentrations were significantly higher in obese children than in normal weight children, whereas there was no difference in FT_4 levels ($p = 0.804$). Lipids did not correlate significantly to thyroid hormones in cross-sectional and longitudinal analyses. FT_3, FT_4, and lipids did not differ significantly in the 43 (17%) children with TSH levels above the normal range from the children with TSH levels within the normal range. Substantial weight loss in 49 obese children led to a significant reduction of TSH ($p = 0.035$) and FT_3 ($p = 0.036$). The 197 obese children without substantial weight loss demonstrated no significant changes of thyroid hormones.
Conclusion: Because FT_3 and TSH were moderately increased in obese children and weight loss led to a reduction, the elevation of these hormones seems to be rather a consequence of obesity than a cause of obesity. Because FT_3 and TSH were both increased in obesity and thyroid hormones were not associated with lipid levels, the authors propose that there is no need for thyroxine treatment in this situation.

This paper, dealing with the clinical impact of the link between central weight regulation and thyroid function, is extremely useful to argue against a thyroxin treatment in obese children with elevated TSH. Most physicians tend to treat obese children with moderately elevated TSH despite normal T_4 and T_3; the parents are convinced that the 'gland' is responsible for obesity. However, the data available so far about the interrelation of central leptin function and proTRH expression were very suggestive that the elevated TSH in obese children is the consequence and not the cause of obesity. The authors could demonstrate that the elevated TSH normalize after weight reduction efforts which proves the consequence concept rather the cause concept. We have now at least one citable paper to argue against the widespread use of LT_4 in obese children. Less eating and more moving remain as the only options. The topic of euthyroid TSH elevation as touched in this paper becomes increasingly relevant based on the discussion of the normal upper limit of TSH. One informative review about this discussion appeared in 2006 and is included in the following section.

To treat or not to treat: a European statement on the upper limit of normal TSH values

Is there a need to redefine the upper normal limit of TSH?

Brabant G, Beck-Peccoz P, Jarzab B, Laurberg P, Orgiazzi J, Szabolcs I, Weetman AP, Wiersinga WM
Abteilung Gastroenterologie, Hepatologie und Endokrinologie, Medizinische Hochschule, Hannover, Germany
georg.brabant@manchester.ac.uk
Eur J Endocrinol 2006;154:633–637

Background: Mild forms of hypothyroidism – subclinical hypothyroidism – have recently been discussed as being a risk factor for the development of overt thyroid dysfunction and for a number of clinical disorders. The diagnosis critically depends on the definition of the upper normal limit of serum TSH as, by definition, free thyroxine serum concentrations are normal. Cut-off levels of 4–5 mU TSH/l have been conventionally used to diagnose an elevated TSH serum concentration. Recent data from large population studies have suggested a much lower TSH cut-off with an upper limit of 2.0–2.5 mU/l, but application of strict criteria for inclusion of subjects from the general population studies aiming at assessing TSH reference intervals (no personal or family history of thyroid disease, no thyroid antibodies and a normal thyroid on ultrasonography) did not result in an unequivocal upper limit of normal TSH at 2.0–2.5 mU/l.
Result: When summarizing the available evidence for lowered upper TSH cut-off values and their potential therapeutic implications, there is presently insufficient justification to lower the upper normal limit of TSH and, for practical purposes, it is still recommended to maintain the TSH reference interval of 0.4–4.0 mU/l.
Conclusion: Classifying subjects with a TSH value between 2 and 4 mU/l as abnormal, as well as intervening with thyroxine treatment in such subjects, is probably doing more harm than good.

This review discusses the questionable indication to treat patients with 'borderline' TSH in the range of 2–4 mU/l as it is increasingly propagated from different groups in the USA. The main message is that most likely treatment of these patients will result in a large number of borderline hyperthyroid patients with suppressed TSH. This iatrogenic condition is more harmful than the borderline hypothyroid condition as a large number of studies suggest, especially in older patients with heart disease. Since we are faced with an increasing demand of treating children with borderline elevated TSH (see previous paper on obese children) the cited references and the argumentation of the paper are also relevant for pediatric endocrinologists. Even more in children, borderline TSH might represent a variant and not a disease and a lifelong treatment with LT_4 will most likely be even more harmful compared to adults.

New mechanisms: a pathfinder function of cervical arteries for the developing thyroid gland

Arteries define the position of the thyroid gland during its developmental relocalization

Alt B, Elsalini OA, Schrumpf P, Haufs N, Lawson ND, Schwabe GC, Mundlos S, Grüters A, Krude H, Rohr KB
Institute for Developmental Biology, University of Cologne, Cologne, Germany
Development 2006;133:3797–3804

Background: During vertebrate development, the thyroid gland undergoes a unique relocalization from its site of induction to a distant species-specific position in the cervical mesenchyme.
Results: The authors have analyzed thyroid morphogenesis in wild-type and mutant zebrafish and mice, and find that localization of growing thyroid tissue along the anteroposterior axis in zebrafish is linked

to the development of the ventral aorta. In grafting experiments, ectopic vascular cells influence the localization of thyroid tissue cell non-autonomously, showing that vessels provide guidance cues in zebrafish thyroid morphogenesis. In mouse thyroid development, the midline primordium bifurcates and two lobes relocalize cranially along the bilateral pair of carotid arteries. In hedgehog-deficient mice, thyroid tissue always develops along the ectopically and asymmetrically positioned carotid arteries, suggesting that, in mice (as in zebrafish), co-developing major arteries define the position of the thyroid.

Conclusion: The similarity between zebrafish and mouse mutant phenotypes further indicates that thyroid relocalization involves two morphogenetic phases, and that variation in the second phase accounts for species-specific differences in thyroid morphology. Moreover, the involvement of vessels in thyroid relocalization sheds new light on the interpretation of congenital thyroid defects in humans.

The 22q11 deletion syndrome candidate gene Tbx1 determines thyroid size and positioning

Fagman H, Liao J, Westerlund J, Andersson L, Morrow BE, Nilsson M
Department of Medical Chemistry and Cell Biology, Institute of Biomedicine, Sahlgrenska Academy at Goteborg University, Goteborg, Sweden
henrik.fagman@anatcell.gu.se
Hum Mol Genet 2007;16:276–285

Background: Thyroid dysgenesis is the major cause of congenital hypothyroidism in humans. The underlying molecular mechanism is in most cases unknown, but the frequent co-incidence of cardiac anomalies suggests that the thyroid morphogenetic process may depend on proper cardiovascular development. The T-box transcription factor TBX1, which is the most probable gene for the 22q11 deletion syndrome (22q11DS/DiGeorge syndrome/velo-cardio-facial syndrome), has emerged as a central player in the coordinated formation of organs and tissues derived from the pharyngeal apparatus and the adjacent secondary heart field from which the cardiac outflow tract derives.

Results: The authors show that Tbx1 impacts greatly on the developing thyroid gland, although it cannot be detected in the thyroid primordium at any embryonic stage. Specifically, in Tbx1$^{-/-}$ mice, the downward translocation of Titf1/Nkx2.1-expressing thyroid progenitor cells is much delayed. In late mutant embryos, the thyroid fails to form symmetric lobes but persists as a single mass approximately one-fourth of the normal size. The hypoplastic gland mostly attains a unilateral position resembling thyroid hemiagenesis. The data further suggest that failure of the thyroid primordium to re-establish contact with the aortic sac is a key abnormality preventing normal growth of the midline anlage along the third pharyngeal arch arteries. In normal development, this interaction may be facilitated by Tbx1-expressing mesenchyme filling the gap between the pharyngeal endoderm and the detached thyroid primordium.

Conclusion: The findings indicate that Tbx1 regulates intermediate steps of thyroid development by a non-cell-autonomous mechanism. Thyroid dysgenesis related to Tbx1 inactivation may explain an overrepresentation of hypothyroidism occurring in patients with the 22q11DS.

Most children with congenital hypothyroidism are affected by a developmental defect of the thyroid gland, summarized as thyroid dysgenesis. In the last 10 years we have become familiar with several genes identified as key transcription factors during early steps of thyroid development, e.g. TITF1/NKX2.1, FOXE1/TTF2 and PAX8, which all act in a cell-autonomous way. These two new papers describe a mechanism how the developing thyroid gland is guided through the complex pharyngeal field to reach its proper position in anterior neck which is far away from the origin of the thyroid primordium in the pharyngeal endoderm. In the first paper the zebrafish was instructive as a model for thyroid development where cervical arteries could be identified in several genetic models to be responsible for the relocalization of thyroid follicles in the fish head region. Based on these fish data, a detailed description of the three-dimensional orientation of the developing mouse thyroid revealed a complex co-development of the gland with the cervical arteries, mainly the aortic arch during a first phase of caudal migration and in later stages during cranial relocalization with the carotid arteries. Disturbed artery development in a sonic hedgehog-deficient mouse model confirmed a causal link between cervical artery and thyroid development.

The second paper focused on the observation that in the 22q11 deletion syndrome, aortic arch malformations are associated with some thyroid alterations in up to 20% of patients. Reinvestigation of the Tbx1 knockout mouse, which resembles most of the 22q11 deletion human phenotypes, revealed a constant asymmetric hypoplastic thyroid defect. The authors concluded that the thyroid defect most likely is a consequence of the surrounding field defect because Tbx1 is not expressed in the developing thyroid itself and further speculated that the cervical arteries might attract the thyroid bud by soluble growth factors.

Together these papers open the search for additional external growth factors in the developing pharyngeal field which are similarly relevant for normal thyroid development as the cell-autonomously acting so far known transcription factors. Signal molecules sent out by the arteries to stimulate and position the gland seem to be attractive candidates in this view. This brings us to some clinically relevant papers about congenital hypothyroidism summarized in the next section.

How to manage congenital hypothyroidism: a US consensus and a European innovation

Update of newborn screening and therapy for congenital hypothyroidism

Rose SR, Brown RS, Foley T, Kaplowitz PB, Kaye CI, Sundararajan S, Varma SK
American Academy of Pediatrics, Section on Endocrinology and Committee on Genetics, American Thyroid Association, Public Health Committee, and Lawson Wilkins Pediatric Endocrine Society, Dallas, Tex., USA
Pediatrics 2006;117:2290–2303

Unrecognized congenital hypothyroidism leads to mental retardation. Newborn screening and thyroid therapy started within 2 weeks of age can normalize cognitive development. The primary thyroid-stimulating hormone screening has become standard in many parts of the world. However, newborn thyroid screening is not yet universal in some countries. An initial dosage of 10–15 µg/kg L-thyroxine is recommended. The goals of thyroid hormone therapy should be to maintain frequent evaluations of total thyroxine or free thyroxine in the upper half of the reference range during the first 3 years of life and to normalize the serum thyroid-stimulating hormone concentration to ensure optimal thyroid hormone dosage and compliance. Improvements in screening and therapy have led to improved developmental outcomes in adults with congenital hypothyroidism who are now in their 20s and 30s. Thyroid hormone regimens used today are more aggressive in targeting early correction of thyroid-stimulating hormone than were those used 20 or even 10 years ago. Thus, newborn infants with congenital hypothyroidism today may have an even better intellectual and neurologic prognosis. Efforts are ongoing to establish the optimal therapy that leads to maximum potential for normal development for infants with congenital hypothyroidism. Remaining controversy centers on infants whose abnormality in neonatal thyroid function is transient or mild and on optimal care of very low birth weight or preterm infants. Of note, thyroid-stimulating hormone is not elevated in central hypothyroidism. An algorithm is proposed for diagnosis and management. Physicians must not relinquish their clinical judgment and experience in the face of normal newborn thyroid test results. Hypothyroidism can be acquired after the newborn screening. When clinical symptoms and signs suggest hypothyroidism, regardless of newborn screening results, serum free thyroxine and thyroid-stimulating hormone determinations should be performed.

Recombinant human TSH in the diagnosis of congenital hypothyroidism

Tiosano D, Even L, Shen Orr Z, Hochberg Z
Meyer Children's Hospital, Haifa, Israel
d_tiosano@rambam.health.gov.il
J Clin Endocrinol Metab 2007;92:1434–1437

Background: The modern approach to congenital hypothyroidism requires a definitive diagnosis of the underlying mechanisms; this can be achieved within the first weeks of life. When uncertainty persists, treatment is commenced, and the definitive diagnosis of congenital hypothyroidism is deferred to the age of 3 years. The interruption of thyroid replacement treatment is perceived as risky by parents and physicians. The aim of this pilot study was to test the possibility of a definitive diagnosis during thyroid replacement treatment, utilizing stimulation of thyroid tissue by rhTSH.

Results: Eight patients, 3 boys and 5 girls, aged 5–15 years, mean 9.5 ± 3.7 years, with congenital hypothyroidism who had been diagnosed by the neonatal screening program and a verified diagnosis between 3 and 4 years of age were re-evaluated while on thyroid replacement therapy. Patients received i.m. 0.6 mg/m^2 rhTSH (Thyrogen, Genzyme) on 2 consecutive days. rhTSH pharmacokinetics, C_{max}, $t_{1/2}$ and AUC in children were different as compared to adults. In the patients with intact TSH receptors, FT_4 levels decreased after the first and the second injection of rhTSH (p = 0.0137, p = 0.0149). All 8 children showed identical scintigraphy after rhTSH administration, as compared to thyroid replacement withdrawal.

Conclusions: The use of rhTSH is effective for definitive diagnosis of congenital hypothyroidism during thyroid replacement treatment and no safety issues were encountered.

Almost 30 years after the initiation of newborn screening for congenital hypothyrodism in the USA, this paper summarizes the actual diagnostics and treatment consensus of the American Academies involved in the treatment of patients with congenital hypothyrodism. The consensus is quite openly formulated when dealing with the controversial topics of thyroid imaging at diagnosis, treatment of hyperthyrotropinemia and the LT_4 dose, and the authors leave it to the decision of individual physicians. However, the more conservative US habits in imaging studies might not find an equal European counterpart, because the statement that scintigraphy is more recommended than ultrasound because an ectopic gland might be overseen is not outcome relevant in the view of adequate higher doses and does need to be performed in every child. Also the question of LT_4 dose, which was traditionally lower in the USA compared with Europe, is slowly moving towards higher doses and the authors now recommend 10–15 μg/kg, but state that the 'higher' dose of 50 μg will make an evaluation of cognitive outcome important to recognize overtreatment. In a normal-weight newborn of ca. 3.5 kg, 50 μg LT_4 corresponds with 15 μg/kg and with the recommendations made. Moreover, since the US market only offers LT_4 tablets and no LT_4 solution, the only practical alternatives are 50 or 37.5 μg and the latter dose was shown to be less efficient to reach normal IQ according to the two prospective ongoing studies [1]. Statistically significant differences of 5 IQ points with 37 vs. 50 μg might have a lifelong impact in the affected child and the future debate in this field will clearly focus on such minor differences in dose recommendations. The second paper approaches a new diagnostic procedure in thyroid imaging in congenital hypothyrodism adopted from post-surgery cancer treatments in adolescents. The authors suggest avoiding the withdrawal of LT_4 treatment in the confirmatory phase of diagnosis after at least 2 years of treatment by stimulation thyroid function with exogenous recombinant TSH rather than endogenous TSH. They show in 8 patients a reliable scintigraphy image under this regimen. However, in most cases nowadays of 'the modern approach to congenital hypothyrodism', the withdrawal will be mainly indicated in those children with normal-appearing thyroid tissue in ultrasound at birth and only mild hypothyroidism to exclude a transient form of congenital hypothyrodism. The recombinant TSH approach will not help to exclude a mild hypothyroidism with a normal gland in place, since for this diagnosis the endogenous increase of TSH is the key diagnostic feature and not the image of the gland.

The syndrome of the year . . .

Mutations in GLIS3 are responsible for a rare syndrome with neonatal diabetes mellitus and congenital hypothyroidism

Senee V, Chelala C, Duchatelet S, Feng D, Blanc H, Cossec JC, Charon C, Nicolino M, Boileau P, Cavener DR, Bougneres P, Taha D, Julier C
Institut Pasteur, Génétique des Maladies Infectieuses et Autoimmunes, Paris, France
Nat Genet 2006;38:682–687

Background: The authors recently described a new neonatal diabetes syndrome associated with congenital hypothyroidism, congenital glaucoma, hepatic fibrosis and polycystic kidneys.

Results: Now they show that this syndrome results from mutations in GLIS3, encoding GLI-similar 3, a recently identified transcription factor. In the original family, they identified a frameshift mutation predicted to result in a truncated protein. In two other families with an incomplete syndrome, they found that affected individuals harbor deletions affecting the 11 or 12 5′-most exons of the gene. The absence of a major transcript in the pancreas and thyroid (deletions from both families) and an eye-specific transcript (deletion from one family), together with residual expression of some GLIS3 transcripts, seems to explain the incomplete clinical manifestations in these individuals. GLIS3 is expressed in the pancreas from early developmental stages, with greater expression in β cells than in other pancreatic tissues.

Conclusion: These results demonstrate a major role for GLIS3 in the development of pancreatic β cells and the thyroid, eye, liver and kidney.

Careful clinical observations in one consanguineous family defined this new syndrome with the two endocrine features of congenital diabetes and hypothyroidism and the luck of appearance of two further informative consanguineous families opened the way to identify the molecular basis for this disease with only 3 familial cases. Two large deletions with a likely effect on the GLIS3 gene expression and one intragenic insertion mutation were enough to identify GLIS3 as the gene involved. The spectrum of the syndrome can vary and the different deletions might differentially affect the expression in different tissues, which demonstrate a very nice example of a molecular mechanism for a variable phenotype in a monogenic disease. The thyroid phenotype was described in the first clinical description of the syndrome by the same authors [2] and it seems that at least in 1 patient a normally located gland was shown by ultrasound while TSH was elevated with a low FT_4 and elevated thyroglobulin, suggesting a functional rather than a developmental thyroid defect. It will be of great interest to learn more about the role of GLIS3 for normal thyroid function, especially the target genes of this transcription factor.

Sodium/iodide symporter (NIS) gene expression is the limiting step for the onset of thyroid function in the human fetus

Szinnai G, Lacroix L, Carre A, Guimiot F, Talbot M, Martinovic J, Delezoide AL, Vekemans M, Michiels S, Caillou B, Schlumberger M, Bidart JM, Polak M

Faculty of Medicine René Descartes, Paris V, Site Necker, Institut National de la Sante et de la Recherche Médicale Equipe Mixte 0363, Pediatric Endocrine Unit, Assistance Publique-Hôpitaux de Paris (AP-HP), Hôpital Necker Enfants-Malades, Paris, France

J Clin Endocrinol Metab 2007;92:70–76

Background: Terminal differentiation of the human thyroid is characterized by the onset of follicle formation and thyroid hormone synthesis at 11 gestational weeks (GW). This study aimed to investigate the ontogeny of thyroglobulin (Tg), thyroid peroxidase (TPO), sodium/iodide symporter (NIS), pendrin (PDS), dual oxidase 2 (DUOX2), thyroid-stimulating hormone receptor (TSHR), and thyroid transcription factor 1 (TITF1), forkhead box E1 (FOXE1), and paired box gene 8 (PAX8) in the developing human thyroid. Thyroid tissues from human embryos and fetuses (7–33 GW; n = 45) were analyzed by quantitative PCR to monitor mRNA expression for each gene and by immunohistochemistry to determine the cellular distribution of TITF1, TSHR, Tg, TPO, NIS, and the onset of T_4 production.

Results: TITF1, FOXE1, PAX8, TSHR, and DUOX2 were stably expressed from 7 to 33 GW. Tg, TPO, and PDS expression was detectable as early as 7 GW and was correlated with gestational age (all $p < 0.01$), and the slope of the regression line was significantly different before and after the onset of T_4 synthesis at 11 GW (all $p < 0.01$). NIS expression appeared last and showed the highest fit by the broken-line regression model of all genes (correlation age $p < 0.0001$, broken-line regression $p < 0.0001$). Immunohistochemical studies detected TITF1, TSHR, and Tg in unpolarized thyrocytes before follicle formation. T_4 and NIS labeling were only found in developing follicles from 11 GW onwards.

Conclusion: These results imply a key role of NIS for the onset of human thyroid function.

The extraordinary role of iodine for the synthesis of thyroid hormone has been known for a long time. Now it seems that also during development the supply of the already built thyroid follicles with iodine is the key step of onset of thyroid function during embryogenesis. This ethically sensible study in human fetuses demonstrates that all other genes necessary for thyroid hormone production are already expressed but that just in the moment when thyroid hormone secretion begins expression of the iodine symporter, NIS is initiated. For future studies these data give much food to think about because now the question needs to be answered how this orchestrated expression pattern of the functionally relevant genes in thyroid development is regulated, especially which transcription factor might be the critical specific one to initiate the expression of NIS at that later time point when all other factors which are known so far are already expressed but are obviously not yet sufficient to induce NIS expression.

Assessment of iodine status using dried blood spot thyroglobulin: development of reference material and establishment of an international reference range in iodine-sufficient children

Zimmermann MB, de Benoist B, Corigliano S, Jooste PL, Molinari L, Moosa K, Pretell EA, Al-Dallal ZS, Wei Y, Zu-Pei C, Torresani T
Laboratory for Human Nutrition, Swiss Federal Institute of Technology, Zurich, Switzerland
michael.zimmermann@ilw.agrl.ethz.ch
J Clin Endocrinol Metab 2006;91:4881–4887

Background: Thyroglobulin (Tg) may be a valuable indicator of improving thyroid function in children after salt iodization. A recently developed Tg assay for use on dried whole blood spots (DBS) makes sampling practical, even in remote areas. The study aim was to develop a reference standard for DBS-Tg, establish an international reference range for DBS-Tg in iodine-sufficient children, and test the standardized DBS-Tg assay in an intervention trial. Serum Tg reference material of the European Community Bureau of Reference (CRM-457) was adapted for DBS and its stability tested over 1 year. DBS-Tg was determined in an international sample of 5- to 14-year-old children (n = 700) who were euthyroid, anti-Tg antibody-negative, and residing in areas of long-term iodine sufficiency. In a 10-month trial in iodine-deficient children, DBS-Tg and other indicators of iodine status were measured before and after introduction of iodized salt.

Results: Stability of the CRM-457 Tg reference standard on DBS over 1 year of storage at −20 and −50°C was acceptable. In the international sample of children, the third and 97th percentiles of DBS-Tg were 4 and 40 μg/l, respectively. In the intervention, before introduction of iodized salt, median DBS-Tg was 49 μg/l, and more than two-thirds of children had DBS-Tg values >40 μg/l. After 5 and 10 months of iodized salt use, median DBS-Tg decreased to 13 and 8 μg/l, respectively, and only 7 and 3% of children, respectively, had values >40 μg/l. DBS-Tg correlated well at baseline and 5 months with urinary iodine and thyroid volume.

Conclusion: The availability of reference material and an international reference range facilitates the use of DBS-Tg for monitoring of iodine nutrition in school-age children.

A brief summary of the findings would be helpful. This methodological paper opens new perspectives for the general feasibility of iodine measurement based on screening filter paper. The implementation of newborn screening makes it very attractive to measure additional parameters in the blood spots with the chance to generate population-based data of a variety of parameters – although this is of some ethical concern too. This paper started with the general proof that Tg levels mirror iodine status in schoolchildren as measured in DBS on filter paper and supplied us with the reference ranges for Tg in this material. They also showed that Tg is stable in DBS after 1 year of storage at −20°C. Measurement of Tg in screening blood samples might have additional indications in the differential diagnosis of positive screening results, e.g. to discriminate iodine exposure, dysgenesis and dyshormonogenesis.

Selenium and goiter prevalence in borderline iodine sufficiency

Brauer VF, Schweizer U, Kohrle J, Paschke R
Third Department of Medicine, University of Leipzig, Leipzig, Germany
Eur J Endocrinol 2006;155:807–812

Background: Selenium (Se) is required for the biosynthesis of selenocysteine-containing proteins. Several selenoenzymes, e.g. glutathione peroxidases and thioredoxin reductases, are expressed in the thyroid.

Selenoenzymes of the deiodinase family regulate the levels of thyroid hormones. For clinical investigators, it is difficult to determine the role of Se in the etiology of (nodular) goiter, because there are considerable variations of Se concentrations in different populations as reflected by dietary habits, bioavailability of Se compounds, and racial differences. Moreover, most previous clinical trials which investigated the influence of Se on thyroid volume harbored a bias due to the coexistence of severe iodine deficiency in the study populations. Therefore, the authors investigated the influence of Se on thyroid volume in an area with borderline iodine sufficiency.

Methods: The authors investigated randomly selected probands for urinary iodine and creatinine excretion in spot urine samples and determined the prevalence of goiter and thyroid nodules by high-resolution ultrasonography as well as urinary Se excretion in probands with goiter and matched probands without goiter.

Results: The mean urinary Se excretion and urinary iodine rates of all 172 probands were 24 µg Se/l or 27 µg Se/g creatinine and 96 µg iodine/l or 113 µg iodine/g creatinine indicating borderline Se (20–200 µg/l) and iodine (100–200 µg/l) sufficiency of the study population. Probands with goiter (n = 89) showed significantly higher urinary Se levels than probands with normal thyroid volume (n = 83; $p < 0.05$). Urinary Se rates were not influenced by present smoking or pregnancy.

Conclusion: Urinary Se is not an independent risk factor for the development of goiter. The higher urinary Se in probands with goiter in comparison with probands with normal thyroid volume is most likely a coincidence. Se does not significantly influence thyroid volume in borderline iodine sufficiency because the iodine status is most likely the more important determinant.

There is a hype of the role of Se in several aspects of human physiology and pathology. However, this paper, at least for the thyroid, brings it down to reality. The authors searched for a role of Se deficiency as an additional factor for the development of goiter in a borderline iodine-sufficient area. In contrast to the expectation, urinary Se excretion was higher in patients with goiter compared with normal thyroid individuals, suggesting that Se deficiency is not the key factor in the pathogenesis of thyroid enlargement. It seems that the good old trace element iodine is by far the more relevant element in terms of goiter development.

Effect of iodine intake on thyroid diseases in China

Teng W, Shan Z, Teng X, Guan H, Li Y, Teng D, Jin Y, Yu X, Fan C, Chong W, Yang F, Dai H, Yu Y, Li J, Chen Y, Zhao D, Shi X, Hu F, Mao J, Gu X, Yang R, Tong Y, Wang W, Gao T, Li C
Department of Endocrinology and Metabolism, First Affiliated Hospital, China Medical University, Shengyang, China
twpendocrine@yahoo.com.cn
N Engl J Med 2006;354:2783–2793

Background: Iodine is an essential component of thyroid hormones; either low or high intake may lead to thyroid disease. The authors observed an increase in the prevalence of overt hypothyroidism, subclinical hypothyroidism, and autoimmune thyroiditis with increasing iodine intake in China in cohorts from three regions with different levels of iodine intake: mildly deficient (median urinary iodine excretion, 84 µg/l), more than adequate (median, 243 µg/l), and excessive (median, 651 µg/l). Participants were enrolled in a study in 1999, and during the 5-year follow-up through 2004, the effect of regional differences in iodine intake on the incidence of thyroid disease was examined. Of the 3,761 unselected subjects who were enrolled at baseline, 3,018 (80.2%) participated in this follow-up study. Levels of thyroid hormones and thyroid autoantibodies in serum, and iodine in urine, were measured and B-mode ultrasonography of the thyroid was performed at baseline and follow-up.

Results: Among subjects with mildly deficient iodine intake, those with more than adequate intake, and those with excessive intake, the cumulative incidence of overt hypothyroidism was 0.2, 0.5, and 0.3%, respectively; that of subclinical hypothyroidism, 0.2, 2.6, and 2.9%, respectively, and that of autoimmune thyroiditis, 0.2, 1.0, and 1.3%, respectively. Among subjects with euthyroidism and antithyroid antibodies at baseline, the 5-year incidence of elevated serum thyrotropin levels was greater among those with more than adequate or excessive iodine intake than among those with mildly deficient iodine intake. A baseline serum thyrotropin level of 1.0–1.9 mIU/l was associated with the lowest subsequent incidence of abnormal thyroid function.

Conclusion: More than adequate or excessive iodine intake may lead to hypothyroidism and autoimmune thyroiditis.

This impressive and highest impact factor clinical paper in the thyroid field this year unambiguously demonstrates that too much iodine might be harmful for the wellbeing of the thyroid. By comparing three different areas in northeast China with three different iodine intake habits as mildly deficient, more than adequate and excessive (it remains unclear why a whole region ingested very high amounts of iodine in drinking water), the authors compared alterations of thyroid function. The prospective observation of more than 3,500 individuals enabled the authors to show that too much iodine causes a status of subclinical hypothyroidism as well as thyroid autoimmune phenomena. However, the incidences increased from mild deficiency to more than adequate and excessive iodine from 0.2 to 2.6 and 2.9 for subclinical hypothyroidism and from 0.2 to 1.0 and 1.3 for autoimmunity. Compared to the hazard resulting from iodine deficiency, these numbers are more reason to reassure rather than to be concerned. Compared with these incidences, the ten times higher rates of goiter development in severe iodine deficiency and the negative impact of maternal iodine deficiency for the mental outcome of the offspring seems to be much more dangerous. Nevertheless, care should be taken to prevent overdosing a population with iodine. However, providing an individualized iodine supplementation program fitting personal needs is not a feasible task worldwide.

At the end (of the chapter) but probably not the end (of the problem) – course and treatment of Hashimoto's thyroiditis in childhood

The natural history of euthyroid Hashimoto's thyroiditis in children

Radetti G, Gottardi E, Bona G, Corrias A, Salardi S, Loche S
Department of Pediatrics, Regional Hospital, Bolzano, Italy
giorgio.radetti@asbz.it
J Pediatr 2006;149:827–832

Background: The natural history of Hashimoto's thyroiditis (HT) in children and factors predictive of thyroid dysfunction have not been described in many studies so far. The authors evaluated 160 children (43 males and 117 females, mean age 9.10 ± 3.6 years, with HT and normal (group 0; 105 patients) or slightly elevated (group 1; 55 patients) serum thyroid-stimulating hormone (TSH) concentrations. The patients were assessed at presentation and then followed for at least 5 years if they remained euthyroid or if their TSH did not rise twofold over the upper normal limit.

Results: At baseline, age, sex, thyroid volume, free thyroxine, free triiodothyronine, thyroid peroxidase antibody (TPOab), and thyroglobulin antibody (TGab) serum concentrations were similar in the two groups. During follow-up, 68 patients of group 0 remained euthyroid, and 10 patients moved from group 0 to group 1. In 27 patients, TSH rose twofold above the upper normal limit (group 2), and 9 of these patients developed overt hypothyroidism. Sixteen patients of group 1 ended up in group 0, 16 remained in group 1, and 23 moved to group 2. A comparison of the data of the patients who maintained or improved their thyroid status with those of the patients whose thyroid function deteriorated revealed significantly increased TGab levels and thyroid volume at presentation in the latter group. However, none of these parameters alone or in combination were of any help in predicting the course of the disease in a single patient.

Conclusion: The presence of goiter and elevated TGab at presentation, together with progressive increase in both TPOab and TSH, may be predictive factors for the future development of hypothyroidism. At 5 years of follow-up, more than 50% of the patients remained or became euthyroid.

Hashimoto's disease is the most frequent thyroid disease in childhood with little reliable prospective data. Therefore, these two retrospective studies are included in this chapter. Taken together, this retrospective 5-year follow-up study confirms the course of the disease in patients with positive thyroid antibodies with resolution in a few patients and deterioration in a large number. The well-organized Italian pediatric endocrinologists have brought together 20 centers to collect data from more than 150 patients. However, the data calls for a prospective study to clarify if thyroxin treatment will improve thyroid function in the long term. However, most patients in this study have an additional condition including diabetes, celiac disease or Turner syndrome and the conclusion might not apply to other patient groups with Hashimoto's thyroiditis.

L-Thyroxine in euthyroid autoimmune thyroiditis and type 1 diabetes: a randomized, controlled trial

Karges B, Muche R, Knerr I, Ertelt W, Wiesel T, Hub R, Neu A, Klinghammer A, Aufschild J, Rapp A, Schirbel A, Boehm BO, Debatin KM, Heinze E, Karges W

Division of Pediatric Endocrinology and Diabetes, University Children's Hospital Ulm; Institute of Biometrics, University of Ulm; University Children's Hospital Erlangen; Children's Hospital Heidenheim; Children's Hospital Datteln; University Children's Hospital Tubingen; Children's Hospital Chemnitz; Department of Nuclear Medicine, University of Wurzburg; Division of Endocrinology, Clinic for Internal Medicine I, University of Ulm, and Division of Endocrinology and Diabetes, RWTH Aachen University, Germany

J Clin Endocrinol Metab 2007 Feb 13 [Epub ahead of print]

Background: Patients with type 1 diabetes (T1D) have an increased risk of autoimmune thyroiditis (AIT). The authors determined whether LT_4 treatment prevents the clinical manifestation of AIT in euthyroid subjects with T1D in a prospective, randomized, open, controlled clinical trial in six tertiary care centers for pediatric endocrinology and diabetes including 611 children and adolescents with T1D.

Results: 89 individuals (14.5%) were identified with positive thyroid peroxidase antibodies (TPOAb), thyreoglobulin antibodies (TgAb), or both. Of these, 30 patients (age 13.3 ± 2.1 years) met the inclusion criteria and were randomized to receive LT_4 (16 patients) or no treatment (14 patients). Intervention: LT_4 (1.3 μg/kg daily) was given for 24 months in the treatment group, followed by an additional observation period of 6 months in both groups. Thyroid gland volume (as determined by ultrasound), serum levels of thyrotropin, thyroid hormones, TPOAb, and TgAb were assessed every 6 months for 30 months. Mean thyroid volume decreased in the treatment group after 24 months (−0.60 standard deviation score, SDS) and increased in the observation group (+1.11 SDS, p = 0.0218). Serum thyrotropin, FT_4, TPOAb, and TgAb levels were not significantly different in both groups during the entire study period. Hypothyroidism developed in 3 individuals treated with LT_4 and in 4 untreated patients (conversion rate, 9.3% per year).

Conclusions: In this study in euthyroid patients with AIT and T1D, LT_4 treatment reduced thyroid volume but had no effect on thyroid function and serum autoantibody levels.

The authors tried to search for an effect of LT_4 treatment in euthyroid patients affected with DM1 and Hashimoto's thyroiditis. Within an unfortunately small group of 30 patients they performed a randomized prospective study with a follow-up of 30 months. No significant change of the thyroid function parameters after the treatment period was found between the treated and non-treated groups. However, although a few patients per group were included and the study concerned patients with Hashimoto's thyroiditis and diabetes, this study is important because it tries to resolve the important question of thyroid hormone treatment in euthyroid Hashimoto's thyroiditis. In this patient population, treatment with thyroid hormone did not improve thyroid function after 24 months. Obviously, further studies with longer treatment durations, more patients in various age groups and with isolated Hashimoto's thyroiditis are needed. Given the widespread use of thyroid hormones in euthyroid Hashimoto's thyroiditis, these preliminary results stress the need for these studies.

References
1. Krude H: Thyroid: Physiology and Disease; in Carel JC, Hochberg Z (eds): Yearbook of Pediatric Endocrinology 2006. Basel, Karger, 2007, pp 19–32.
2. Taha D, Barbar M, Kanaan H, Balfe W: Neonatal Diabetes Mellitus, congenital hypothyroidism, hepatic fibrosis, polycystic kidneys and congenital glaucoma. Am J Med Gen A 2003;122–273.

Growth and Growth Factors

Evelien F Gevers[a,b], Peter C Hindmarsh[a] and Mehul T Dattani[a]

[a]Developmental Endocrine Research Group, Clinical and Molecular Genetics Unit, Institute for Child Heath, London, UK
[b]Division of Molecular Neuroendocrinology, National Institute for Medical Research, London, UK

The past year was once again a fruitful year regarding research into growth and growth factors. Exciting new developments include new mutations causing Noonan syndrome, all of which increase RAS signalling, as well as studies succeeding in altering imprinting of IGF-2 in tumor cells and studies shedding light on regulation of a network of imprinted genes that is involved in embryonic growth. Long-range control of gene transcription was studied in detail for the growth hormone (GH) and *SHOX* genes and the importance of such regulation was suggested by the presence of deletions downstream of the SHOX-coding region in patients with Leri-Weill dyschondrosteosis. We have learnt more about GH signalling; the importance of negative regulation of cytokine signalling by SOCS2 and JAK2, and the intricate relations between Stats and hepatic nuclear factors that are important for gene transcription in response to GH. Several new animal models were born, including mice overexpressing IGFBP-1 or IGF-1 in the liver, and nude mice transduced with adenoviral vectors containing luciferase reporter genes for Stat5. Clinical trials have suggested efficacy of GH treatment in patients with *SHOX* mutations, but contradicting results were reported regarding the response to GH treatment in patients carrying the exon-3-deleted variant of the GH receptor. Last, but not least, important data from cohort studies were published regarding the long-term follow-up of children with IUGR and SGA.

Mechanism of the year
Noonan syndrome

Germline KRAS mutations cause Noonan syndrome

Schubert S, Zenker M, Rowe SL, Boll S, Klein C, Bollag G, van der Burgt I, Musante L, Kalscheuer V, Wehner LE, Nguyen H, West B, Zhang KYJ, Sistermans E, Rauch A, Niemeyer CM, Shannon K, Kratz CP
Department of Pediatrics, University of California, San Francisco, Calif., USA
christian.kratz@uniklinik-freiburg.de
Nat Genet 2006;38:331–336

Background: Noonan syndrome, a disorder characterized by short stature, facial dysmorphism and cardiac defects, has previously been linked to gain-of-function mutations in *PTPN11*, a gene which encodes SHP-2, a non-receptor protein tyrosine phosphatase. However, mutations in this gene account for ~50% of cases of Noonan syndrome. The aim of this study was to establish whether mutations in *KRAS*, another component of the RAS-signalling pathway, could contribute to the etiology of Noonan syndrome.

Methods: Mutational screening of 174 individuals with Noonan syndrome and 12 patients with cardio-facio-cutaneous (CFC) syndrome. Mutations identified were then studied further using intrinsic and GAP-stimulated GTP hydrolysis assays, retroviral transduction and hematopoietic progenitor assays and Ras-GTP assays.

Results: Three different heterozygous mutations (T58I, V14I and D153V) were identified in 5 patients with Noonan syndrome; a P34R mutation was identified in a patient with CFC syndrome. The functional consequences of the V14I and T58I were studied, and the proteins showed defective intrinsic GTPase activity and impaired responsiveness to GAPs. Additionally, the two mutations rendered primary hematopoietic progenitors hypersensitive to growth factors and deregulated signal transduction in a cell-lineage-specific manner.

Conclusion: These studies and those previously published showing the role of *SHP-2* mutations in Noonan syndrome suggest that hyperactive Ras is a critical biochemical lesion in Noonan syndrome.

Gain-of-function *SOS1* mutations cause a distinctive form of Noonan syndrome

Tartaglia M, Pennacchio LA, Zhao C, Yadav KK, Fodale V, Sarkozy A, Pandit B, Oishi K, Martinelli S, Shackwitz W, Ustaszewska A, Martin J, Bristow J, Carta C, Lepri F, Neri C, Vasta I, Gibson K, Curry CJ, Siguero JPL, Digilio MC, Zampino G, Dallapiccola B, Bar-Sagi D, Gelb BD
Dipartimento di Biologia Cellulare e Neuroscienze, Istituto Superiore di Sanita, Rome, Italy
bruce.gelb@mssm.edu
Nat Genet 2007;39:75–79

Background: The ligand-dependent conversion of RAS-GDP to RAS-GTP is a critical step in the activation of the RAS-MAPK pathway. This reaction is catalyzed by the RAS-specific guanine nucleotide exchange factor (GEF) Son of Sevenless (SOS). SOS1, one of two human SOS proteins, is basally autoinhibited owing to complex regulatory intra- and intermolecular interactions. This study established whether *SOS1* mutations contribute to the etiology of Noonan syndrome.

Methods: 129 patients with Noonan syndrome in whom no mutation had been identified in the established genes associated with the syndrome were screened for mutations in *SOS1*.

Results: Mutations were identified in 22 of 129 individuals. The mutations led to aminoacid substitutions at residues implicated in the maintenance of SOS1 in its autoinhibited form. Functional studies performed on two of the mutants revealed enhanced RAS and ERK activation. Although the phenotype associated with *SOS1* mutations is within the Noonan spectrum, the patients manifest generally normal development and linear growth. However, there is a high incidence of pulmonary valve anomalies and ectodermal abnormalities such as facial keratosis pillaris and curly hair.

Conclusion: Gain-of-function mutations in *SOS1* are associated with upregulation of the RAS pathway and consequent Noonan syndrome.

About half of the patients with Noonan-syndrome carry mutations in *PTPN11*, a protein tyrosine phosphatase that functions in the RAS pathway. The Ras-signalling system centers on Ras proteins like H-RAS, K-RAS and N-RAS (fig. 1). RAS proteins are intermediates in a signal transduction pathway that initiates with phosphorylation of a tyrosine kinase receptor in response to an extracellular signal. The phosphorylated tyrosine kinase receptor forms protein complexes with GEFs (guanine nucleotide exchange factors) and GAPs (GTPase-activating proteins) which respectively activate and inactivate RAS. Activated RAS (RAS-GTP) stimulates the mitogen-activated protein kinase (MAPK)-signalling pathway which is involved in cell proliferation. *PTPN11* mutations found in Noonan syndrome result in prolonged signal flux through the RAS-MAPK pathway. Several research groups argued that mutations of other components of the RAS pathway may also result in Noonan syndrome or cardio-facio-cutaneous (CFC) syndrome of which the features overlap with those of Noonan syndrome. Indeed, the first paper, and a similar paper by Carta et al. [1] shows that mutations in *K-RAS* are found in Noonan syndrome and CFC syndrome. The mutations result in an increased active RAS-GTP state and a decreased sensitivity for GAPs, thus resulting in increased RAS-MAPK signalling. Tartaglia et al. found *SOS-1* mutations in patients with Noonan syndrome. Son-of-Sevenless (SOS) proteins are GEFs that catalyze activation of RAS (RAS-GTP) and so activate MAPK signalling. The *SOS-1* mutations found by Tartaglia, and also by Roberts et al. [2], are gain-of-function mutations resulting in increased RAS activation and MAPK signalling. Mutations in both *K-RAS* and *SOS-1* together with *PTPN11* in total account for up to 60% of patients with Noonan syndrome. Mutations in other components of this pathway will probably account for the remainder of cases. Linear growth of patients with *SOS1* mutations is often normal linear but they have more pulmonary valve abnormalities. It will be of clinical importance to further evaluate genotype-phenotype correlations in order to give patients with Noonan syndrome and related syndromes optimal care. Activating *PTPN11* mutations activate RAS-MAPK signalling but inhibit GH signalling by interacting with the GH receptor and result in mild GH resistance. Mutations in *K-RAS* and *SOS-1* are less likely to affect JAK-Stat signalling directly [3].

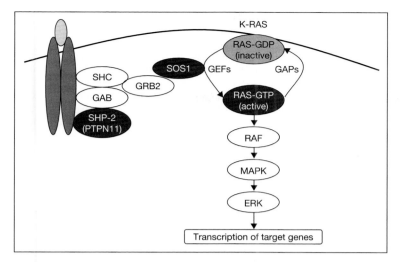

Fig. 1. Simplified schematic diagram showing the RAS-MAPK signal transduction pathway. Mutations resulting in Noonan/cardio-facio-cutaneous syndrome are shown in dark grey. The grey ovals and light grey oval represent a ligand-bound tyrosine kinase receptor. The mutations shown result in overactivation of the Ras-signalling pathway. SHP-2 = Src homology-2-containing tyrosine phosphatase; GAB = Grb-associated binding protein; Shc = SHC (Src homology-2 domain-containing)-adaptor protein; GRB2 = growth factor receptor-bound protein-2; SOS1 = Son-of-Sevenless-1; GEFs = guanine nucleotide exchanging factors; GAPs = GTPase-activating proteins; RAF = raf oncogen; MAPK = mitogen-activated protein kinase; ERK = extracellular regulated MAP kinase. Figure adapted from Gelb et al. [11].

**New paradigms
Long-range gene regulation**

Locus control region transcription plays an active role in long-range gene activation

Ho Y, Elefant F, Liebhaber SA, Cooke NE
Department of Genetics, University of Pennsylvania School of Medicine, Philadelphia, Pa., USA
necooke@mail.med.upenn.edu
Mol Cell 2006;23:365–375

Background: Remote chromatin determinants can regulate the activation of eukaryotic genes such as the *hGH* gene, which is activated by a 5′-remote locus control region (LCR). Pituitary-specific DNase I hypersensitive site I (HSI) is the dominant *hGH* LCR element, and is separated from the *hGH-N* promoter by a 14.5-kb region that contains the B-lymphocyte-specific *CD79b* gene.

Results: Site-specific inactivation of HSI results in loss of acetylation throughout the domain, with a 20-fold reduction in *hGH-N* expression. A non-coding domain of Pol II transcription in pituitary somatotropes includes the *hGH* LCR and adjacent *CD79b* locus. This entire 'LCR domain of transcription' is HIS-dependent and terminates 3′ to *CD79b*. Insertion of a Pol II terminator within the LCR blocks CD79b transcription and represses hGH-N expression. mRNA levels of CD79b are high but not translated.

Conclusion: Removal of HSI reveals a marked repression of transcription throughout the hGH LCR and adjacent CD79b. Thus the hGH LCR is transcribed and the domain of transcription extends to include CD79b. Transcription of the entire region is pituitary-specific and HSI-dependent. The robust HSI-dependent LCR domain of transcription is therefore complex – bidirectional 5′ of *CD79b*, but in the 'sense' orientation through *CD79b*.

Transcription of genes is often regulated by binding of factors to the promoter region, thereby enhancing or repressing transcription of the downstream gene. However, it has become apparent that gene transcription can also be regulated by DNA elements far away from the coding region of the gene. This means that aberrant gene transcription (and thus protein production), for example abnormal GH production, cannot only result from mutations in coding regions of the gene, or mutations in the promoter, but even from mutations in DNA much further upstream or downstream. The region of DNA involved in regulation of transcription of the gene is the 'locus control region' (LCR). This elegant study has given new insights into the role of the LCR in regulating GH expression; the data presented suggest that the LCR and the adjacent gene CD79b are transcribed, and form a domain of transcription. The process is dependent upon the presence of an intact HSI; when this site is inactivated, acetylation of DNA decreases which results in a decrease of both GH and CD79b transcription. Such knowledge of the regulation of the GH gene will help in identifying new causes of aberrant GH production.

Transactivation function of an ~800-bp evolutionarily conserved sequence at the *SHOX* 3' region: implication for the downstream enhancer

Fukami M, Kato F, Tajima T, Yokoya S, Ogata T
Department of Endocrinology and Metabolism, National Research Institute for Child Health and Development, Tokyo, Japan
mfukami@nch.go.jp
Am J Hum Genet 2006;78:167–170

Background: The human *SHOX* gene is one of the major genes contributing to longitudinal growth, and mutations resulting in haploinsufficiency have been reported in patients with isolated short stature and Leri-Weill dyschondrosteosis (LWD). *SHOX* lies in the pseudoautosomal region (PAR) 1 on both sex chromosomes, and deletions downstream of *SHOX* have been identified in LWD patients with intact *SHOX*-coding regions. These data suggest the presence of a downstream enhancer for *SHOX* transcription.
Methods: Analysis of the *SHOX* 3' region in five Japanese families in which the proband and one of the parents had variable degrees of LWD in the presence of two copies of intact *SHOX*-coding exons. The smallest region of overlapping deletion was delineated using the Japanese patients as well as the previously published patients, and within this region, the presence of evolutionarily conserved sequences (ECS) was investigated. Transcriptional activity of the ECS was examined using the human *SHOX* promoter on exon 2 in a dual-luciferase reporter assay system.
Results: Seven ECS regions were identified, but luciferase activity increased only when ECS4 was co-transfected with the *SHOX* promoter.
Conclusion: The results suggest that the ~800-bp ECS4 harbors the putative downstream enhancer for SHOX transcription.

Long-range conserved non-coding *SHOX* sequences regulate expression in developing chicken limb and are associated with short stature phenotypes in human patients

Sabherwal N, Bang F, Roth R, Weiss B, Jantz K, Tiecke E, Hinkel GK, Spaich C, Hauffa BP, van der Kemp H, Kapelier J, Tickle C, Rappold G
Department of Molecular Human Genetics, University of Heidelberg, Heidelberg, Germany
gudrun_rappold@med.uni-heidelberg.de
Hum Mol Genet 2007;16:210–222

Background: Deletions downstream of *SHOX* have been identified in patients with Leri-Weill dyschondrosteosis (LWD) with intact *SHOX*-coding regions. These data suggest the presence of a downstream enhancer for *SHOX* transcription.
Methods: Analysis of four families with LWD with deletions in the pseudoautosomal region of the sex chromosomes, but with an intact *SHOX*-coding region, using the techniques of fluorescence in situ hybridization, single nucleotide polymorphism analysis, and comparative genomic analysis. Enhancer potential of candidate regions was performed in chicken embryos by in ovo electroporation of the limb bud, using a green fluorescent protein reporter construct driven by the β-globin promoter.

Results: An interval of ~200 kb that was deleted in all tested affected family members but retained in unaffected members as well as 100 control individuals was identified. Eight highly conserved non-genic elements were identified between 48 and 215 kb downstream of the *SHOX* gene. Of these, *cis*-regulatory activity was observed in three elements in the developing limbs.

Conclusion: These data suggest that the deleted regions in these families contain several distinct elements that regulate *SHOX* expression in the developing limb. The deletions are associated with a phenotype that is apparently indistinguishable from those patients with mutations in the *SHOX*-coding region.

This paper is similar to the work by Ho et al. in that it concerns regulation of gene transcription by pieces of DNA a long distance away from the coding region of the gene. These two studies suggest that deletions of downstream enhancers of *SHOX* may account for some short stature phenotypes. The incidence of *SHOX* mutations/deletions accounts for around 50–70% of patients with LWD, and approximately 3–15% of patients with idiopathic short stature. It appears likely that a further percentage of these phenotypes might be accounted for by mutations/deletions of downstream enhancers of *SHOX*. These data have wider implications for other monogenic disorders, disorders for which one gene mutation is responsible, as well; mutations should not only be sought in coding regions of DNA or gene promoters, but also in enhancers or repressors further up- or downstream of the gene.

New hope
Correction of abnormal IGF-2 imprinting

Correction of aberrant imprinting of IGF-2 in human tumors by nuclear transfer-induced epigenetic reprogramming

Chen HL, Li T, Qiu XW, Wu J, Ling JQ, Sun ZH, Wang W, Chen W, Hou A, Vu TH, Hoffman AR, Hu JF
Medical Service, VA Palo Alto Health Care System, Palo Alto, Calif., USA
jifan@stanford.edu
EMBO J 2006;25:5329–5338

Background: Loss of genomic imprinting of insulin-like growth factor-2 (IGF-2) is a hallmark of many human neoplasms. The authors aimed to correct this aberrant epigenotype in tumor cells.

Methods and Results: Nuclei from human tumor cells that showed loss of IGF-2 imprinting were transferred into enucleated mouse and human fibroblasts that had maintained normal IGF-2 imprinting. After nuclear transfer, the abnormal biallelic expression of IGF-2 in tumor nuclei transiently converted to normal monoallelic imprinted expression in the reconstructed diploid cells. In tetraploid hybrid cells normal IGF-2 imprinting was permanently restored in the tumor genome. Cyclohexamide inhibits the synthesis of putative *trans*-imprinting factors and led to loss of IGF-2 imprinting in normal cultured fibroblasts, suggesting that normal cells produce proteins that act in *trans* to induce or maintain genomic imprinting.

Conclusion: Abnormal tumor epigenotype can be corrected by in vitro reprogramming, suggesting that loss of imprinting is associated with the loss of activity of *trans*-imprinting factor(s) that are either inactivated or mutated in tumors.

Loss of genomic imprinting of IGF-2 is a hallmark of many human neoplasms. In theory, correction of this aberrant epigenotype should be possible. Genomic imprinting is the feature of genomes in which only one set of a pair of genes present on homologous chromosomes is expressed, the second gene being silenced by methylation. Additionally, methylation of imprinting control regions can control transcription. IGF-2 is an imprinted gene that is expressed only from the paternal allele in a tissue-, promoter- and development-specific manner. Loss of IGF-2 imprinting results in biallelic expression and abnormally high IGF-2 production, and has been found in many human neoplasms, for example in Wilms' tumor. Control of IGF-2 imprinting is complex and in this paper the authors tried to normalize IGF-2 imprinting in tumor cells. Tumor cells with loss of IGF-2 imprinting were used and their nuclei were transferred to normal cells that had their nuclei removed. This resulted in normalization of IGF-2 imprinting so that IGF-2 was only transcribed from one gene; however, this effect was only transient and DNA methylation was not altered. The authors speculated that this was the case because enzymes necessary for genomic imprinting were not being produced by the nuclei from the tumor cells. In the next experiment therefore, hybrid cells were made by fusing tumor cells with normal cells. In these hybrid tetraploid cells, IGF-2 imprinting was normalized and monoallelic IGF-2 expression was permanent and the authors suggest that the presence of cytoplasmic active 'trans-imprinting' factors are involved in the maintenance of normal imprinting. This work is an important step in understanding and altering abnormal gene imprinting in tumor formation.

New animal models
GH action

In vivo imaging of hepatic GH signalling

Frank S, Wang X, He K, Yang N, Fang P, Rosenfeld RG, Hwa V, Chaudhuri TR, Deng L, Zinn KR
Department of Medicine, University of Alabama at Birmingham, Ala., USA
sjfrank@uab.edu
Mol Endocrinol 2006;20:2819–2830

Background: This study aimed to develop a mouse model system to non-invasively and repeatedly image in vivo hepatic GH signalling.

Methods: Nude mice were used for adenoviral mediated delivery of STAT5-dependent GH response element luciferase reporter to detect GH signalling serially by bioluminescence imaging.

Results: Female nude mice were injected with Ad-GHRE-luc and 3 days later fasted for 16 h. They were then anesthetized and injected with i.p. luciferin for a baseline image, and then injected with i.v. hGH. They received another injection of i.p. luciferin 1, 3, 5 and 7 h later. Bioluminescence images were collected 10 min after each luciferin injection. Luminescence was detected 1 h after hGH injection and was most intense 3 h after hGH stimulation, and was mostly in the region of the liver.

Conclusion: This system allows for in vivo analysis of Stat5-dependent signalling.

Luciferase reporters have been used for many years to quantify gene activation in vitro, but Frank et al. have generated a system to detect and quantify Stat5-induced luciferase activity in live animals. They created an adenoviral vector composed of the firefly luciferase gene driven by a promoter with eight repeats of the STAT5-dependent GH-response element of Spi2.1 (Ad-GHRE-luc) and injected it into nude mice. Adenovirus primarily targets the liver and therefore vector injection should result in enhanced expression of the reporter in the liver. Using a tail vein injected HA-labelled GHR adenoviral vector and in vivo injected radioactive antibodies to HA, the authors very elegantly showed that indeed the adenoviral vector mainly targeted the liver. Once the authors had established this, they continued to visualize the response to hGH. To do this, female mice were injected with the Ad-GHRE-luciferase vector. Stimulation by GH will result in Stat5 production and activation, which will then bind to the GHRE-luciferase DNA and as a result luciferase will be transcribed. The injected luciferin will give rise to a bioluminescence signal, which can be measured and is dependent on the amount of luciferase produced. The authors used a sensitive imaging system that was able to measure the bioluminescence signal in live animals. The authors also found that fasting increased the sensitivity to exogenous GH when mice received adenoviral GHRE-Luc in combination with adenoviral GHR. In conclusion, this is a very useful system for the in vivo analysis of cytokine induced Stat5 signalling that may also be used in other rodent models and will increase our understanding of the regulation of GH signalling.

Elevated circulating insulin-like growth factor-binding protein-1 is sufficient to cause fetal growth restriction

Watson CS, Bialek P, Anzo M, Khosravi J, Yee S-P, Han VKM
Samuel Lunenfeld Research Institute, Mount Sinai Hospital, Toronto, Ont., Canada
watson@mshri.on.ca
Endocrinology 2006;147:1175–1186

Background: Circulating IGF-binding protein-1 (IGFBP-1) is elevated in newborns and experimental animals with fetal growth restriction (FGR) and it is known that IGFBP-1 can inhibit actions of IGF-1. The aim of this study was to study a possible causal relationship between high circulating IGFBP-1 and FGR. *Methods:* Transgenic mice overexpressing human IGFBP-1 (hIGFBP-1) driven by mouse α-fetoprotein gene promoter in the fetal liver were generated. *Results:* Transgenic mice (AFP-BP-1) expressed hIGFBP-1 mainly in the fetal hepatocytes, starting at embryonic day 14.5 (E14.5) and peaking at 1 week postnatally. At birth, AFP-BP-1 pups were 18% smaller, and mice did not demonstrate any postnatal catch-up growth. The placentas of the AFP-BP-1 mice were larger than WT from E16.5 onwards. *Conclusion:* High concentrations of circulating IGFBP-1 are sufficient to cause FGR.

Insulin-like growth factor-binding protein (IGFBP-1) involvement in intrauterine growth retardation: study on IGFBP-1 overexpressing transgenic mice

Ben Lagha N, Seurin D, Le Bouc Y, Binoux M, Berdal A, Menuelle P, Babajko S
Laboratoire de Biologie Oro-faciale et Pathologie, INSERM Unit 714, Institut Biomédical des Cordeliers, Paris, France
Sylvie.Babajko@bhdc.jussieu.fr
Endocrinology 2006;147:4730–4737

Background: In this work, the authors wished to establish the impact of circulating IGFBP-1 on body growth associated to bone mineralization and carbohydrate resources. *Methods:* Transgenic mice used in this work overexpressed human IGFBP-1, driven from the human α₁-antitrypsin promoter, in liver from embryonic day (E)14.5, concomitantly to the appearance of ossification centers, through to adulthood. *Results:* Growth retardation was observed as early as E17.5 in homozygous mice, which were 20% smaller at birth. The mice exhibited pleiotropic defects of several skeletal units in the appendicular and axial skeleton. IGFBP-1 overexpression contributed to decreased fetal hepatic glycogen and neonatal circulating glucose levels. *Conclusion:* Overexpression of fetal human IGFBP-1 is related to antenatal growth retardation and delayed bone mineralization in transgenic mice.

There is a large body of evidence from animal experiments and clinical observation implicating the IGF system in modulating fetal growth. Both the ligand (IGF-1) and receptor are involved in the process. Less is known of the role for the IGF-binding proteins in the modulation of fetal growth. These two complementary papers demonstrate that animals in which IGFBP-1 has been overexpressed are 18–20% smaller than the wild-type animals. Altered bone size and mineralization accompanied the loss of IGFBP-1 along with a reduction in fetal hepatic glycogen and blood glucose concentration. Of interest was the observation that placental size was increased although the components of the placenta responsible for this change were not characterized. Postnatal growth was normal in both overexpressing and wild-type animals so catch-up growth was not observed.

Codependence of growth hormone-responsive, sexually dimorphic hepatic gene expression on signal transducer and activator of transcription 5b and hepatic nuclear factor 4α

Holloway MG, Lax EV, Waxman DJ
Division of Cell and Molecular Biology, Boston University, Boston, Mass., USA
djw@bu.edu
Mol Endocrinol 2006;20:647–660

Background: Stat5 deficiency results in decreased expression in male mouse liver of male-predominant cytochrome P_{450} CYP2d enzymes and an increase of female-predominant Cyp2b proteins.

Methods: This study characterized the effects of Stat5b deficiency on 15 individual Cyp RNAs, and assessed the effect of Stat5b deficiency, HNF4α deficiency and GH regulation (by hypophysectomy, pulsatile GH treatment, continuous GH treatment).

Results and Conclusion: All 7 male-specific RNAs were decreased to female levels in Stat5b-deficient male liver, whereas 5 of 8 female-specific RNAs (designated class I) were increased in expression up to 200-fold. Stat5b deficiency had a much more modest effect on the expression of these genes in females. The female-specific genes could be designated to two groups: class I mRNAs that were affected by Stat5b deficiency and class II mRNAs that were not affected by Stat5b deficiency. Hypophysectomy and GH treatment studies showed positive GH pulse regulation of all 7 male RNAs and negative GH pulse regulation of class I but not class II female RNAs in male mice. Many of the gender-specific genes responded in parallel to the loss of Stat5b and the loss of HNF4α suggesting that Stat5b and HNF4α may coregulate gender-specific gene expression. Continuous GH treatment of intact male mice induced expression of class I female RNAs in 4–7 days but of class II RNAs not until 7–14 days. Given the slow response of all 15 genes to changes in GH status, the authors propose that regulation of gender-specific CYP expression is indirect and mediated by Stat5b- and HNF4α-dependent factors that may include repressors of female-specific Cyps and other targets of GH action.

Sex-dependent liver gene expression is extensive and largely dependent upon signal transducer and activator of transcription 5b (Stat5b): Stat5b-dependent activation of male genes and repression of female genes revealed by microarray analysis

Clodfelter KH, Holloway MG, Hodor P, Park S-H, Ray WJ, Waxman DJ
Division of Cell and Molecular Biology, Boston University, Boston, Mass., USA
djw@bu.edu
Mol Endocrinol 2006;20:1333–1351

Background: Sexual dimorphism in mammalian liver contributes to gender differences in physiology and many sex-dependent liver genes are regulated by GH and Stat5b.

Methods: A large-scale gene expression study was conducted to characterize sex differences in liver gene expression and their dependence on Stat5b. Male and female, wild-type and Stat5b-deficient mice were used.

Results: 850 genes were more highly expressed in males and 90% were decreased in Stat5b deficiency. 753 genes were female-predominant of which 61% were upregulated in Stat5b-deficient males. However, 90% of the gender-dependent genes were unaffected by Stat5b deficiency in females.

Conclusion: Stat5b is essential for sex-dependent liver gene expression, equalling 4% of the genome. Male-predominant liver gene expression requires Stat5b or Stat5b-dependent factors. Many female-predominant liver genes are repressed in males in a Stat5b-dependent manner.

The main signalling transduction pathway for GH is the JAK2-STAT5 pathway and activation of this pathway is differentially affected by 'male' and 'female' GH secretory patterns (fig. 2). A pulsatile 'male-like' GH pattern stimulates Stat5b activation to a greater extent than a more continuous 'female-like' GH pattern. Stat5b-deleted mice are small, especially the males, and have altered hepatic

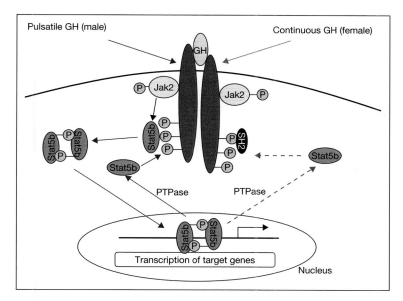

Fig. 2. Sexual dimorphism in GH-activated Stat5b phosphorylation. GH binding to dimerized GH receptors (GHR) results in proximity of GHR-associated tyrosine kinase JAK2 molecules, resulting in autophosphorylation and tyrosine phosphorylation of GHR residues, generating docking sites for Stat5b and other SH2 domain-containing proteins. After binding to these sites, Stat5b undergoes JAK2 catalyzed tyrosine phosphorylation, followed by dimerization, nuclear translocation and induction of transcription of target genes. Stat5b is then deactivated by phosphotyrosine phosphatases (PTPase), and Stat5b may then be reactivated in subsequent cycles of docking and phosphorylation. In females, the Stat5b is much less activated and the Stat5b cycle is more rapidly terminated. Jak2 = Janus kinase 2; P = phosphate; Stat5b = signal transducer and activator of transcription 5b; PTPase = phosphotyrosine phosphatase; SH2 = Scr homology-2-containing protein. Figure redrawn from Waxman and O'Connor [4].

gene expression. The papers above describe two extensive studies regarding the regulation of gender-specific hepatic gene expression. Many of these genes were found to be affected by Stat5b deficiency in males, but not necessarily in females. Several of the Stat5b-dependent male genes encode transcriptional repressors; these may include direct Stat5b targets that repress female-predominant genes in male liver. Several female-predominant repressors were elevated in Stat5b-deficient males; these may contribute to the major loss of male gene expression seen in the absence of Stat5b. The involvement of Stat5b in the regulation of sex-dependent genes is therefore not straightforward. HNF4α also contributes to gender specificity of liver gene expression through positive regulation of male-specific Cyp genes and negative regulation of female-specific Cyp genes. The authors showed that many genes are co-dependent on Stat5b and HNF4α and suggest that Stat5b and HNF4α act in concert, by an indirect mechanism, to affect expression of sexually dimorphic hepatic genes. Figure 3 shows a hypothesis of gender-specific hepatic gene regulation based on these findings. Since 4% of the genome is affected by Stat5b deficiency, responsible for gender differences in fat, carbohydrate, steroid and drug metabolism, it is important to elucidate underlying mechanisms and these studies help in doing so. An excellent review by Waxman and O'Connor [4] discusses this matter further.

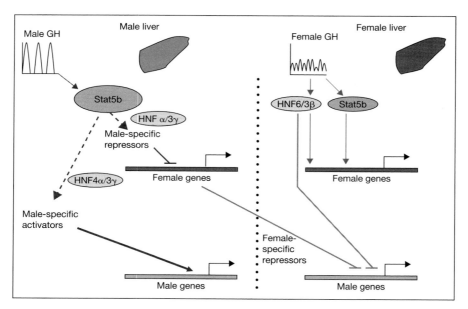

Fig. 3. Hypothetical mechanism for indirect regulation of sex-specific genes by liver Stat5b and hepatic nucleic factors (HNFs). Male GH pulse-activated Stat5b is proposed to activate male-specific activators and male-specific repressors, which then respectively induce male-specific genes and repress female-specific genes. The female-specific genes will include female repressors that inhibit the expression of male-specific genes in female liver. The low Stat5 activity found in female liver may act directly or indirectly (via HNF6 and/or HNF3β) to induce female gene expression. HNF6 can inhibit transcription of male-specific genes. HNF4α is required for transcription of a subset of Stat5b induced male-specific genes, as observed in the co-dependence of gender-specific gene expression on Stat5b and HNF4α. Figure adapted from Waxman and O'Connor [4].

> **Continuing debate**
> **Liver-produced IGF-1**

Liver-specific overexpression of the insulin-like growth factor-1 enhances somatic growth and partially prevents the effects of growth hormone deficiency

Liao L, Dearth RK, Zhou S, Britton OL, Lee AV, Xu J
Department of Molecular and Cellular Biology, Baylor College of Medicine, Houston, Tex., USA
jxu@bcm.tmc.edu
Endocrinology 2006;147:3877–3888

Background: Since the role and importance of circulating IGF-1 in body growth remains unclear, the authors wished to create an animal model that secreted supraphysiological amounts of IGF-1 from the liver. *Methods:* Mice carrying a transthyretin enhancer-promoter-IGF-1 transgene were created. *Results:* Mice transcribed transgene IGF-1 solely in the liver and had a 50–60% increase in circulating IGF-1 levels. Transgenic (TG) mice had increased body weight and body length compared with wild-type (WT) mice. Lean body mass was increased due to increased number and thickness of skeletal muscle fibers. Treatment with GH antagonist Pegvisomant caused a severe growth deficit in WT mice but Pegvisomant also reduced body growth in TG mice. Glucose tolerance was slightly improved in TG mice compared to WT mice. *Conclusion:* Higher circulating levels of IGF-1 stimulate somatic growth and lean body mass modestly and improve glucose tolerance slightly.

This is a nice study in which the authors created a mouse strain that could be seen as the mirror model of the liver induced IGF-1-deficient (LID) mice. LID mice have a 75% reduction in circulating IGF-1 levels but normal growth, suggesting that liver-generated IGF-1 does not play a major role in the promotion of growth, although several aspects of this model have been criticized [5, 6]. The mouse model created by Liao et al. has a liver-specific overexpression of mouse IGF-1 resulting in a modest 50–60% increase in circulating IGF-1 levels. These mice have a modestly increased body weight of ca. 10% and bone length (5%) that reaches statistical significance at the age of 8–9 weeks. This suggests that supraphysiological IGF-1 production is able to increase growth modestly, in line with response to IGF-1 treatment in GHD rodents and humans. The increase in muscle mass in these mice was much more impressive, with a 30% increase in soleus thickness, muscle fiber number and fiber thickness. Blockade of GH signalling with Pegvisomant (from 21 to 56 days of age) resulted in a reduction of body growth in both TG and WT mice to a similar extent. Although transgene IGF-1 expression was unaffected by Pegvisomant, reduction of endogenous IGF-1 transcription and reduction of ALS production resulted in a 50% reduction of IGF-1 levels in the TG mice. Therefore, the mechanism of GHR blockade-induced reduction of growth is still unclear and can be due to either a blockade of direct GH action in peripheral tissues or reduced stimulation by IGF-1. Cross-breeding of these mice with mice harboring other defects in the GH-IGF-1 axis may take us a step further.

Important for clinical practice
Small children growing up

Growth trajectories of extremely low birth weight infants from birth to young adulthood: a longitudinal, population-based study

Saigal S, Stoskopf B, Streiner D, Paneth N, Pinelli J, Boyle M
Department of Pediatrics, McMaster University, Hamilton, Ont., Canada
saigal@mcmaster.ca
Pediatr Res 2006;60:751–758

Background: The outcome of growth attainment of children born with extremely low birth weight (ELBW) is not well known and the authors therefore aimed to study this in a population-based cohort.
Methods: Growth attainment of a population-based cohort of ELBW (<1,000 g) and a cohort of sociodemographically comparable normal birth weight (NBW) was compared at young adulthood, and the pattern of growth trajectories and correlates of growth at ages 1, 2, 3, and 8 years, and teen and young adulthood were compared.
Results: The proportion considered small for gestational age was ELBW 25% versus NBW 3%. Weight for age z-scores for ELBW showed substantial decline to age 3 years, with subsequent catch up to adolescence and smaller gains to adulthood.
Conclusion: ELBW children showed growth failure during infancy, followed by accelerated weight gain and crossing of BMI percentiles at adolescence.

Long-term growth outcomes for ELBW infants are not common, so this comparison from a population of 147 ELBW (<1,000 g) and 131 sociodemographically comparable normal birth weight (NBW) cases at young adulthood is of value. Weight for age z-scores for ELBW showed substantial decline to age 3 years, with subsequent significant catch up to adolescence and smaller gains to adulthood. Height for age z-scores showed both sexes of ELBW were disadvantaged at every age compared with NBW and their expected mid-parental height. The BMI z-scores for ELBW showed a sustained incline from age 3 years to adulthood, where both sexes normalized to above zero, and were comparable to their peers. These patterns of growth may be particularly important in the ELBW children, as in other studies it has been associated with an increased risk of insulin resistance and coronary heart disease.

The influence of head growth in fetal life, infancy, and childhood on intelligence at the ages of 4 and 8 years

Gale CR, O'Callaghan FJ, Bredow M, Martyn CN
Medical Research Council Epidemiology Resource Centre, University of Southampton, Southampton, UK
crg@mrc.soton.ac.uk
Pediatrics 2006;118:1486–1492

Background: The relation between head growth and cognitive function is not clear and in this work, the authors studied the effects of head growth prenatally, during infancy, and during later periods of development on cognitive function at the ages of 4 and 8 years.

Methods: 633 term-born children from the Avon Longitudinal Study of Parents and Children cohort were followed and their cognitive function was assessed at the age of 4 and 8 years.

Results: At 4 years, full-scale IQ increased by an average of 2.41 points for each 1 SD increase in head circumference at birth and 1.97 points for each 1 SD increase in head growth during infancy, conditional on head size at birth. At 8 years, head circumference at birth was no longer associated with IQ, but head growth during infancy remained a significant predictor, with full-scale IQ increasing an average of 1.56 points for each 1 SD increase in growth.

Conclusion: This study suggests that the brain volume a child achieves by the age of 1 year helps determine later intelligence. Growth in brain volume after infancy may not compensate for poorer earlier growth.

Impact of prenatal and/or postnatal growth problems in low birth weight preterm infants on school-age outcomes: an 8-year longitudinal evaluation

Casey PH, Whiteside-Mansell L, Barrett K, Bradley RH, Gargus R
Department of Pediatrics, University of Arkansas for Medical Sciences, Little Rock, Ark., USA
CaseyPatrickH@uams.edu
Pediatrics 2006;118:1078–1086

Background: The objective of this study was to assess the 8-year growth, cognitive, behavioral status, health status, and academic achievement in low birth weight preterm infants who had failure to thrive only, were small for gestational age only, had failure to thrive plus were small for gestational age, or had normal growth.

Methods: A total of 985 infants were evaluated until age 8; 180 infants met the criteria for failure to thrive between 4 and 36 months' gestational corrected age.

Conclusion: Low birth weight preterm infants who had postnatal growth problems, particularly when associated with prenatal growth problems, demonstrated lower physical size, cognitive scores, and academic achievement at age 8. When postnatal growth was adequate, there was no independent effect of small for gestational age status on cognitive status and academic achievement.

Poor head growth occurs in a number of situations, particularly in severe intrauterine growth restriction and in the babies of mothers who smoke during pregnancy. These two papers demonstrate that (Gale et al.) when the influence of head growth was distinguished for different periods, only prenatal growth and growth during infancy were associated with subsequent IQ. These observations pertain to the general population but are largely echoed in the study (Casey et al.) in low birth weight infants assessed at the age of 8 years. In this situation, children who were both small for gestational age and had failure to thrive were the smallest in all growth variables at age 8, and also demonstrated the lowest cognitive and academic achievement scores. The children with failure to thrive only were significantly smaller than the children with normal growth in all growth variables and had significantly lower IQ scores. Those who were small for gestational age only did not differ from those with normal growth in any cognitive or academic achievement measures. These observations suggest that the brain volume a child achieves by the age of 1 year helps determine later intelligence and growth in brain volume after infancy may not compensate for poorer earlier growth particularly in situations where postnatal growth is also compromised.

Evidence for hypermetabolism in boys with constitutional delay of growth and maturation

Han JC, Balagopal P, Sweeten S, Darmaun D, Mauras N
Division of Endocrinology, Nemours Children's, Jacksonville, Fla., USA
nmauras@nemours.org
J Clin Endocrinol Metab 2006;91:2081–2086

Background: The authors hypothesized that an imbalance between energy intake and expenditure may contribute to the pathogenesis of constitutional delay of growth and maturation (CDGM) and therefore compared differences in nutrition, body composition and energy expenditure in boys with CDGM and controls.

Methods: Observational, cross-sectional study of 36 boys (8–17 years): 12 with CDGM (short stature, delayed bone age and puberty, and no other pathology) and 12 height-matched (pre- or early pubertal) and 12 age-matched (pubertal) healthy controls.

Results: Nutritional markers were comparable among the groups. CDGM subjects had bone mineral density lower than age-matched controls ($p < 0.01$) but comparable with height-matched controls. Even though resting energy expenditure did not differ between groups, CDGM subjects had 25% higher caloric intake adjusted for fat-free mass (FFM) than height-matched controls ($p < 0.05$) and 78% higher caloric intake per kilogram FFM compared with age-matched controls ($p < 0.00001$). CDGM subjects had 46% ($p < 0.05$) and 91% ($p < 0.001$) higher total energy expenditure per kilogram FFM than height- and age-matched controls, respectively.

Conclusions: Boys with CDGM have higher rates of overall energy expenditure compared with age- and size-matched controls. This increased metabolism may result in impaired tempo of growth.

Children with CDGM tend to be thin and it has been suggested their growth pattern is reminiscent of nutritional insufficiency. Using doubly labelled water studies, serum nutritional/hormonal markers, dual-energy x-ray absorptiometry, dietary analysis, and indirect calorimetry values were compared between patients with CDGM and height- or age-matched controls. Even though resting energy expenditure did not differ between groups, CDGM subjects had 25% higher caloric intake adjusted for FFM than height-matched controls and 78% higher caloric intake per kilogram FFM compared with age-matched controls. IGF-1 and testosterone were by definition lower than age-matched controls. Although it was suggested that augmenting nutrition to match energy needs (with or without hormonal therapy) might improve linear and ponderal growth, given that adult outcomes for this group of individuals is no different from the general population, it is difficult to see the advantage of such an approach.

Clinical trials, new treatment

Growth hormone is effective in treatment of short stature associated with short stature homeobox-containing gene deficiency: two-year results of a randomized, controlled, multicenter trial

Blum WF, Crowe BJ, Quigley CA, Jung H, Cao D, Ross JL, Braun L, Rappold GJ
Lilly Research Laboratories, Eli Lilly & Co., Bad Homburg, Germany
Blum_Werner@Lilly.com
J Clin Endocrinol Metab 2007;92:219–228

Background: The human *SHOX* gene is one of the major genes contributing to longitudinal growth, and mutations resulting in haploinsufficiency have been reported in patients with isolated short stature and Leri-Weill syndrome (LWS). The aim of this study was to determine the efficacy of GH in treating short stature associated with SHOX deficiency (SHOX-D).

Methods: Randomized trial with a GH-treated and untreated group of patients with short stature and proven SHOX-D. Comparisons were made with a GH-treated group of patients with Turner syndrome. 1,608 samples from children with idiopathic short stature or LWS were analyzed for abnormalities of the *SHOX* gene. First- and second-year height velocity, height SD score and height gain (cm) were com-pared between the groups.

Results: The GH-treated SHOX-D group had a significantly greater first-year height velocity than the untreated control group (mean ± SE: 8.7 ± 0.3 vs. 5.2 ± 0.2 cm/year; p < 0.001) and similar first-year height velocity to GH-treated subjects with TS (8.9 ± 0.4 cm/year; p = 0.592). Second-year height velocity (7.3 ± 0.2; vs. 5.4 ± 0.2 cm/year; p < 0.001) and second-year height SDS (−2.1 ± 0.2 vs. −3 ± 0.2; p < 0.001) were all significantly greater in GH-treated subjects than controls and were com-parable to second-year height velocity (7.0 ± 0.2 cm/year) and second-year height SDS (−2.6 ± 0.2) in the GH-treated girls with Turner syndrome.

Conclusion: GH treatment increased height velocity and height SDS over a 2-year treatment period in patients with SHOX-D, and this effect was similar to that observed in TS.

This is a good study size with 52 prepubertal patients with short stature (height <3rd percentile or <10th percentile and HV <25th percentile) and a molecularly proven *SHOX* gene defect that were either treated with hGH or not. *SHOX* gene abnormalities were found in 67 of 1,608 patients with ISS or LWS, and comprised gene deletions, partial gene deletions and point mutations, and randomiza-tion was stratified by these different gene abnormalities, the presence of LWS and gender. SHOX-D is believed to contribute significantly to the growth retardation associated with Turner syndrome and therefore comparison was also made with 26 patients with Turner syndrome treated with GH. All patients were treated for 2 years with a dose of 50 µg/kg/day (equalling ca. 1.3 mg/m²/day). This study shows the beneficial effects of GH treatment in SHOX-D patients treated with GH over a 2-year period. The height SDS improvement was approximately +1 SDS in 2 years and was comparable to the benefit of GH in Turner syndrome. It is therefore not unlikely that final height improvements will be in a sim-ilar range as those found in Turner syndrome. Interestingly, the effect of GH treatment seemed some-what larger in ISS compared to LWS, but it is unclear from this work whether that is due to genotype differences or whether end-organ response to GH treatment is different between these groups.

New mechanisms
GH action and regulation of signalling

Growth hormone promotes skeletal muscle cell fusion independent of insulin-like growth factor-1 upregulation

Sotiropoulos A, Ohanna M, Kedzia C, Menon RK, Kopchick JJ, Kelly PA, Pende M
INSERM, Faculté de Médicine Necker-Enfants Malades, Paris, France
sotiropoulos@necker.fr
Proc Natl Acad Sci USA 2006;103:7315–7320

Background: The growth retardation of double GHR/IGF-1 mutants is more severe than that observed with single mutants. It is therefore likely that GH exerts specific and direct actions and the aim of this paper was to identify these GH-specific actions on muscle.

Methods: GHR$^{-/-}$ mice were studied and primary muscle cell cultures from these mice were used.

Results: The mass of skeletal muscles lacking GHR is reduced because of a decrease in myofiber size, whereas myofiber number is normal. GH has no effect on size, proliferation and differentiation of myoblast precursors, but controls the size of differentiated myotubes in a cell-autonomous manner. The GH hypertrophic action leads to increased myonuclear number, suggesting that GH facilitates fusion of myoblasts with nascent myotubes. This action is independent of IGF-1 but depends on NFATC2, a transcription factor that regulates myoblast-myotube fusion. This effect of GH occurs without an increase in local IGF-1 and also without increasing Stat5.

Conclusion: The effects of GH and IGF-1 on muscle are distinct and additive, and rely on different sig-nalling transduction pathways.

It is well established that GHRs are present in many peripheral tissues and indeed also in muscle, but nevertheless the direct effect of GH on these cells remains unclear. In this study the authors aimed to unravel GH-specific actions in muscle. GHR deficiency caused a switch from oxidative slow type I fibers to glycolytic fast type II fibers, consistent with an increase in type I fibers in mice overexpressing hGH [3]. GHD however decreased muscle fiber size by 40% in both type I and type II fibers. It was shown that this was not due to altered proliferation or differentiation of myoblasts but that GH increases the size of myotubes by promoting fusion of myotubes with myoblasts. Muscle cells are multinucleated cells and muscle hypertrophy occurs through fusion of cells, and this process is stimulated by GH. This is an important paper since it suggests a new concept of the mechanism of GH action.

Functional cross-modulation between SOCS proteins can stimulate cytokine signalling

Piessevaux J, Lavens D, Montoye T, Wauman J, Catteeuw D, Vandekerckhove J, Belsham D, Peelman F, Tavernier J
Flanders Interuniversity Institute for Biotechnology, Ghent University, Ghent, Belgium
jan.tavernier@ugent.be
J Biol Chem 2006;281:32953–32966

Background: SOCS (suppressors of cytokine signalling) are negative regulators of cytokine signalling that function primarily at the receptor level. Interestingly, SOCS2 can have both inhibitory and stimulatory effects on GH signalling. Other SOCS proteins can also inhibit GH signalling and therefore this study examined direct cross-modulation between SOCS proteins.

Methods: Cell culture, transfection with labelled SOCS constructs, cytokine receptors and luciferase reporters, Western blotting and co-immunoprecipitation.

Results: The authors demonstrated that SOCS2 interfered with the negative regulatory effects of SOCS1 and SOCS3 via direct interaction, possibly due to degradation of the targeted SOCS proteins. SOCS2 can interact with all members of the SOCS family and not only affects GH signalling but also interferon and leptin signalling. These observations were extended to SOCS6 and SOCS7.

Conclusions: SOCS2, SOCS6 and SOCS7 are capable of controlling SOCS protein stability and thus altering cytokine sensitivity.

Negative control of cytokine signalling occurs at many levels and involves, amongst others, inhibition of Stat activation by SOCS proteins. The SH2 domain of SOCS2 inhibits Stat activation by competition with Stats for binding to phosphorylated receptor-docking sites necessary for Stat phosphorylation. In accordance, SOCS2 knockout mice display overgrowth and have increased sensitivity to GH, but interestingly overexpression of SOCS2 also results in gigantism. This study aids in the explanation of the underlying physiological mechanism and shows that SOCS2 plays a pivotal role in the regulation of cytokine sensitivity. Expression of SOCS1 and SOCS3 was able to completely abolish GH signalling in vitro and co-expression of SOCS2 counteracted this effect. This was not only the case for GH signalling but also for IFN-γ and leptin signalling. The authors showed that SOCS2 directly interacted with elongin BC complex after which the complex bound to SOCS1 and SOCS3. The elongin BC complex is part of a complex that marks proteins for degradation, and indeed the authors showed that SOCS1 was degraded by increasing levels of SOCS2. These results suggest that SOCS2, but also SOCS6 and SOCS7, regulates multiple cytokine-signalling pathways. So even though SOCS2 is mainly associated with inhibiting GH signalling, it can increase signalling of IFN-γ and leptin, and possibly other cytokines, through increased degradation of SOCS1 and SOCS3 that normally inhibit IFN-γ and leptin signalling. This may be of help in defining underlying mechanisms for alterations of cytokine signalling in states of GH deficiency, insensitivity or overproduction.

Clinical and biochemical characteristics of a male patient with a novel homozygous Stat5b mutation

Vidarsdottir S, Walenkamp MJE, Pereira AM, Karperien M, Van Doorn J, Van Duyvenvoorde HA, White S, Breuning MH, Roelfsema F, Kruithof MF, Van Dissel J, Janssen R, Wit JM, Romijn JA
Department of Endocrinology and Metabolic Diseases, Leiden University Medical Center, Leiden, The Netherlands
m.j.e.walenkamp@lumc.nl
J Clin Endocrinol Metab 2006;91:3482–3485

Background: Recently, 2 females with severe short stature and pulmonary and immune abnormalities were found to have homozygous mutations in the *Stat5b* gene. This paper describes a new *Stat5b* mutation in a male with severe short stature.
Methods: Genotyping of Stat5 cDNA and Western blotting for Stat5b in cultured fibroblasts before and after GH stimulation.
Results: A homozygous frameshift mutation in the DNA-binding domain of *Stat5b* gene was found in a patient with severe short stature (-5.9 SDS), delayed puberty, and no history of pulmonary or immunological problems. Plasma prolactin was elevated. IGF-1, IGFBP-3 and ALS were extremely low (-6.9, -12 and -7.5 SDS).
Conclusion: This report confirms the essential role of Stat5b in GH signalling and growth in the human, in both males and females, and suggests that pulmonary and immunological abnormalities are not necessarily part of the phenotype.

This is an interesting paper showing that human *Stat5b* mutations are not confined to the female gender. In mice, Stat5b deficiency affects growth of males more than that of females, possibly related to the more pulsatile fashion of GH secretion in males. In humans the distinction between genders regarding GH secretion is not as pronounced as it is in rodents and this may underlie the fact that the severity of the growth defect in this male patient is similar to that described in the 2 females. However, a greater number of affected patients are required to assess possible gender differences. The second interesting observation is that this patient lacks pulmonary or immunological pathology. In addition, this patient differs from other patients with *Stat5b* mutations in that he did not have elevated GH secretion, even though he did have enhanced prolactin secretion. The pathophysiological mechanism of the pulmonary abnormalities is still unclear but in the patient described by Kofoed et al. [7], Stat1 and Stat3 signalling was increased and this may contribute to altered immune function and we do not know whether that is the case in this patient. We now know of 2 more patients (siblings) with a *Stat5b* mutation (a homozygous splice site mutation in exon 13) who do not suffer from pulmonary disease but 1 of whom has juvenile idiopathic arthritis, also suggesting disordered immune function [8].

Novel mutations in known genes: acid-labile subunit

Total absence of functional-acid labile subunit, resulting in severe insulin-like growth factor deficiency and moderate growth failure

Hwa V, Haeusler G, Pratt KL, Little BM, Frisch H, Koller D, Rosenfeld RG
Department of Pediatrics, Oregon Health and Science University Portland, Oreg., USA
hwav@ohsu.edu
J Clin Endocrinol Metab 2006;91:1826–1831

Background: IGF-1 circulates as part of a ternary complex with IGF-binding protein (IGFBP)-3 and acid-labile subunit (ALS) and may mediate the growth-promoting effects of GH. Another patient with inactivation of the ALS gene has been described [9], but due to the absence of family history and delayed puberty, the impact on growth was unproven.

Methods: A patient in which serum IGF-1 and IGFBP-3 were abnormally low (−5.8 and −7.2 SDS), but growth failure was modest (−2.1 SDS at 15.5 years), was investigated.

Results: A novel homozygous missense mutation was identified in the ALS gene, which resulted in undetectable levels of serum ALS.

Conclusions: ALS is critical for maintaining normal serum concentrations of IGF-1 and IGFBP-3. ALS deficiency can be associated with moderate growth failure, and does not seem to affect the onset and progression of puberty.

IGF-1 circulates as ternary complex with IGFBP-3 and an ALS. This paper reports a patient with a novel homozygous missense mutation in the ALS gene resulting in undetectable ALS. Despite this, growth was minimally affected although the circulating concentrations of IGF-1 and IGFBP-3 were very low. This observation mirrors the phenotype of ALS-deficient mice [10] and confirms the phenotype of ALS deficiency in humans [9] and argues for a modest role for the ternary complex in the regulation of stature.

Reviews

Endocrine regulation of human fetal growth: the role of the mother, placenta, and fetus

Murphy VE, Smith R, Giles WB, Clifton VL
Mother and Baby Research Centre, Hunter Medical Research Institute, University of Newcastle, N.S.W., Australia
vicki.clifton@newcastle.edu.au
Endocr Rev 2006;27:141–169

The environment in which the fetus develops is critical for its survival and long-term health. The regulation of normal human fetal growth involves many multidirectional interactions between the mother, placenta, and fetus. The mother supplies nutrients and oxygen to the fetus via the placenta and the fetus influences the provision of maternal nutrients via the placental production of hormones that regulate maternal metabolism. Endocrine regulation of fetal growth involves interactions between the mother, placenta, and fetus, and these effects may program long-term physiology.

This is an excellent overview of current concepts of the endocrinology of human fetal growth. It draws on both clinical observation, placental physiology and incorporates as appropriate animal data to support the contention that the endocrine system plays a greater role than hitherto thought.

Food for thought
Exon-3-deleted growth hormone receptor

Growth hormone (GH) pharmacogenetics: influence of GH receptor exon-3 retention or deletion on first year growth response and final height in patients with severe GH deficiency

Jorge AA, Marchisotti FG, Montenegro LR, Carvalho LR, Mendonca BB, Arnhold IJP
Hospital das Clinicas, Laboratorio de Hormonios, São Paulo, Brazil
alexj@usp.br
J Clin Endocrinol Metab 2006;91:1076–1080

Background: A polymorphism in the gene encoding the GH receptor (*GHR*) that results in the exclusion of exon-3 (*GHRd3*) with the consequent removal of 22 amino acids is associated with better first- and second-year growth responses to recombinant human growth hormone (rhGH) in patients with idiopathic short stature or those who were born small-for-gestational [8]. The aim of this study was to study the effect of GHR-exon-3 genotype on the short- and long-term response to GH treatment in children with GHD.

Methods: Genotype and retrospective data collection was performed on 75 children with GHD. Patients were divided into two groups based on the genotype: full-length (*fl*) and exon-3-deleted (*d3*, homozygous and heterozygous) alleles. First-year growth velocity (n = 58, prepubertal) and adult height (n = 44) after 7.5 ± 3.0 years of treatment were the main outcome measures.

Results: Patients carrying at least one *GHRd3* allele had a significantly better growth velocity in the first year of GH treatment (12.3 ± 2.6 vs. 10.6 ± 2.3 cm/year; p < 0.05) and achieved a taller adult height (final height SDS −0.8 ± 1.1 vs. −1.7 ± 1.2; p < 0.05) when compared with patients homozygous for *GHRfl* alleles.

Conclusion: In this study, patients with GHD who were homozygous for *GHR exon-3-fl* responded less well to rhGH treatment.

The growth hormone (GH) response to GH treatment in children with isolated GH deficiency is independent of the presence of the exon-3-minus isoform of the GH receptor

Blum WF, Machinis K, Shavrikova EP, Keller A, Stobbe H, Pfaeffle RW, Amselem S
Lilly Research Laboratories, Eli Lilly & Co., Bad Homburg, Germany
Blum_Werner@Lilly.com
J Clin Endocrinol Metab 2006;91:4171–4174

Background: The aim of this study was to examine the impact of the *GHR* genotype on the phenotype and growth response in patients with isolated GH deficiency (IGHD) treated with GH.

Methods: A retrospective, multinational, multicenter observational study of 107 patients with IGHD. Genotypes (*fl-GHR/fl-GHR*, *fl-GHR/d3-GHR*, or *d3-GHR/d3-GHR*) were correlated with height SDS, height velocity, height velocity SDS at baseline and 1 year of GH treatment, and the changes in these parameters over 1 year of treatment.

Results: No statistically significant differences were observed between patients with the *d3-GHR* allele (n = 48) and patients who were homozygous for the *fl-GHR* allele (n = 59). The mean serum IGF-1 concentration was lower in the *fl/fl* group, but this did not reach statistical significance.

Conclusion: The data suggest that the presence of the *d3-GHR* allele does not influence response to standard replacement doses of rhGH in a cohort of GHD children.

These two studies evaluating the effect of the presence of the *d3-GHR* allele on response to rhGH treatment in a cohort of patients with GHD appear to contradict each other. The reasons for this discrepancy remain open to speculation. Blum et al. suggest that the impact of the *GHR* genotype on GH responsiveness may be a dose-dependent phenomenon, and may be apparent only when supraphysiological doses of rhGH are used in SGA and Turner syndrome. Further studies will be required to clarify these issues.

References
1. Carta C, Pantaleoni F, Bocchinfuso G, Stella L, Vasta I, Sarkozy A, et al: Germline missense mutations affecting KRAS isoform B are associated with a severe Noonan syndrome phenotype. Am J Hum Genet 2006;79:129–135.
2. Roberts AE, Araki T, Swanson KD, Montgomery KT, Schiripo TA, Joshi VA, et al: Germline gain-of-function mutations in SOS1 cause Noonan syndrome. Nat Genet 2007;39:70–74.
3. Binder G, Wittekindt N, Ranke MB: Noonan syndrome: genetics and responsiveness to growth hormone therapy. Horm Res 2007;67(suppl 1):45–49.
4. Waxman DJ, O'Connor C: Growth hormone regulation of sex-dependent liver gene expression. Mol Endocrinol 2006;20:2613–2629.
5. Yakar S, Liu JL, Stannard B, Butler A, Accili D, Sauer B, et al: Normal growth and development in the absence of hepatic insulin-like growth factor-1. Proc Natl Acad Sci USA 1999;96:7324–7329.
6. Sjogren K, Liu JL, Blad K, Skrtic S, Vidal O, Wallenius V, et al: Liver-derived insulin-like growth factor 1 (IGF-1) is the principal source of IGF-1 in blood but is not required for postnatal body growth in mice. Proc Natl Acad Sci USA 1999;96:7088–7092.
7. Kofoed EM, Hwa V, Little B, Woods KA, Buckway CK, Tsubaki J, et al: Growth hormone insensitivity associated with a STAT5b mutation. N Engl J Med 2003;349:1139–1147.
8. Hwa V, Camacho-Hubner C, Little BM, David A, Metherell LA, El-Khatib N, et al: Growth hormone insensitivity and severe short stature in siblings: a novel mutation at the exon 13-intron 13 junction of the STAT5b gene. Horm Res 2007;68:218–224.

9. Domene HM, Bengolea SV, Martinez AS, Ropelato MG, Pennisi P, Scaglia P, et al: Deficiency of the circulating insulin-like growth factor system associated with inactivation of the acid-labile subunit gene. N Engl J Med 2004;350:570–577.
10. Ueki I, Ooi GT, Tremblay ML, Hurst KR, Bach LA, Boisclair YR: Inactivation of the acid-labile subunit gene in mice results in mild retardation of postnatal growth despite profound disruptions in the circulating insulin-like growth factor system. Proc Natl Acad Sci USA 2000;97:6868–6873.
11. Gelb BD, Tartaglia M: Noonan syndrome and related disorders: dysregulated RAS-mitogen activated protein kinase signal transduction. Hum Mol Genet 2006;15(Spec No 2):R220–R226.

Growth Plate, Bone and Calcium

Dionisios Chrysis[a], Terhi Heino[b], and Lars Sävendahl[b]

[a]Endocrinology Unit, Department of Pediatrics, Medical School, University of Patras, Greece
[b]Pediatric Endocrinology Unit, Department of Woman and Child Health, Karolinska Institutet, Stockholm, Sweden

Growth plate and bone are highly organized structures with a complex cellular biology. Studies have been limited by the relative lack of relevant experimental models. Thanks to new technologies, e.g. targeted deletions of genes, the knowledge is rapidly expanding. The first paper selected representing the **mechanism of the year** describes a new cause of autosomal recessive hypophosphatemia. Under **new paradigms**, we chose two papers showing that FSH directly regulates bone mass. The possibility to transplant mesenchymal stem cells and/or autologous tissue-engineered composites gives **new hope** for the therapeutic intervention of growth plate injuries. Another new hope comes from a report of growth plate-sparing effects of a new selective glucocorticoid receptor modulator. A **new concern** is the increasing amount of reports of bisphosphonate-induced osteonecrosis of the jaws. **Concepts revised or re-centered** are represented by a paper suggesting that the skeletal benefits from calcium supplementation are limited. **Important observation for clinical practice** is represented by a report of reduced bone mineral density and increased bone metabolism in young adults with 21-hydroxylase deficiency. A paper by Kollet et al. was selected to describe a **new mechanism** of osteoclasts to be involved in the mobilization of hematopoietic progenitor cells. In the section **new genes**, a paper identifying a new cause of recessive lethal osteogenesis imperfecta is discussed. The **review** of the year entitled 'C-type natriuretic peptide (CNP) in growth: A new paradigm' elegantly discusses the critical role of CNP in the regulation of linear bone growth not only in mice but also in humans. Finally, we selected two papers supplying some **food for thought**.

Mechanism of the year

Loss of DMP1 causes rickets and osteomalacia and identifies a role for osteocytes in mineral metabolism

Feng JQ, Ward LM, Liu S, Lu Y, Xie Y, Yuan B, Yu X, Rauch F, Davis SI, Zhang S, Rios H, Drezner MK, Quarles LD, Bonewald LF, White KE
Oral Biology, University of Missouri-Kansas City, Kansas City, Mo., USA
dquarles@kumc.edu
Nat Genet 2006;38:1310–1315

Background: Dentin matrix protein 1 (DMP1) is highly expressed in osteocytes and plays an important role in bone remodeling. Knockout mice for DMP1 have hypomineralized bones. Dmp1 null mice and humans with autosomal recessive hypophosphatemic rickets have rickets and osteomalacia with isolated renal phosphate wasting, associated elevated fibroblast growth factor-23 (FGF23) levels and normocalciuria. Thus the authors investigated whether this gene regulates bone mineralization not only directly but also through the regulation of phosphate homeostasis.

Results: Mutational analyses in two families with autosomal recessive hypophosphatemic rickets revealed two different mutations in the DMP1 gene. One mutation affected the start codon, and the other was a 7-bp deletion disrupting the highly conserved DMP1 C-terminus. Studies in DMP1 null mice demonstrated defective osteocyte maturation and increased FGF23 expression leading to pathological changes in bone mineralization.

Conclusion: These results suggest that a bone-renal axis is necessary for proper bone mineral metabolism.

DMP1 mutations in autosomal recessive hypophosphatemia implicate a bone matrix protein in the regulation of phosphate homeostasis

Lorenz-Depiereux B, Bastepe M, Benet-Pages A, Amyere M, Wagenstaller J, Muller-Barth U, Badenhoop K, Kaiser SM, Rittmaster RS, Shlossberg AH, Olivares JL, Loris C, Ramos FJ, Glorieux F, Vikkula M, Juppner H, Strom TM
Institute of Human Genetics, GSF National Research Center for Environment and Health, Munich-Neuherberg, Germany
TimStrom@gsf.de
Nat Genet 2006;38:1248–1250

Background: Hypophosphatemic rickets is a genetically heterogeneous disease.
Results: The autosomal recessive form was mapped to chromosome 4q21. In addition, homozygous mutations in DMP1 (dentin matrix protein 1) were identified, encoding a non-collagenous bone matrix protein expressed in osteoblasts and osteocytes. Furthermore, the phosphaturic protein FGF23 was elevated in the plasma of 2 of 4 affected individuals.
Conclusion: The data provide a possible explanation for the phosphaturia and inappropriately normal 1α,25-dihydroxyvitamin D_3 [1,25(OH)$_2$D$_3$] levels and suggest that DMP1 may regulate FGF23 expression.

Over the last years a big progress has been made in our understanding of the molecular basis of the different forms of hypophosphatemic rickets. The common denominator has been FGF23, a protein with phosphaturic action. The enzyme Phex inactivates FGF23 by cleavage. In X-linked hypophosphatemic rickets the Phex gene is mutated (inactive), whereas in the autosomal dominant form, FGF23 is mutated in the Phex cleavage site. These two articles clarify the etiology of autosomal recessive hypophosphatemic rickets (ARHR). Both research groups identified mutations in dental matrix acidic phosphoprotein 1 (DMP1) gene in patients with ARHR. ?he mechanism how DMP1, a bone matrix protein involved in mineralization, causes hypophosphatemia is still unknown. From these studies, PHEX does not seem to be involved. More interestingly, as in X-linked hypophosphatemic rickets, many patients have elevated serum levels of FGF23 or in the upper normal range. Furthermore, the paper by Feng et al. suggests that osteocyte has an important functional role in regulating mineral metabolism. Despite big steps in our understanding of phosphorus homeostasis in recent last years, much still remains unknown. The treatment of hypophosphatemic rickets is not optimal, with side effects, and often linear growth does not improve. A better understanding of phosphorus homeostasis and related pathways could help us to develop a better treatment in the future. The amazing message is that it is the bone that through several mechanisms coordinates systemic phosphate balance. After all, the bone contains 85% of all body phosphate.

New paradigms

FSH directly regulates bone mass

Sun L, Peng Y, Sharrow AC, Iqbal J, Zhang Z, Papachristou DJ, Zaidi S, Zhu LL, Yaroslavskiy BB, Zhou H, Zallone A, Sairam MR, Kumar TR, Bo W, Braun J, Cardoso-Landa L, Schaffler MB, Moonga BS, Blair HC, Zaidi M
Mount Sinai Bone Program, Department of Medicine and Department of Orthopedics, Mount Sinai School of Medicine, New York, N.Y., USA
mone.zaidi@mssm.edu
Cell 2006;125:247–260

Background: Postmenopausal osteoporosis is traditionally explained by decreased estradiol levels due to a decline in ovarian function. However, at the same time, FSH (follicle-stimulating hormone) levels increase dramatically. It has previously been shown that while ovariectomy itself induces bone loss, the response is blunted in hypophysectomized animals. This suggests that FSH may directly affect bone metabolism.
Methods: Measurements of bone mineral density and bone histomorphometry were performed in FSH receptor and FSH null mice. Serum FSH was measured by RIA and serum TRAP and osteocalcin by ELISAs. Osteoclastogenesis of mouse bone marrow cells, macrophages and human monocytes was studied in the presence of FSH. The resorptive activity of human monocyte-derived osteoclasts was detected by number and size of resorption pits formed on dentine. The effect of FSH on the formation of osteoblastic cells was also examined.

Results: Hypogonadal FSHR and FSH null mice were surprisingly observed not to lose bone and heterozygotic FSH$^{+/-}$ mice even had a slight increase in BMD. FSH receptors were expressed on the osteoclast surface and FSH increased osteoclast differentiation and bone resorption in vitro. FSH signaling in osteoclasts was mediated via the MEK/Erk, NF-κB and Akt pathways. However, FSH did not have any effect on osteoblasts.

Conclusion: FSH stimulates the formation and function of osteoclasts in vitro and in vivo. Despite the normal estrogen levels, haploinsufficiency of circulating FSH increases bone mass by reducing osteoclastic bone resorption. This indicates a direct estrogen-independent action of FSH on bone metabolism.

Follicle-stimulating hormone stimulates TNF production from immune cells to enhance osteoblast and osteoclast formation

Iqbal J, Sun L, Kumar TR, Blair HC, Zaidi M
Mount Sinai Bone Program, Department of Medicine and Department of Orthopedics, Mount Sinai School of Medicine, New York, N.Y., USA
mone.zaidi@mssm.edu
Proc Natl Acad Sci USA 2006;103:14925–14930

Background: It is well known that declining estrogen production after menopause causes osteoporosis in which the bone resorption exceeds the increase in bone formation, thus leading to net bone loss. However, a recent study suggests that FSH would also be an important direct, estrogen-independent regulator of bone mass. This study aimed at studying the possible involvement of TNF-α and ascorbic acid in FSH-induced bone loss.

Methods: TNF-α levels in FSH-deficient mice were measured by ELISA. TNF-α production was studied in bone marrow granulocytes and macrophages in vitro and different cell populations were identified by flow cytometry. A mathematical model of bone metabolism was used to understand how elevations in TNF-α contributed to high-turnover bone loss. Osteoclast and osteoblast formation assays were performed in the presence of TNF-α and ascorbic acid.

Results: FSH-deficient mice were shown to have low circulating levels of TNF-α compared to littermate controls. In parallel, the exposure of bone marrow cells to recombinant FSH caused an increase in TNF-α secretion. Macrophages and granulocytes were the main cell populations responsible for this effect. By applying a mathematical model and in vitro studies, it was concluded that the TNF-α-induced increase in osteoclast number accounted for most of the observed high-turnover bone loss. Interestingly, ascorbic acid reversed the stimulatory action of TNF-α on osteoclast precursors.

Conclusion: The reported effects of FSH on bone mass are partially exerted via TNF-α production by bone marrow macrophages and granulocytes. Furthermore, ascorbic acid may prevent FSH-induced bone loss in hypogonadal states by modulating the pro-resorptive actions of TNF-α.

These two papers suggest a new role for follicle-stimulating hormone (FSH) in the central regulation of bone mass. The authors report observations from which they conclude that high circulating FSH levels, and not declining estrogen levels, would be responsible for the bone loss observed in hypogonadal states, and that this bone loss would be partially mediated by immune cell-derived TNF-α. In the report by Sun et al., the deletion of FSH receptors (FSHR) had unexpectedly no effect on bone mass despite the presence of low serum estrogen levels. Surprisingly, also in the absence of FSH, there was no bone loss and even some gain. The most intriguing finding was that FSH heterozygous mice, despite having normal estrogen levels and 50% reduction in FSH levels, had decreased bone resorption. Half a year later, the same group published new data partially in the same animals. This time, Iqbal et al. focused on the possible involvement of TNF-α and immune cells in FSH-induced bone loss. They demonstrated that FSH null mice, despite low estrogen levels, have unexpectedly low levels of TNF-α. They furthermore showed that FSH stimulates TNF-α secretion from macrophages and granulocytes in vitro. A mathematical model was used to demonstrate that TNF-α actions mainly target osteoclast precursors and in vitro studies were used to confirm that this stimulatory effect was reversed by ascorbic acid, suggesting that vitamin C supplementation might be useful in the treatment of postmenopausal osteoporosis. Both reports have been criticized by some scientists working within the bone field [1–3]. Their main criticism focused on lack of data on circulating levels of estrogen and especially testosterone in these animals. It has previously been shown that FSHR null mice have high levels of testosterone, and thus it is possible that testosterone itself or its further aromatization

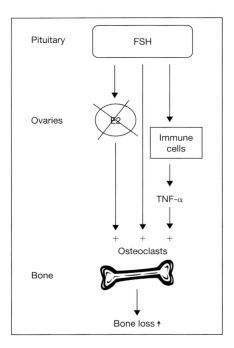

Fig. 1. Novel paradigm of hormonal control of bone mass. Under decreased gonadal function (menopause), estradiol levels are decreased and FSH levels are increased. This leads to increased activity of osteoclasts, both directly and indirectly via increased TNF-α production by immune cells.

into estrogen is sufficient to prevent bone loss in these animals. Thus at this point it may be better to conclude that both estrogen and FSH are important in regulating the bone response to menopause and gonadectomy as outlined in figure 1. Most likely, further studies with proper measurement of sex steroids and LH, as well as studies on combined effects of FSH with anti-estrogens, androgen receptor blockers or aromatase inhibitors are needed before this new mechanism will be generally accepted. However, the paper by Iqbal et al. brings a new nutritional aspect for the treatment of postmenopausal osteoporosis. They demonstrated that ascorbic acid (vitamin C) reversed the actions of TNF-α on both osteoclasts and osteoblasts, suggesting that supplementation with vitamin C might be a beneficial tool for the prevention of low bone mass and risk of fractures.

New hope

RANKL inhibition: a novel strategy to decrease femoral head deformity after ischemic osteonecrosis

Kim HK, Morgan-Bagley S, Kostenuik P
Center for Research in Skeletal Development and Pediatric Orthopedics, Shriners Hospitals for Children, Tampa, Fla., USA
hkim@shrinenet.org
J Bone Miner Res 2006;21:1946–1954

Background: Legg-Calve-Perthes disease is a juvenile form of osteonecrosis of the femoral head which can produce permanent femoral head deformity and premature osteoarthritis. Femoral head deformity is characterized by a predominance of bone resorption that produces a fragmented appearance and finally collapse of the femoral head. Inhibition of interaction between RANK and RANKL by osteoprotegerin (OPG-Fc) is a potential therapeutic strategy to prevent this condition.

Methods: Ischemic osteonecrosis was surgically induced in 18 male piglets by disrupting the blood flow to the right femoral head. Two weeks later, OPG-Fc or saline was administered subcutaneously to 9 animals per group for 6 weeks. The left femoral heads from the animals treated with saline served as normal, non-disease controls. At 8 weeks, radiographic, histomorphometric, and immunohistochemical analyses were performed.

Results: Radiography showed significantly better preservation of the femoral head structure and higher ratio of epiphyseal height to diameter in the OPG-Fc group compared with the saline group. Histomorphometry revealed a significant reduction in the number of osteoclasts present in the treated group, and trabecular bone parameters (volume, number and separation) were significantly better preserved in the OPG-Fc group. No significant difference in femoral length was observed. By immunohistochemistry, OPG-Fc was observed only within the blood vessels, with no apparent staining of bone matrix or trabecular bone surfaces.

Conclusion: RANKL inhibition decreases bone resorption and femoral head deformity after ischemic osteonecrosis. Because RANKL inhibitors, such as OPG-Fc, do not bind to bone, their effects on resorption are reversible. This is very appealing when treating pediatric bone diseases such as Legg-Calve-Perthes disease, where the resorptive stage of the disease lasts for 1–2 years.

Interactions between osteoblasts and osteoclasts via the RANK-RANKL-OPG system play a major role in bone metabolism. This paper describes a new treatment strategy of ischemic femoral head deformity (Perthes disease) based on the inhibition of RANKL. The authors report for the first time that RANK-RANKL interaction plays a role in pathological bone resorption in femoral head deformity. This interaction can be targeted by soluble RANKL inhibitor and thus there exists a possibility to preserve femoral head and epiphyseal trabecular bone after ischemic osteonecrosis. Previous animal studies have suggested that bisphosphonates would be the treatment of choice to decrease femoral head deformity and prevent disease progression. However, the long-term effects of bisphosphonates on the growing skeleton are not known. Thus, for pediatric conditions, the reversible nature of RANKL inhibition as a therapeutic strategy is appealing. However, this study has some limitations. Only the short-term results were analyzed and it is not clear whether the effects will prevail. Furthermore, to counteract the effects of porcine-derived neutralizing antibodies against human OPG-Fc, the dosing in this study was two times higher than in a previous clinical study [4]. More importantly, it is well known that RANK-RANKL interaction also plays a role in regulating T-cell/dendritic cell communications and lymph node formation [for review, see 5]. It is thus possible that RANKL inhibition may have some immunological consequences and thus detailed investigations on possible side effects are needed before this new treatment strategy can be used in clinical practice.

Orally bioavailable GSK-3α/β dual inhibitor increases markers of cellular differentiation in vitro and bone mass in vivo

Kulkarni NH, Onyia JE, Zeng Q, Tian X, Liu M, Halladay DL, Frolik CA, Engler T, Wei T, Kriauciunas A, Martin TJ, Sato M, Bryant HU, Ma YL
Lilly Research Laboratories, Eli Lilly & Co., Lilly Corporate Center, Indianapolis, Ind., USA
jeo@lilly.com
J Bone Miner Res 2006;21:910–920

Background: Glycogen synthase kinase-3 (GSK-3) is a component of canonical Wnt signaling. Inactivation of GSK-3 leads to stabilization, accumulation and translocation of β-catenin into the nucleus and further activation of downstream Wnt genes. The effects of the small molecule inhibitor of GSK-3 (603281-31-8) on pre-osteoblastic cells and osteopenic rats were studied.

Methods: Mouse mesenchymal cells were treated with GSK-3 inhibitor and assayed for β-catenin levels, Wnt-responsive promoter activation, as well as for osteogenic and adipogenic markers. In vivo, GSK-3 inhibitor was administered daily for 60 days to ovariectomized rats. Treatment was started 1 month after ovariectomy. At the end of treatment, bone mineral density, bone histomorphometry, biomechanical strength and the expression of osteoblast-related genes were measured.

Results: Treatment of mouse mesenchymal cells with GSK-3 inhibitor increased the levels of β-catenin followed by Wnt-responsive promoter activation. Markers for osteogenic differentiation (bone sialoprotein, collagens type I and V, osteocalcin, alkaline phosphatase and runx2) were upregulated. Ovariectomized rats treated with GSK-3 inhibitor had significant increases in bone mineral content and bone mineral density. This was associated with increased bone strength. Histomorphometric analysis revealed increased bone formation but no effect on bone resorption. The mRNA levels for collagens, biglycan, osteonectin and runx2 increased in response to GSK-3 inhibition in rat femur.

Conclusion: The GSK-3 inhibitor is capable of inducing osteoblast differentiation and increasing bone formation markers in vitro. After oral administration to ovariectomized rats, this small molecule increased markers for bone formation and improved bone mass and strength.

Besides many morphogenic growth factor- and hormone-signaling pathways, the canonical wingless (Wnt) pathway plays an essential role in the development of the skeleton and formation of bone tissue. In mesenchymal progenitor cells, the Wnt-signaling pathway is critical for the differentiation of the progenitors into osteoblasts and chondrocytes. Wnt functions through a co-receptor (LRP-5) and Frizzled receptor that transduce the signal through either the canonical β-catenin pathway or the non-canonical pathway. Following the discovery that Wnt/LRP-5/β-catenin signaling is anabolic for bone, there have been continuous efforts in finding new anabolic agents acting on this pathway. One potential target is GSK-3, an enzyme that is a part of the β-catenin inactivation complex. Lithium chloride has previously been demonstrated to inhibit GSK-3 and thus increase bone mass [6]. Here the authors demonstrate that GSK-3 inhibition increased the levels of β-catenin and activated Wnt signaling in stem cell-like pluripotent cells. This was followed by a decrease in proliferation, a biphasic increase in osteogenic markers and a decrease in adipogenic markers. This indicates that GSK-3 inhibition predisposes mesenchymal stem cells to osteoblast commitment instead of adipogenic differentiation, thus acting in a 'pro-bone, anti-fat' way. The most interesting results in this study were obtained with ovariectomized rats fed with the GSK-3 inhibitor, where the GSK-3 inhibition maintained bone mineral density and improved bone microarchitecture. This suggests that GSK-3 inhibitors are new promising therapeutic compounds that, in the future, may be available for the treatment of osteoporosis and other states of increased bone loss.

The growth plate-sparing effects of the selective glucocorticoid receptor modulator, AL-438

Owen HC, Miner JN, Ahmed SF, Farquharson C
Bone Biology Group, Division of Gene Function and Development, Roslin Institute, Edinburgh, UK
helen.owen@bbsrc.ac.uk
J Mol Cell Endocrinol 2007;264:164–170

Background: It is well known that long-term use of glucocorticoids can cause growth retardation in children, an effect mediated through their actions on growth plate chondrocytes. The non-steroidal anti-inflammatory agent AL-438 acts through the glucocorticoid receptor and is known to retain full anti-inflammatory efficacy while having reduced negative effects on osteoblasts compared to those elicited by prednisolone or dexamethasone.

Methods: The murine chondrogenic ATDC5 cell line was used to compare the effects of AL-438 with those of dexamethasone and prednisolone on chondrocyte dynamics. The effects on bone growth were evaluated in cultured fetal mouse metatarsal bones.

Results: Dexamethasone and prednisolone caused a reduction in cell proliferation and proteoglycan synthesis, whereas exposure to AL-438 had no effect. Fetal mouse metatarsals grown in the presence of dexamethasone were shorter than control bones whereas AL-438-treated metatarsals paralleled control bone growth.

Conclusion: The data suggest that AL-438 has a reduced side effect profile on chondrocytes and bone growth compared to other glucocorticoids. This could prove important in the search for new anti-inflammatory treatments for children.

Glucocorticoids are the most effective anti-inflammatory agents known. However, in children, their long-term use leads to growth retardation through a combination of glucocorticoid-mediated effects on the systemic GH/IGF-1 axis, negative calcium metabolism, as well as direct effects on the growth plate. The search for a selective glucocorticoid receptor modulator that has the anti-inflammatory properties of conventional steroids without one or more of the side effects has been a longstanding goal. The mechanism of action of the non-steroidal anti-inflammatory agent AL-438 is based on the hypothesis that many genes involved in undesirable side effects are upregulated (such as enzymes in lipid and muscle metabolism), whereas many proinflammatory genes (i.e. IL-1, IL-6 and TNF-α) are repressed. The authors used a well-established model of cultured fetal mouse metatarsals and were able to demonstrate that bones treated with AL-438 grow parallel to control bones while dexamethasone-treated bones were shorter. Furthermore, the authors confirmed that AL-438 maintains a similar anti-inflammatory efficacy as dexamethasone which was important and proved that AL-438 was still fully efficacious as an anti-inflammatory agent. Thereby the 'proof of principle' exists, i.e. that a non-steroidal anti-inflammatory agent is capable to selectively maintain its anti-inflammatory effects without negatively affecting bone growth. However, it should be emphasized that this conclusion is based on results from in vitro studies in mouse tissues. Therefore, it still remains to be shown if this approach will work in real life.

Treatment of rabbit growth plate injuries with an autologous tissue-engineered composite

Jin X-B, Luo Z-J, Wang J
Orthopedics Institute, Xijing Hospital, Fourth Military Medical University, Xian, PR China
zjluo@fmmu.edu.cn
Cells Tissues Organs 2006;183:62–67

Background: Growth plate injuries could potentially be treated by tissue engineering. The authors attempted to investigate if it is possible to use autologous tissue-engineered composites in the treatment of growth plate injuries.

Methods: Chondrocytes were obtained from iliac crest epiphyseal growth plate cartilage taken from immature New Zealand rabbits. After proliferating in monolayer culture in vitro for 3 weeks, the cells were harvested and seeded onto a demineralized bone matrix scaffold to construct an autologous tissue-engineered composite. The composites were implanted into a defect in the proximal right tibiae growth plate created in 12 rabbits (group A underwent the operation after obtaining chondrocytes 3 weeks beforehand), another 12 rabbits were implanted with only the demineralized bone matrix scaffold (group B), and the defects in group C (12 rabbits) were not implanted. The left tibias of all animals were left undone as the normal control.

Results: When examined by x-ray 2 weeks after the operation, severe shortness and angulation deformity of the right tibia were gradually observed in groups B and C. However, there were no obvious changes in group A and there were significant differences between group A and groups B and C after 4, 8, and 16 weeks. Histological examination after 16 weeks revealed that the defects of the right tibias in group A had restored to almost the normal growth plate structure.

Conclusion: Tissue-engineered composites established by the combination of autologous growth plate chondrocytes and demineralized bone matrix has the potential to be used to prevent the formation of bone bridges and restore growth after growth plate injuries.

Repair of full-thickness cartilage defects with cells of different origin in a rabbit model

Yan H, Yu C
Institute of Sports Medicine, Third Hospital, Peking University, Beijing, PR China
YCL123@vip.sina.com
Arthroscopy 2007;23:178–187

Background: The purpose was to evaluate the repaired tissues formed in full-thickness cartilage defects in a rabbit model implanted with four types of chondrogenic cells.

Methods: Articular derived chondrocytes, mesenchymal stem cells (MSCs), and fibroblasts were isolated from 6-week-old New Zealand rabbits, and human umbilical cord blood stem cells were isolated from the umbilical cord blood of newborn children. The cells were cultured in vitro and embedded in polylactic acid matrices. Full-thickness defects were produced in the femoral trochlear grooves of both knees in adult rabbits. Cell/polylactic acid composites were transplanted into the cartilage defects.

Results: Full-thickness cartilage defects treated with chondrocyte or MSC transplantation were repaired with hyaline-like cartilage tissue, and repair was significantly better than in tissues treated with fibroblasts and human umbilical cord blood stem cells, as well as in the control group. Repaired tissues treated with MSCs had better cell arrangement, subchondral bone remodeling, and integration with surrounding cartilage than did repaired tissues generated by chondrocyte implantation.

Conclusion: MSCs might be the most suitable cell source for cartilage repair. Further investigation into human umbilical cord blood stem cell transplantation is needed. In this study performed in rabbits, MSCs supplied the most promising cell source for cartilage repair.

The shortening and angulation of limbs caused by the bone bridge between the epiphysis and metaphysis is one of the big problems encountered by many orthopedists. Traditional methods, such as bone bridge cutting and fat packing, have many shortcomings. Progress in cell biology and biomaterial technology has led to the possibility of therapeutic applications of tissue engineering for the repair of cartilage defects. In the paper by Jin et al., an attempt was made to treat long bone growth plate injuries in rabbits by using an autologous tissue-engineered composite established in vitro. Although complete prevention of an angular and shortening deformity was not possible, the study demonstrates the potential of the method in treating growth plate injuries. It is important to emphasize that the graft can only efficiently prevent bone bridge formation in acutely injured rabbit models. The second paper by Yan et al. aimed to compare different cell sources for their potential to repair growth plate defects. Full-thickness cartilage defects treated with articular chondrocytes or MSC transplantation were repaired with hyaline-like cartilage tissue, and repair was significantly better than in tissues treated with fibroblasts and human umbilical cord blood stem cells. Damaged growth plates repaired with MSCs had the best histomorphology and integration with surrounding cartilage. The evaluation was pure histological and the follow-up time was only 12 weeks, a timepoint when many patients have not yet been diagnosed with growth plate injuries. Although the data in both these reports are promising, there still exists a big challenge to establish a treatment protocol for patients who have suffered from growth plate injuries over a long period of time and obviously already have developed a deformity of the limbs.

New concerns

Systematic review: bisphosphonate-induced osteonecrosis of the jaws

Woo SB, Hellstein JW, Kalmar JR
Brigham and Women's Hospital and Harvard School of Dental Medicine, Boston, Mass., USA
Ann Intern Med 2006;144:753–761

Background: Bisphosphonates are used to treat osteoporosis, Paget disease of bone and other metabolic bone diseases, multiple myeloma and skeletal events associated with metastases. In pediatrics, their use is restricted mainly to patients with osteogenesis imperfecta. Their primary mechanism of action is to inhibit osteoclastic bone resorption. Within the past years, many articles have suggested the possible involvement of bisphosphonates in the development of osteonecrosis of the jaws. This review discusses the clinical manifestations, current treatment strategies, possible mechanisms and need for research in the future.

Methods: All published case reports and case series of patients with bisphosphonate-associated osteonecrosis of the jaws were reviewed. Through direct communication with some authors, it was confirmed that some patients were included in multiple reports. When this occurred, data only from the larger, more recent publication was used.

Results/Conclusion: This paper summarizes 368 reported cases of bisphosphonate-associated osteonecrosis of the jaw. Most cases manifested the bone of mandible only (65%), approximately one third of lesions were painless, and there was a slight female predilection among all reported cases. Importantly, 60% of cases occurred after dental surgery procedure. Patients with multiple myeloma and bone metastases who are receiving intravenous, nitrogen-containing bisphosphonates (primarily pamidronate and zoledronic acid) were observed to be at greatest risk for osteonecrosis of the jaws; these patients represented 94% of published cases. The remaining patients were taking oral bisphosphonates for osteoporosis or Paget disease of bone. The most important predisposing factors for the development of bisphosphonate-associated osteonecrosis of the jaws were the type and total dose of bisphosphonate and history of trauma, dental surgery, or dental infection.

Bisphosphonates are drugs that powerfully inhibit bone resorption. They are incorporated into the bone matrix and are thus remarkably persistent drugs. We have had a quick touch on the trigger, but have no indications for how long to treat. It has been noted that prolonged use of bisphosphonates may suppress bone turnover to the point that microdamages cannot be repaired, leading to decreased biomechanical properties. Furthermore, continuing mineralization may yield a hard, brittle bone with an osteopetrotic appearance and an increased risk for fractures. Osteonecrosis of the jaws is a recently described side effect of bisphosphonate therapy, and not a rare one. This review gives an excellent overview based on all reported cases and summarizes current treatment strategies, as well as discusses possible mechanisms of etiology and pathogenesis. Clinical trials are needed to address many issues, e.g. could alternative dosing schedules or monitoring bone turnover markers reduce the incidence? Additional risk factors that may predispose the patient to the development of this condition also need to be studied. The most effective and still safe treatment protocol for these patients still needs to be defined. It should be noted that, e.g., pediatric patients with severe forms of osteogenesis imperfecta often have dental problems, which may require implant surgery. Concurrently, these patients are treated with intravenous pamidronate, which may predispose them for the development of osteonecrosis of the jaws. Thus, constant follow-up of dental health of patients treated with bisphosphonates is required.

Concepts revised or re-centered

Skeletal benefits from calcium supplementation are limited in children with calcium intakes near 800 mg daily

Iuliano-Burns S, Wang X-F, Evans A, Bonjour J-P, Seeman E
Department of Endocrinology, Austin Health, University of Melbourne, West Heidelberg, Vic., Australia
sandraib@unimelb.edu.au
Osteoporos Int 2006;17:1794–1800

Background: It is still controversial if calcium supplementation improves bone mineral density in children. The authors tested the hypothesis that calcium from milk minerals (MM) but not calcium carbonate (CC) will be beneficial for bone health after discontinuation of supplementation.
Methods: The study included 99 prepubertal boys and girls 5–11 years old who received 800 mg/day of calcium from MM or CC, or a placebo in a 10-month double-blind study. The patients were then followed for 12 months. Total body and regional bone mineral content, and femoral shaft bone dimensions were measured using dual-energy x-ray absorptiometry. Group differences were determined using ANCOVA.
Results: No group differences were observed with regards to increments in bone mineral content or bone dimensions during and after supplementation. Children who remained prepubertal had sustained a greater gain in pelvis bone mineral content in the MM group than controls (37.9 vs. 29.3% respectively, $p < 0.02$).
Conclusion: Calcium supplementation in healthy children already consuming about 800 mg calcium daily does not improve skeletal health. In prepubertal children, calcium supplementation could have a beneficial effect on the pelvis but its biological significance and longevity has to be determined.

Osteoporosis is a major health problem and more than 90% of the peak bone mass is attained by the age of 18 years [7]. Thus, any intervention before that age in order to optimize peak bone mass could have beneficial effects preventing osteoporosis later in life or have a more immediate benefit. A public health intervention could be targeted to diet and/or physical activity. Calcium supplementation has been used in post-menopausal women to improve bone mineral density although only a small positive effect was reported (1.13–2.05%) [8]. Data concerning calcium supplementation in children have not helped us to clarify whether there is a benefit in healthy children already receiving the recommended daily intake, and whether any benefit is sustained after supplementation. The authors conducted a randomized double-blind placebo-controlled trial which shows no benefit of calcium supplementation on bone mineral content except in the pelvis of prepubertal children, a finding of questionable biological meaning. In support of this work, a recent meta-analysis confirms that calcium supplementation has little effect on skeletal health in healthy children (reviewed in the chapter 'evidence based medicine' of this book) [9]. Therefore, the general belief endorsed by many primary care physicians and mass media that calcium supplementation in children makes bones stronger is not totally right. Our efforts have to be focused on ensuring that all children receive 800 mg calcium per day, and most importantly – vitamin D. Remember, one glass of milk contains 200 mg of calcium. Physical activity is by all means more important than any of the supplements.

Important observations for clinical practice

Reduced bone mineral density and increased bone metabolism rate in young adult patients with 21-hydroxylase deficiency

Sciannamblo M, Russo G, Cuccato D, Chiumello G, Mora S
Laboratory of Pediatric Endocrinology and Department of Pediatrics, San Raffaele Scientific Institute, Vita-Salute S. Raffaele University, Milan, Italy
mora.stefano@hsr.it
J Clin Endocrinol Metab 2006;91:4453–4458

Background: Patients with congenital adrenal hyperplasia (CAH) are on long-term glucocorticoid therapy. On the other hand, glucocorticoid therapy is the most frequent cause of drug-induced osteoporosis. This study aimed at evaluating bone mineral density (BMD) and bone metabolism in young adult CAH patients.
Methods: A cross-sectional observational study was conducted at a referral center for pediatric endocrinology. Thirty young patients with the classical form of CAH (aged 16.4–29.7 years) treated with glucocorticoid from diagnosis (duration of treatment 16.4–29.5 years) and 138 healthy controls (aged 16.0–30.0 years) were enrolled. BMD in the lumbar spine and whole body was measured by dual-energy x-ray absorptiometry (DXA). Biochemical markers for bone formation (BALP) and resorption (CTX) were measured in serum.
Results: Height was significantly lower in CAH patients than in controls (women −6.8 and men −13.3 cm). Therefore, several different methods were used to correct for the effect of this difference on BMD measurements. In CAH patients, whole-body BMD measurements were significantly lower than in controls (p < 0.03), after correcting for height. No differences were found in lumbar spine BMD. The biochemical markers of bone metabolism were higher in CAH patients than in control subjects (p < 0.04). No significant correlations were observed in BMD measurements or bone markers with the actual glucocorticoid dose or mean dose over the previous 7 years.
Conclusion: Young adult patients with the classical form of CAH, receiving continuous glucocorticoid treatment from the very first months of their lives, are shorter and have decreased BMD. Furthermore, their bone metabolism rate is higher. This may put them at risk of developing osteoporosis later in life.

Life-dependent long-term glucocorticoid therapy in CAH patients could potentially cause bone loss and bone fragility. Previous reports of bone mass in CAH patients on glucocorticoid-therapy have showed contradictory results (increased, decreased or normal BMD) [10–12]. Thus, the authors of this paper aimed to measure bone mass and metabolism in young adult patients with the classical form of CAH. Their results demonstrate that CAH patients were significantly shorter than controls. It is well known that DXA measurements are greatly influenced by bone size, and there will be an overestimation of bone deficits in children if the height is not taken into account. Thus, the authors used different methods to account for the height differences. Different approaches yielded that the observed lower total body BMD in CAH patients was real and not size-dependent. Increased levels of biochemical markers for bone metabolism also indicated a high bone turnover state, leading to a low bone mass. However, no correlation was observed between the glucocorticoid dose and BMD/bone markers, suggesting other underlying mechanisms. Premature growth plate fusion, commonly seen in CAH patients, may shorten the time for bone accrual and lead to lower peak bone mass. Therefore, it is possible that the low peak bone mass, rather than glucocorticoid treatment per se, predisposes these patients to osteoporosis later in life. Longitudinal studies are needed to elucidate this issue.

Osteoclasts degrade endosteal components and promote mobilization of hematopoietic progenitor cells

Kollet O, Dar A, Shivtiel S, Kalinkovich A, Lapid K, Sztainberg Y, Tesio M, Samstein RM, Goichberg P, Spiegel A, Elson A, Lapidot T

Department of Immunology, Weizmann Institute of Science, Rehovot, Israel

tsvee.lapidot@weizmann.ac.il

Nat Med 2006;12:657–664

Background: Bone remodeling is a tightly regulated process involving the coordinated actions of bone-resorbing osteoclasts and bone-forming osteoblasts. These actions are carried out on the endosteal bone surface, which is close to the microenvironment, or niche, of hematopoietic stem cells (HSCs). The majority of stem cells are located within the bone marrow but a small population is constitutively released to the circulation. However, the mechanisms of this release are unknown. The aim of this study was to investigate the potential role of osteoclasts in homeostasis and stress-induced mobilization of hematopoietic precursors.

Methods: Balb/c, C57BL/6 and protein tyrosine phosphatase ε (PTPε) knockout mice were bled or injected with stromal cell-derived factor 1 (SDF-1), hepatocyte growth factor (HGF), lipopolysaccharide (LPS) or receptor activator of NFκB ligand (RANKL) to induce mobilization and the bones were stained for TRAP which is a phosphatase produced by active osteoclasts. Peripheral blood precursors and white blood cells were counted and analyzed with FACS. Levels of SDF-1 and stromal cell factor (SCF) were measured and osteoclast precursor formation was assayed ex vivo.

Results: Appearance of bone-resorbing osteoclasts along the endosteal surfaces was observed by two different types of physiological stress: mild bleeding and LPS administration mimicking bacterial inflammation. This process was associated with mobilization of hematopoietic progenitors from bone marrow to the circulation. A similar effect was observed by in vivo administration of SDF-1 or HGF. Furthermore, progenitor mobilization was reduced in the presence of calcitonin (known osteoclast inhibitor) but induced with administration of RANKL (known osteoclast stimulator). RANKL administration in vivo was associated with increased expression of MMP-9 and cathepsin K, which in turn reduced the components of the endosteal niche, such as osteopontin and SCF, allowing the release of progenitors. SDF-1 and SCF were demonstrated to be cleaved by cathepsin K in vitro. Interestingly, PTPε-deficient mice, which have a defect in osteoclast adhesion and bone resorption capacity, had lower levels of progenitors and stem cells in their blood. RANKL did not induce progenitor mobilization in these mice.

Conclusion: Osteoclasts have a unique role in the regulation of stress-induced recruitment and release of bone marrow progenitors. Osteoblast-osteoclast balance may be the major regulator of hematopoiesis and turnover of the stem cell niche. Furthermore, RANKL could be considered as a potential agent for clinical transplantation protocols.

A new function for the osteoclast – to mediate stem cells mobilization. HCSs reside in the bone marrow, in specialized microenvironmental domains of the endosteal surfaces, which are called niches. Niches provide HSCs with signals required for a stationary (quiescent) state, during which very few HSCs are released to the circulation. However, the levels of circulating precursors are dramatically increased in response to chemotherapy, irradiation, cytokine stimulation and other stress signals. The authors of this elegant paper demonstrate a new participant in the endosteal niche of HSCs, the bone-resorbing osteoclast. They observed that bleeding or LPS induced stem cell mobilization was associated with increased numbers of osteoclasts on the endosteal surfaces. RANKL, which is a potent osteoclastogenic factor, not only increased osteoclastogenesis (as expected) but also induced stem cell mobilization. This was accompanied by increased expression of osteoclastic proteases, such as MMP-9 and cathepsin K, as well as decreased expression of osteopontin and SCF. The link between osteoclast activation and HSC mobilization was strengthened by experiments with PTPε-deficient mice, which have dysfunctional osteoclasts. These mice had fewer precursors in their bloodstream and bone marrow stem cells were not mobilized in response to RANKL. In summary, it seems that remodeling of bone tissue and remodeling of bone marrow niches are closely coupled. The authors demonstrate that activation of osteoclasts and mobilization of stem cells overlap and depend on the same signals. It is possible that anti-bone resorptive treatments impair progenitor cell mobilization and thus have clinical implications on bone marrow transplantation procedures. We used to think of the osteoclast-osteoblast unit. The new unit now includes stem cells.

Vitamin D receptor in chondrocytes promotes osteoclastogenesis and regulates FGF23 production in osteoblasts

Masuyama R, Stockmans I, Torrekens S, Van Looveren R, Maes C, Carmeliet P, Bouillon R, Carmeliet G
Laboratory of Experimental Medicine and Endocrinology, Katholieke Universiteit Leuven, Leuven, Belgium
geert.carmeliet@med.kuleuven.be
JCI 2006;116:3150–3159

Background: $1\alpha,25$-dihydroxyvitamin D_3 [$1,25(OH)_2D_3$] is crucial for calcium homeostasis and therefore for normal bone metabolism, mainly through actions in the intestine, kidneys and bone. The direct role of the vitamin D receptor (VDR) in bone metabolisms is questionable since calcium supplementation rescues hypocalcemia and hyperparathyroidism and restores bone mineralization both in patients and mice with loss of VDR function. Based on that, using mice with conditional inactivation of the VDR in chondrocytes, the authors studied whether the VDR is involved in growth-plate development and endochondral bone formation.

Results: The lack of VDR in chondrocytes had no effect on growth-plate development but vascular invasion was impaired and osteoclast number was reduced in young mice resulting in increased trabecular bone mass. In vitro experiments revealed that VDR signaling in chondrocytes directly regulate osteoclastogenesis by inducing the expression of receptor activator of NF-κB ligand (RANKL). Despite that the VDR was specifically inactivated in chondrocytes, mineral homeostasis in young mice, in whom growth-plate activity is important, was also affected since serum phosphate and $1,25(OH)_2D_3$ levels were increased. Further experiments clarified the mechanism: VDR inactivation in chondrocytes decreased the expression of FGF23 by osteoblasts and subsequently increased renal expression of 1α-hydroxylase and of the sodium phosphate cotransporter type IIa.

Conclusion: This study shows that VDR signaling in chondrocytes is not essential for growth-plate development but it is important for osteoclast formation during bone development and for the endocrine action of bone in phosphate homeostasis.

$1,25(OH)_2D_3$ is one of the major regulators of calcium homeostasis mainly through actions in intestine and kidneys, whereas its actions on bone are controversial. Despite in vitro data in the literature, indicating that VDR has actions on bone, the controversy has risen from patients and mice with loss of VDR function. Calcium supplementation has been shown to rescue hypocalcemia and hyperparathyroidism and to restore bone mineralization in both patients and mice [13, 14]. In addition, mice lacking VDR had growth-plate abnormalities before the onset of hypocalcemia, suggesting a role of VDR signaling in endochondral bone formation. Several findings in this article are surprising and very interesting. A new role of the growth plate was revealed; the growth plate as a co-player in the endocrine regulation of bone. Thus, the growth-plate chondrocytes, especially in young rapidly growing mice, contribute to the endocrine negative feedback loop between $1,25(OH)_2D_3$ and FGF23. Moreover, the findings support the existence of a soluble chondrocyte-derived factor inducible by $1,25(OH)_2D_3$ which stimulates FGF23 production by osteoblasts. Further research is needed to confirm the paracrine role of the growth plate in the regulation of bone metabolism and also to define the underlying mechanisms.

FGF18 is required for early chondrocyte proliferation, hypertrophy and vascular invasion of the growth plate

Liu Z, Lavine KJ, Hung IH, Ornitz DM
Department of Molecular Biology and Pharmacology, Washington University School of Medicine, St. Louis, Mo., USA
dornitz@wustl.edu
Dev Biology 2007;302:80–91

Background: Fibroblast growth factor-18 (FGF18) has been shown to regulate chondrocyte proliferation and differentiation by signaling through FGF receptor-3 (FGFR3) and to regulate osteogenesis by signaling through other FGFRs. Fgf18$^{-/-}$ mice have an apparent delay in skeletal mineralization that is not seen in Fgfr3$^{-/-}$ mice and thus, this delay in mineralization cannot be simply explained by FGF18 signaling to osteoblasts.

Methods: Skeletal explants of Fgf18$^{-/-}$ mice were studied. Bone mineralization, growth plate morphology and expression patterns were studied by immunohistochemistry and in situ hybridization.

Results: A delayed mineralization in Fgf18$^{-/-}$ mice was shown to be closely associated with delayed initiation of chondrocyte hypertrophy, decreased proliferation at early stages of chondrogenesis, delayed skeletal vascularization and delayed osteoclast and osteoblast recruitment to the growth plate. FGF18 was found to be necessary for the expression of vascular endothelial growth factor (VEGF) in hypertrophic chondrocytes and perichondrium, and be sufficient to induce VEGF expression in skeletal explants.

Conclusion: The findings support a model in which FGF18 regulates skeletal vascularization and subsequent recruitment of osteoblasts/osteoclasts through regulation of early stages of chondrogenesis and VEGF expression. FGF18 thus coordinates neovascularization of the growth plate with chondrocyte and osteoblast growth and differentiation.

We barely adopted FGF23, and here comes another family member. The authors demonstrate delayed ossification in Fgf18$^{-/-}$ mice which is closely associated with delayed initiation of chondrocyte hypertrophy, skeletal vascularization and osteoclast recruitment, and decreased chondrocyte proliferation. The findings support a model in which FGF18 regulates skeletal vascularization and osteoclast recruitment through regulation of VEGF signaling. The data presented also support a role for FGF18 to regulate chondrocyte proliferation and differentiation by signaling via FGFR3 (gain of function in achondroplasia) in proliferating chondrocytes and osteogenesis by signaling via FGFR1 and/or FGFR2 in the perichondrium/periosteum. It can be concluded that FGF18 functions in coordinating the critical developmental stages of endochondral ossification by balancing the developmental timing of chondrogenesis, osteogenesis and vascularization. The functional consequences of disturbed FGF18 function in humans remains to be described. If you have a child with delayed bone mineralization and poor growth, you might have a case of mutated FGF18!

New genes

Deficiency of cartilage-associated protein in recessive lethal osteogenesis imperfecta

Barnes AM, Chang W, Morello R, Cabral WA, Weis M, Eyre DR, Leikin S, Makareeva E, Kuznetsova N, Uveges TE, Ashok A, Flor AW, Mulvihill JJ, Wilson PL, Sundaram UT, Lee B, Marini JC
National Institute of Child Health and Human Development, National Institutes of Health, Bethesda, Md., USA
oidoc@helix.nih.gov
N Engl J Med 2006;355:2757–2764

Background: The classic form of osteogenesis imperfecta (OI) is caused by mutations in the genes for type I collagen. A recessive form of OI has long been suspected in some cases, where unaffected parents have more than one child with severe bone dysplasia. Since loss of cartilage-associated protein (CRTAP) causes severe osteoporosis in mice, the possible role of the CRTAP gene in lethal or severe OI was studied.

Methods: Dermal fibroblasts from 10 children with lethal (type II) or very severe (type III) OI were sampled and CRTAP mRNA levels were determined by RT-PCR. These children had normal primary structure of type I collagen with excess post-translational modifications in the helical region of the α-chain. Several different controls were also examined. Three children with decreased CRTAP mRNA levels were screened for 7 CRTAP exons and surrounding intronic sequences. Western blot of CRTAP protein and analysis of collagen modifications were performed.

Results: In 3 infants (1, 2 and 3) CRTAP mRNA levels were 0–25% of the normal value. The parents of infants 1 and 3 had normal levels of CRTAP mRNA, indicating that there was more than one defective allele involved. The exons and surrounding introns of infants 1, 2 and 3 were sequenced, and mutations were identified. Mutations led to premature termination of translation, triggering intracellular destruction of the mutant mRNA transcripts. At the protein level, no intracellular CRTAP was detectable in fibroblasts from infants 1, 2 and 3, and prolyl 3-hydroxylation of type I collagen was minimal.

Conclusion: Three of 10 children with lethal or severe OI without primary collagen defects were found to have a recessive condition resulting in CRTAP deficiency. CRTAP deficiency led to no or minimal Pro986 hydroxylation near the C-terminus of type I collagen, and the spectrum of mutations suggests that prolyl 3-hydroxylation is crucial for normal bone formation. It is possible that this process is important for other organs as well, contributing to the lethal outcome.

The clinical picture of OI patients is heterogeneous with symptoms extending from mild to perinatal lethality. Most cases are caused by mutations in type I collagen gene, and the pathogenesis is related to quantitative and qualitative abnormality of collagen. OI is usually autosomal dominant, and a recessive form has long been suspected but candidate genes have yet not been identified. Morello et al. demonstrated that loss of CRTAP in mice causes an osteochondrodysplasia which is characterized by severe osteoporosis, decreased osteoid production and decreased prolyl 3-hydroxylation of collagens in bone and cartilage [15]. Furthermore, Morello et al. [15] demonstrated that in humans, CRTAP mutations were associated with a clinical spectrum of recessive OI. Complete loss of CRTAP led to more severe forms of OI. These findings were partially confirmed by Barnes et al., who screened skin samples from 10 children with lethal or severe OI with normal primary structure of type I collagen. They were able to identify null mutations in the CRTAP gene leading to a lethal condition with death occurring within the first year of life. In summary, variable loss of CRTAP function and prolyl 3-hydroxylation seem to be a mechanism for recessive OI and may contribute to new cases, whose previous diagnosis has only been based on alterations in type I collagen. Indeed, the involvement of the prolyl 3-hydroxylase gene (LEPRE1) in a recessive metabolic bone disorder resembling lethal or severe OI has recently been published [16]. The authors present 5 cases resulting from LEPRE1 null alleles, whose phenotypes overlap with severe OI but also have distinctive features, such as lack of blue sclerae, a round face and a short chest. Taken together, these findings suggest that the classification and genetical diagnosis of OI and related disorders is far from complete.

Functional characterization of heterogeneous nuclear ribonuclear protein C1/C2 in vitamin D resistance

Chen H, Hewison M, Adams JS
Division of Endocrinology, Diabetes and Metabolism, Burns and Allen Research Institute, Cedars-Sinai Medical Center, UCLA School of Medicine, Los Angeles, Calif., USA
adamsj@cshs.or
J Biol Chem 2006;281:39114–39120

Background: Almost all of the cases with hereditary vitamin D-resistant rickets (HVDRR) are caused by homozygous mutations (loss of function) in the vitamin D receptor (VDR). In 2003, the authors described a patient with the classical HVDRR phenotype but normal VDR function [17]. This patient was hormone-resistant because of a constitutive overexpression of the heterogeneous nuclear ribonucleoprotein (hnRNP) which competed with a normally functioning VDR-retinoid X receptor dimer for binding to the vitamin D response element (VDRE). In the present study the authors purified, cloned, and further clarified the function of this competitive response element-binding protein (REBiP) hnRNP C1/C2 causing vitamin D resistance.

Results: The authors purified and cloned the overexpressed VDRE from their HVDRR patient (with no VDR mutation). It was a competitive response element-binding protein (REBiP) hnRNP C1/C2. This gene produces two alternatively spliced translated products (hnRNP C1 and C2). Then, cDNAs for hnRNP C1 and hnRNP C2 inhibited VDR-VDRE-directed transactivation when they were overexpressed in vitamin D-responsive cells. In addition, overexpression of hnRNP C1/C2 exerted a dominant-negative effect on $1,25(OH)_2D_3$-driven VDRE promoter activity. In the presence of 1,25-dihydroxyvitamin D, a cyclical movement of VDR and VDRE starts association-dissociation. The authors found that these receptor response element cycling events happened due to the competitive presence of the REBiP at the VDRE. The temporal and reciprocal pattern of VDR and hnRNP C1/C2 interaction with the VDRE was lost in HVDRR cells overexpressing the hnRNP C1/C2 REBiP.

Conclusion: The data indicate that REBiP is a component of the multiprotein complex involved in the regulation of vitamin D-mediated transcription and most likely REBiP is guiding the cyclical on-off equilibrium between VDR and VDRE.

Most cases of steroid hormone resistance are caused by end-organ resistance due to inactivating mutations of genes encoding their receptors. At least one case has been reported with a mutation not in the receptor but in one of those accessory proteins [18]. A patient with androgen insensitivity syndrome had an intact receptor but an abnormal coactivator protein which interacts with the AF-1 domain of the androgen receptor [18]. The authors of the present article have described another patient with the classical phenotype of HVDRR but normal VDR. In their previous attempt to find out the mechanism they discovered that this patient overexpressed hnRNPs which competed with a normally functioning VDR-retinoid X receptor dimer for binding to the VDRE. Now the authors went one step further. They cloned this protein and elucidated the mechanism of action. This protein is hnRNP C1/C2, a ribonucleoprotein which also functions as a competitive response element-binding protein. $1,25(OH)_2D_3$ initiates a cyclical movement of the VDR being associated and dissociated from the VDRE. hnRNP C1/C2 competes with the VDR for VDRE occupancy and therefore overexpression of hnRNP C1/C2 prevents the VDR to bind to the VDRE. Since VDR-VDRE association is necessary for VDR signaling, the result is resistance to VDR. These findings could also apply to other steroid and nuclear receptors since coactivators, corepressors and response element binding proteins play a key role in their proper function. As has been mentioned, there are patients with androgen resistance with no mutations in the androgen receptor, patients with resistance to multiple steroid hormones, or with a thyroid hormone resistance phenotype but no mutations in the thyroid hormone receptors [19]. These patients could have mutations of elements important for the proper function of their respective receptors.

New hormones/Reviews

C-type natriuretic peptide in growth: a new paradigm

Olney RC
Division of Pediatric Endocrinology, Nemours Children's Clinic, Jacksonville, Fla., USA
rolney@nemours.org
Growth Horm IGF Res 2006;16:S6–S14

Background: C-type natriuretic peptide (CNP), acting through its receptor, natriuretic peptide receptor-B (NPR-B), plays a critical role in linear growth. Knockout mice for CNP and NPR-B are dwarfed, and transgenic mice overexpressing CNP are overgrown. CNP has a direct regulatory effect on growth plate chondrocytes, acting primarily to promote terminal differentiation and hypertrophy.
Results: In humans, homozygous NPR-B mutations are the cause of acromesomelic dysplasia, Maroteaux type (AMDM). A patient with AMDM and the NPR-B knockout mouse both have low IGF-1 levels, suggesting an interaction between these regulatory systems. Heterozygous carriers of NPR-B mutations also have reduced stature, but no other abnormalities. Hence, heterozygous NPR-B mutations are another cause of 'idiopathic' short stature.
Conclusion: The CNP–NPR-B system has only recently been found to be an important regulator of human growth, and abnormalities in this system have clinical implications. Considerable work is needed to further understand this new paradigm of human growth regulation.

Data from mouse models and in vitro studies have shown that CNP, acting through its receptor NPR-B, plays a critical role in the regulation of the growth plate and hence in linear growth. The recent discovery of NPR-B mutations as a cause for acromesomelic dysplasia, Maroteaux type (AMDM), a severe form of dwarfism in humans, demonstrates that the CNP–NPR-B regulatory system is also critical to human linear growth. Preliminary findings suggest that the CNP-NPR-B system also interacts with the GH-IGF-1 system, which may have an additional, indirect role in linear growth. As discussed in this review, heterozygous carriers of inactivating NPR-B mutations have reduced stature. These carriers lack the skeletal disproportion and abnormal IGF-1 levels of AMDM and would clinically be diagnosed with 'idiopathic' short stature. Since the prevalence of AMDM in the general population is 1 in 2,000,000, the prevalence of heterozygous NPR-B mutation carriers is 1 in 700 (assuming Hardy-Weinberg equilibrium). The authors present data showing that these carriers have a mean height z-score of -1.8. Using the definition of a height z-score of less than -2.25 for 'idiopathic' short stature, about 1 in 30 of these individuals would be carriers of NPR-B mutations. Based on the information given, it can be assumed that heterozygous NPR-B mutations may be a significant cause of 'idiopathic' short stature. Further studies are needed to confirm this and also whether these patients do respond better to GH than other patients with 'idiopathic' short stature.

Food for thought

Regulation of fibroblast growth factor-23 signaling by Klotho

Kurosu H, Ogawa Y, Miyoshi M, Yamamoto M, Nandi A, Rosenblatt KP, Baum MG, Schiavi S, Hu MC, Moe OW, Kuro-o M
Department of Pathology, Pediatrics, and Internal Medicine and Applied Genomics, Genzyme Corp., The University of Texas Southwestern Medical Center, Dallas, Tex., USA
makoto.kuroo@utsouthwestern.edu
J Biol Chem 2006;281:6120–6123

Background: Klotho is a gene suppressing aging and Klotho knockout mice have a variety of aging-like phenotypes, many of them similar to those observed in fibroblast growth factor-23 (FGF23) knockout mice. The authors aimed to study whether Klotho and FGF23 use common signal transduction pathway(s).
Results: Experiments revealed that the Klotho protein directly binds to multiple FGF receptors (FGFRs) and then the Klotho-FGFR complex binds to FGF23 with higher affinity than FGFR or Klotho alone. Furthermore, Klotho increased the ability of FGF23 to induce phosphorylation of FGF receptor substrate and ERK.
Conclusion: The data indicate that Klotho can act as a cofactor important for the activation of FGF signaling by FGF23.

Hypervitaminosis D and premature aging: lessons learned from FGf23 and Klotho mutant mice

Razzaque MS, Lanske B
Department of Developmental Biology, Harvard School of Dental Medicine, Boston, Mass., USA
mrazzaque@hms.harvard.edu
Trends Mol Med 2006;12:298–305

Background: Mice lacking Klotho (K1) or fibroblast growth factor-23 (FGF23) have similar phenotypes concerning aging. In addition, both have increased levels of vitamin D and altered mineralization. On the other hand, it is well known that aging is associated with decreased levels of vitamin D. Based on this knowledge, the authors hypothesized that high levels of vitamin D could limit the aging process.
Results: The article reviews data from human diseases caused by hyper- and hypofunction of FGF23 and genetically modified mice. FGF23 knockout mice have premature aging similarly to Klotho-deficient mice. Both mice have hypercalcemia and increased serum levels of $1,25(OH)_2D_3$. When the activity of vitamin D was eliminated or reduced in K1 and FGF23 knockout mice, the aging process was decelerated with prolonged survival.
Conclusion: Based on the above data in the literature, the authors conclude that increased vitamin D activity could accelerate aging.

The new hormone Klotho was discussed for the first time in our 2006 Yearbook [20]. Both Klotho and FGF23 are related to aging in mice. Experiments with transgenic mice have revealed their involvement in accelerated aging [21]. Most surprisingly, FGF23 and Klotho-deficient mice have similar aging phenotypes indicating that these two proteins may function through a common signaling pathway. Indeed, the article by Kurosu et al. clearly shows that Klotho is a cofactor important for the activation of FGF signaling by FGF23. Klotho binds to FGFR and this complex binds to FGF23 with higher affinity than FGFR or Klotho alone. FGF23 is a phosphaturic protein and it is involved in human diseases of phosphate homeostasis. In addition to phosphorus, FGF23 negatively regulates vitamin D in mice and humans and Klotho in mice. In addition to premature aging, both Klotho and FGF23-deficient mice have increased vitamin D due to increased renal expression of 1α-hydroxylase. The second article by Razzaque and Lanske raises a very interesting question based on data in literature: Is hypervita-minosis D associated with accelerated aging? The question is very important with potential impact on public health since many postmenopausal women are treated with high doses of vitamin D. The authors raised this question based on studies in transgenic FGF23, Klotho, and 1α-hydroxylase mice. They noticed that the common link in FG23 and Klotho-deficient mice is premature aging with increased serum levels of vitamin D. This phenotype was reversed when the 1α-hydroxylase gene was knocked out in addition to FGF23 or when Klotho-deficient mice were on vitamin D-deficient diet. This research area is now very exciting revealing an unexpected role of vitamin D. For sure, we will soon learn more about the role of vitamin D in the regulation of aging.

References

1. Baron R: FSH versus estrogen: who's guilty of breaking bones? Cell Metab 2006;3:302–305.
2. Martin TJ, Gaddy D: Bone loss goes beyond estrogen. Nat Med 2006;12:612–613.
3. Prior JC: FSH and bone – important physiology or not? Trends Mol Med 2007;13:1–3.
4. Bekker PJ, Holloway D, Nakanishi A, Arrighi M, Leese PT, Dunstan CR: The effect of a single dose of osteoprotegerin in postmenopausal women. J Bone Miner Res 2001;16:348–360.
5. Walsh MC, Choi Y: Biology of the TRANCE axis. Cytokine Growth Factor Rev 2003;14:251–263.
6. Clement-Lacroix P, Ai M, Morvan F, Roman-Roman S, Vayssiere B, Belleville C, Estrera K, Warman ML, Baron R, Rawadi G: Lrp5-independent activation of Wnt signaling by lithium chloride increases bone formation and bone mass in mice. Proc Natl Acad Sci USA 2005;102:17406–17411.
7. Bailey DA, McKay HA, Mirwald RL, Crocker PR, Faulkner RA: A six-year longitudinal study of the relationship of physical activity to bone mineral accrual in growing children: the university of Saskatchewan Bone Mineral Accrual Study. J Bone Miner Res 1999;14:1672–1679.
8. Shea B, Wells G, Cranney A, Zytaruk N, Robinson V, Griffith L, Hamel C, Ortiz Z, Peterson J, Adachi J, Tugwell P, Guyatt G: Calcium supplementation on bone loss in postmenopausal women. Cochrane Database Syst Rev 2004: CD004526.
9. Winzenberg T, Shaw K, Fryer J, Jones G: Effects of calcium supplementation on bone density in healthy children: meta-analysis of randomised controlled trials. BMJ 2006;333:775.
10. Arisaka O, Hoshi M, Kanazawa S, Numata M, Nakajima D, Kanno S, Negishi M, Nishikura K, Nitta A, Imataka M, Kuribayashi T, Kano K: Preliminary report: effect of adrenal androgen and estrogen on bone maturation and bone mineral density. Metabolism 2001;50:377–379.
11. Cameron FJ, Kaymakci B, Byrt EA, Ebeling PR, Warne GL, Wark JD: Bone mineral density and body composition in congenital adrenal hyperplasia. J Clin Endocrinol Metab 1995;80:2238–2243.
12. Mora S, Saggion F, Russo G, Weber G, Bellini A, Prinster C, Chiumello G: Bone density in young patients with congenital adrenal hyperplasia. Bone 1996;18:337–340.
13. Amling M, Priemel M, Holzmann T, Chapin K, Rueger JM, Baron R, Demay MB: Rescue of the skeletal phenotype of vitamin D receptor-ablated mice in the setting of normal mineral ion homeostasis: formal histomorphometric and bio-mechanical analyses. Endocrinology 1999;140:4982–4987.
14. Balsan S, Garabedian M, Larchet M, Gorski AM, Cournot G, Tau C, Bourdeau A, Silve C, Ricour C: Long-term noctur-nal calcium infusions can cure rickets and promote normal mineralization in hereditary resistance to 1,25-dihydroxyvitamin D. J Clin Invest 1986;77:1661–1667.
15. Morello R, Bertin TK, Chen Y, Hicks J, Tonachini L, Monticone M, Castagnola P, Rauch F, Glorieux FH, Vranka J, Bachinger HP, Pace JM, Schwarze U, Byers PH, Weis M, Fernandes RJ, Eyre DR, Yao Z, Boyce BF, Lee B: CRTAP is required for prolyl 3-hydroxylation and mutations cause recessive osteogenesis imperfecta. Cell 2006;127:291–304.
16. Cabral WA, Chang W, Barnes AM, Weis M, Scott MA, Leikin S, Makareeva E, Kuznetsova NV, Rosenbaum KN, Tifft CJ, Bulas DI, Kozma C, Smith PA, Eyre DR, Marini JC: Prolyl 3-hydroxylase 1 deficiency causes a recessive metabolic bone disorder resembling lethal/severe osteogenesis imperfecta. Nat Genet 2007;39:359–365.
17. Chen H, Hewison M, Hu B, Adams JS: Heterogeneous nuclear ribonucleoprotein (hnRNP) binding to hormone response elements: a cause of vitamin D resistance. Proc Natl Acad Sci USA 2003;100:6109–6114.
18. Adachi M, Takayanagi R, Tomura A, Imasaki K, Kato S, Goto K, Yanase T, Ikuyama S, Nawata H: Androgen-insensitivity syndrome as a possible coactivator disease. N Engl J Med 2000;343:856–862.
19. Yanase T, Adachi M, Goto K, Takayanagi R, Nawata H: Coregulator-related diseases. Intern Med 2004;43:368–373.
20. Carel J-C, Hochberg Z: Yearbook of Pediatric Endocrinology 2006. Basel, Karger, 2006.
21. Kuro-o M, Matsumura Y, Aizawa H, Kawaguchi H, Suga T, Utsugi T, Ohyama Y, Kurabayashi M, Kaname T, Kume E, Iwasaki H, Iida A, Shiraki-Iida T, Nishikawa S, Nagai R, Nabeshima YI: Mutation of the mouse Klotho gene leads to a syndrome resembling ageing. Nature 1997;390:45–51.

Reproductive Endocrinology

Bruno Ferraz-de-Souza[a], Lin Lin[a], Teresa K Woodruff[b] and John C Achermann[a]

[a]UCL Institute of Child Health, University College London, London, UK
[b]Feinberg School of Medicine, Northwestern University, Chicago, Ill., USA

The past 12 months have seen significant developments in reproductive endocrinology. Several new single gene disorders have been described causing clinical conditions such as 'XX sex reversal' (RSPO1), hypospadias (CXorf6) and Kallmann syndrome (PROK2, PROK2R), and the role of digenic or polygenic influences on phenotypic expression is being increasingly recognized. The past year has also seen exciting advances in our understanding of germ cell differentiation, description of the potential for adult germ cells to function as pluripotent stem cells, and an insightful review on germ cell tumors. Above all, 2006–2007 may well be remembered as the Year of the Consensus with important documents focusing on disorders of sex development, polycystic ovary syndrome, Turner syndrome and testosterone measurement. These reports have produced useful evidence-based guidelines, wherever possible, but have also served to highlight many inadequacies in our current knowledge about the management of these conditions.

Mechanism of the year: an unexpected meiosis-inhibiting factor

Retinoid signaling determines germ cell fate in mice

Bowles J, Knight D, Smith C, Wilhelm D, Richman J, Mamiya S, Yashiro K, Chawengsaksophak K, Wilson MJ, Rossant J, Hamada H, Koopman P
Division of Genetics and Developmental Biology, Institute for Molecular Bioscience, University of Queensland, Brisbane, Qld., Australia
p.koopman@imb.uq.edu.au
Science 2006;312:596–600

Background: Germ cells in the mouse embryo can develop as either oocytes or spermatogonia, but the molecular signals that regulate these processes are poorly understood.
Methods: The effect of retinoic acid on germ cell differentiation was studied.
Results: Retinoic acid, which is produced by mesonephroi of both sexes, causes germ cells in the ovary to enter meiosis and initiate oogenesis. Meiosis is retarded in the fetal testis by the action of the retinoid-degrading enzyme CYP26B1, which ultimately leads to spermatogenesis. In testes of Cyp26b1-knockout mouse embryos, germ cells enter meiosis precociously, as if in a normal ovary.
Conclusion: The concentration of retinoid exposure during fetal gonad development provides a molecular control mechanism that specifies germ cell fate.

The entry of germ cells into meiosis is a key event in oocyte development. Thus, if meiosis begins during fetal development, oogenesis is triggered, whereas germ cells that delay the onset of meiosis until after birth – as occurs in the testis – will be spermatogenic. It is widely believed that fetal germ cells are intrinsically programmed to enter meiosis and initiate oogenesis unless prevented by a 'meiosis-inhibiting factor'. However, the mechanisms that regulate this process are poorly understood. Here, Bowles et al. show that retinoic acid is an important signaling molecule in this process. Retinoic acid is produced by the mesonephros and diffuses into the developing gonad, where it stimulates germ cells to enter meiosis and to develop as oocytes. So, why does this not happen in the developing male? The answer seems to be that the developing male germ cells are not only protected from retinoic acid exposure by virtue of their position in the primary sex cords, but also that the enzyme CYP26B1, which is expressed in the developing testis, breaks down retinoic acid. Male mice deficient in this enzyme show precocious germ cell meiosis. This study highlights beautifully the intricate paracrine interactions involved in early endocrine development, and that the long-sought 'meiosis-inhibiting factor' is actually a cytochrome P_{450} enzyme.

Digenic mutations account for variable phenotypes in idiopathic hypogonadotropic hypogonadism

Pitteloud N, Quinton R, Pearce S, Raivio T, Acierno J, Dwyer A, Plummer L, Hughes V, Seminara S, Cheng YZ, Li WP, Maccoll G, Eliseenkova AV, Olsen SK, Ibrahimi OA, Hayes FJ, Boepple P, Hall JE, Bouloux P, Mohammadi M, Crowley W
Reproductive Endocrine Unit of the Department of Medicine and Harvard Reproductive Endocrine Science Centers, Massachusetts General Hospital, Boston, Mass., USA; Department of Endocrinology and Royal Victoria Infirmary, School of Clinical Medical Sciences, and Institute for Human Genetics, University of Newcastle upon Tyne, Newcastle upon Tyne, UK; Department of Endocrinology, Royal Free Hospital, London, UK; Department of Pharmacology, New York University School of Medicine, New York, N.Y., USA
npitteloud@partners.org
J Clin Invest 2007;117:457–463

Background: Several single gene disorders have now been reported that cause idiopathic hypogonadotropic hypogonadism (IHH) due to defects of gonadotropin-releasing hormone (GnRH) secretion and/or action. However, significant inter- and intrafamilial variability and apparent incomplete phenotypic penetrance is often seen, even within families with the same mutation.

Methods: The effect of modifier loci was studied in two families. Family 1 had Kallmann syndrome (IHH and anosmia) due to a heterozygous FGF receptor 1 (FGFR1) mutation. Family 2 had normosmic IHH due to compound heterozygous mutations in the gonadotropin-releasing hormone receptor (GNRHR). Both kindred varied markedly in phenotypic expressivity within and across families.

Results: Further candidate gene screening revealed a second heterozygous deletion in the nasal embryonic LHRH factor (NELF) gene in pedigree 1 and an additional heterozygous FGFR1 mutation in pedigree 2 that accounted for the considerable phenotypic variability seen.

Conclusions: Different gene defects can synergize to produce a more severe phenotype in IHH families than either alone. This genetic model could account for some phenotypic heterogeneity seen in GnRH deficiency.

A number of single gene disorders have now been described that can cause Kallmann syndrome or IHH, but phenotypic variability is often seen even within families with the same mutation. Although the effect of modifying factors on disease phenotype has been appreciated for some time, a number of concrete examples of digenic (two genes working together) or limited polygenic inheritance have now been described in endocrine conditions [1]. Here, Pitteloud et al. show how changes in two genes (family 1: FGFR1 + NELF; family 2: GNRHR + FGFR1) combine to influence the expression of phenotype in families with hypogonadotropic hypogonadism. So far, these are relatively simple examples. In the next years, identification of the major genes involved in different developing endocrine systems coupled with high-throughput sequencing or re-sequencing strategies and bioinformatic approaches based on systems biology should be able to dissect out the contributions of more complex combinatorial processes on phenotypic expression. Deciphering these networks might also be valuable for predicting disease progression and individualizing treatment strategies. However, at present, demonstrating concrete examples of simple digenic patterns of influence is important. This report also shows that mutations in FGFR1 can be associated with *normosmic* hypogonadotropic hypogonadism as well as anosmic Kallmann syndrome. In fact, FGFR1 mutations have been described in patients with *normosmic* hypogonadotropic hypogonadism in three separate publications in the past year, showing that FGFR1 mutations represent a monogenic autosomal dominant cause of isolated hypogonadotropic hypogonadism as well as of Kallmann syndrome [2–4]. Finally, the discovery of oligogenic traits raises both conceptual and practical issues. If IHH as a paradigm is no longer considered to be solely a monogenic disorder in all cases, the transmission of a trait through families is no longer always synonymous with the transmission of one specific mutant allele. Labeling mutant alleles as dominant or recessive may be an oversimplification in the world of networks.

Pluripotency of spermatogonial stem cells from adult mouse testis

Guan K, Nayernia K, Maier LS, Wagner S, Dressel R, Lee JH, Nolte J, Wolf F, Li M, Engel W, Hasenfuss G
Department of Cardiology and Pneumology, Heart Center, Georg August University of Göttingen, Göttingen, Germany
hasenfus@med.uni-goettingen.de
Nature 2006;440:1199–1203

Background: Embryonic germ cells as well as germline stem cells from neonatal mouse testis are pluripotent. Thus, the germline lineage may retain the ability to generate pluripotent cells similar to embryonic stem cells. However, until now there has been no evidence for the pluripotency and plasticity of adult spermatogonial stem cells (SSCs), which are responsible for maintaining spermatogenesis throughout life in the male.
Methods: SSCs were isolated using genetic selection from adult mouse testis and their ability to acquire embryonic stem cell properties was studied.
Results: A population of multipotent adult germline stem cells (maGSCs) was identified. These cells were able to spontaneously differentiate into derivatives of the three embryonic germ layers in vitro and generate teratomas in immunodeficient mice. When injected into an early blastocyst, SSCs contribute to the development of various organs and show germline transmission.
Conclusion: The capacity to form multipotent cells persists in adult mouse testis. Establishment of human maGSCs from testicular biopsies may allow individual cell-based therapy without the ethical and immunological problems associated with human embryonic stem cells. Furthermore, these cells may provide new opportunities to study genetic diseases in various cell lineages.

Stem cell research holds many promises but is complicated by ethical issues related to the use of stem cells from human embryos as well as potential immunological issues if tissue generated is transplanted into a different host. Finding a source of accessible cells with pluripotency from one's own body would potentially avoid such issues. The identification and isolation of multipotent adult germline stem cells in the testes of mature mice represents a major potential advancement in this field of research. These cells were able to differentiate into derivatives of all three embryonic germ layers. Whilst this is a potential breakthrough, considerable progress is still needed in relation to the isolation, expansion and differentiation of these cells into viable tissue for transplantation. However, the fact that one would effectively be receiving an autotransplantation (i.e. using one's own tissue) means that some of the immunological and ethical issues that are challenging stem cell research at present could be circumvented.

A population-level decline in serum testosterone levels in American men

Travison TG, Araujo AB, O'Donnell AB, Kupelian V, McKinlay JB
New England Research Institutes, Watertown, Mass., USA
ttravison@neriscience.com
J Clin Endocrinol Metab 2007;92:196–202

Background: Although it is well established that mean testosterone (T) concentration declines with chronological age, a potential longitudinal decline in T has also been proposed based on several cohort studies.
Methods: The magnitude of population-level changes in serum T concentrations was studied in a prospective cohort study of health and endocrine function in randomly selected men aged 45–79 years (1,374 men between 1987 and 1999; 906 between 1995 and 1997, and 489 between 2002 and 2004). The relation of T concentrations to relative weight and other factors was assessed.
Results: A substantial age-independent decline in T was observed, which does not appear to be attributable to observed changes in health and lifestyle characteristics such as smoking and obesity. The estimated

population-level declines are greater in magnitude than the cross-sectional declines in T typically associated with age.

Conclusion: These results indicate that there has been a substantial, and as yet unrecognized, age-independent population-level decrease in T in American men. This decline is potentially attributable to birth cohort differences or to health or environmental effects not captured in the potential confounding factors measured here.

A number of reports have shown a potential decline in sperm count and quality in the past few decades, but only a limited number of studies have assessed longitudinal changes in T levels. Here, Travison et al. have measured T levels in men aged 45–79 years over a 17-year time period. An age-independent decrease in T levels was seen in the group, equating to a fall of approximately 1.2% a year. Although the number of individuals participating in each phase of the study varied due to dropout, which may have introduced some bias, this study does raise potentially important questions regarding the etiology and clinical significance of this change. The authors did study several health and lifestyle characteristics (e.g., smoking, obesity, dietary intake) but were unable to identify any strong correlations with the change in T levels. They concluded that as yet unknown environmental or health factors might be responsible for the fall in T seen. So, does it really matter if the middle-aged American male has somewhat lower levels of T? A fall in T may be associated with decreased bone and muscle mass, increased abdominal obesity, reduced cognitive function and mood, and decreased libido, although the risk of prostate cancer may be less. Coupled with potential downward trends in sperm count and increases in the incidence of congenital defects such as hypospadias, any such trends in population T levels must be viewed with some concern, and more data are needed. It would be of interest now to see if a similar decline in peak T values has occurred at puberty and in early adulthood, although of course only cross-sectional cohort studies would be possible and comparable methods for assaying T between groups would be essential (for discussion of the pitfalls of measuring T, see *New hormones*).

Concepts revised: improving communication within the ovary

Ovarian wedge resection restores fertility in estrogen receptor β knockout (ERβ$^{-/-}$) mice

Inzunza J, Morani A, Cheng G, Warner M, Hreinsson J, Gustafsson JA, Hovatta O
Division of Medical Nutrition, Department of Biosciences and Nutrition, Karolinska University Hospital, Karolinska Institutet, NOVUM, Stockholm, Sweden
jan-ake.gustafsson@mednut.ki.se
Proc Natl Acad Sci USA 2007;104:600–605

Background: Ovulation rarely occurs in mice in which the estrogen receptor β (ERβ) gene has been inactivated (ERβ$^{-/-}$ mice). It is unknown whether the defect resides in the ovary itself or in the disturbed endocrinological milieu of these animals.

Methods: ERβ$^{-/-}$ ovaries were transplanted into WT mice and WT ovaries into ERβ$^{-/-}$ mice. Ovarian wedge resection was also performed in some animals.

Results: Upon mating with ERβ$^{-/-}$ males, fertility increased from 20% in the control intact ERβ$^{-/-}$ group to 40% in the WT recipients with ERβ$^{-/-}$ ovaries. The transplantation procedure was not efficient, and when WT ovaries were transplanted into WT mice, fertility was only 36%. Surgical ovarian wedge resection resulted in 100% fertility in ERβ$^{-/-}$ mice. In ERβ$^{-/-}$ mice, as the follicles enlarged, the thecal layer remained very compact and there was no increase in vascularization. In addition, there was an increase in PDGF receptor α (PDGFRα) and a decrease in PDGFβ expression in the granulosa cells, similar to what has been found in follitropin receptor knockout mice. After wedge resection, expression of both smooth muscle actin (a marker of vascularization) and PDGFRs was normalized.

Conclusions: Increased vascularization of the thecal layer is a prerequisite for further follicular growth during normal follicular development. The defect in ERβ$^{-/-}$ mouse ovaries may be a failure of communication between the granulosa and thecal layers. The follicles do not mature because of insufficient blood supply. This problem is overcome by stimulating neovascularization by simple wedge resection of the ovaries. These data may provide insight into the mechanism by which wedge resection improves ovulation in women with polycystic ovarian syndrome.

This study by Inzunza et al. initially set out to determine whether the reduced fertility of ERβ knock-out mice was due to an ovarian or systemic disturbance. Transplanting ERβ knockout ovaries into wild-type animals resulted in an improvement in fertility similar to wild-type/wild-type transplants, but still only 40%. Surprisingly, wedge resection restored fertility in all cases. Wedge resection has been used historically in the treatment of women with polycystic ovary syndrome (PCOS), but few data have been available to explain how this intervention works. In this ERβ mouse model it appears that wedge resection results in neovascularization and improved communication between the granulosa and thecal layers, resulting in an improvement in follicle maturation. Vascularization and local vascular communication is essential for the development and function of almost all endocrine tissues. Ovarian wedge resection or surgical manipulation (e.g., drilling, electrocautery) is still popular in some centers for women who do not conceive on other forms of therapy such as clomiphene (see *Clinical trials, new treatments*). Whether these techniques result in improved vascular communication in PCOS ovaries warrants further detailed investigation.

Heterozygous missense mutations in steroidogenic factor 1 (SF1/Ad4BP, NR5A1) are associated with 46,XY disorders of sex development with normal adrenal function

Lin L, Philibert P, Ferraz-de-Souza B, Kelberman D, Homfray T, Albanese A, Molini V, Sebire NJ, Einaudi S, Conway GS, Hughes IA, Jameson JL, Sultan C, Dattani MT, Achermann JC
UCL Institute of Child Health and Department of Medicine, University College London, London, UK; Service d'Hormonologie du Développement et de la Reproduction, Hôpital Lapeyronie et INSERM U540, CHU Montpellier, France; Department of Medical Genetics and Department of Paediatric Endocrinology, St George's Hospital Medical School, London, UK; Department of Paediatric Endocrinology, Regina Margherita Hospital, Turin, Italy; Department of Paediatric Histopathology, Great Ormond Street Hospital for Children, London, UK; Department of Paediatrics, University of Cambridge, Cambridge, UK; Feinberg School of Medicine, Northwestern University, Chicago, Ill., USA; Unité d'Endocrinologie Pédiatrique, Hôpital Arnaud de Villeneuve, CHU Montpellier, France
j.achermann@ich.ucl.ac.uk
J Clin Endocrinol Metab 2007;92:991–999

Background: Steroidogenic factor-1 (SF1, NR5A1) is a nuclear receptor transcription factor that plays a key role in regulating adrenal and gonadal development, steroidogenesis, and reproduction. Although human mutations in SF1 were described initially in 2 46,XY individuals with female external genitalia, müllerian structures and primary adrenal failure, recent case reports have suggested haploinsufficiency of SF1 may be associated with a testicular phenotype alone.
Methods: The gene encoding SF1 was analyzed in 30 individuals with a phenotypic spectrum of 46,XY gonadal dysgenesis/impaired androgenization (now termed 46,XY disorders of sex development, DSD) with normal adrenal function.
Results: Heterozygous missense mutations in NR5A1 were found in 4 individuals (4/30, 13%) with this phenotype. These mutations showed impaired transcriptional activation through abnormal DNA binding, altered sub-nuclear localization, or through disruption of the putative ligand-binding pocket. Two mutations appeared to be inherited from the mother in a sex-limited dominant manner.
Conclusions: Heterozygous SF1 mutations may be a more frequent cause of impaired fetal and postnatal testicular function than previously reported.

SF1 plays a key role in many aspects of adrenal and reproductive development and function. Although studies of mice and initial reports of patients with SF1 mutations focused on a combined adrenal and reproductive phenotype, some recent case reports have described potential haploinsufficiency of SF1 in individuals with impaired testis development and function but normal adrenals. This report by Lin et al. describes heterozygous SF1 changes in approximately 15% of 46,XY individuals with a phenotype of mild testicular dysgenesis, impaired androgenization but with normal adrenal function. Müllerian remnants may or may not be present. Furthermore, mothers of affected children can carry these heterozygous SF1 changes and transmit them in a sex-limited dominant fashion, which may mimic an X-linked disorder. Thus, SF1 mutations might be worth considering as one of the first genetic tests undertaken in this group of patients, and it would be prudent to monitor adrenal function in the long term until it is known whether this cohort are likely to develop adrenal insufficiency or not.

Important for clinical practice: the art of agreement

Consensus statement on management of intersex disorders

Hughes IA, Houk C, Ahmed SF, Lee PA
Department of Paediatrics, University of Cambridge, Addenbrooke's Hospital, Cambridge, UK
iah1000@cam.ac.uk
Arch Dis Child 2006;91:554–563

Positions statement: criteria for defining polycystic ovary syndrome as a predominantly hyperandrogenic syndrome: an Androgen Excess Society guideline

Azziz R, Carmina E, Dewailly D, Diamanti-Kandarakis E, Escobar-Morreale HF, Futterweit W, Janssen OE, Legro RS, Norman RJ, Taylor AE, Witchel SF
Cedars-Sinai Medical Center and The David Geffen School of Medicine at the University of California, Los Angeles, Calif., USA
azzizr@cshs.org
J Clin Endocrinol Metab 2006;91:4237–4245

Background: The Androgen Excess Society (AES) convened a task force to review all available data and recommend an evidence-based definition for polycystic ovary syndrome (PCOS) to guide clinical diagnosis and future research.

Methods: Expert investigators in the field undertook a systematic review of published peer-reviewed medical literature, followed by consensus discussion and agreement on a final report.

Results and Conclusions: Based on the available data, the AES Task Force concluded that the phenotype of PCOS should be defined based on the original 1990 National Institutes of Health criteria with some modifications, taking into consideration the concerns expressed in the proceedings of the 2003 Rotterdam conference. A principal conclusion was that PCOS should be considered primarily a disorder of androgen excess or hyperandrogenism, although a minority considered the possibility that there may be forms of PCOS without overt evidence of hyperandrogenism. The task force recognized that the definition of this syndrome will evolve over time to incorporate new research findings.

Care of girls and women with Turner syndrome: a guideline of the Turner Syndrome Study Group

Bondy CA
Developmental Endocrinology Branch, National Institute of Child Health and Human Development, National Institutes of Health, Bethesda, Md., USA
bondyc@mail.nih.gov
J Clin Endocrinol Metab 2007;92:10–25

Background: Updated consensus guidelines for the evaluation and treatment of girls and women with Turner syndrome (TS) are lacking.

Methods: A multidisciplinary panel of experts (The Turner Syndrome Consensus Study Group) met to analyze peer-reviewed published literature to form its principal recommendations. Expert opinion was used in the many situations where good evidence was lacking. Breakout groups focused on genetic, cardiological, auxological, psychological, gynecological, and general medical concerns and drafted recommendations for presentation to the whole group.

Results and Conclusions: The study group made several key recommendations, such as: (1) that parents receiving a prenatal diagnosis of TS be advised of the broad phenotypic spectrum and the good quality of life observed in TS in recent years; (2) that magnetic resonance angiography be used in addition to echocardiography to evaluate the cardiovascular system and that patients with defined cardiovascular defects be cautioned regarding pregnancy and certain types of exercise; (3) that puberty should not be delayed to promote statural growth; (4) that a comprehensive educational evaluation is undertaken in early childhood to identify potential attention deficit or non-verbal learning disorders; (5) that caregivers address the prospect of premature ovarian failure in an open and sensitive manner and emphasize the critical importance of estrogen treatment for feminization and for bone health during in adulthood; (6) that individuals with TS require continued monitoring of hearing and thyroid function, and (7) that adults with TS be monitored for aortic enlargement, hypertension, diabetes, and dyslipidemia.

The 'experts' of the world have clearly been working overtime in the past year in order to draft several important *Consensus* documents or guidelines that are relevant to those involved in pediatric endocrine care. The *Consensus statement on management of intersex disorders* provides important recommendations for nomenclature (such as 'intersex' being replaced by 'disorders of sex development (DSD)') and reviewed a number of key areas such as genetics and etiology, investigations and management, and psychosocial consequences. Attempts were made to gather evidence-based long-term outcome data, but in many areas this was not available. The position statement on the *criteria for defining polycystic ovarian syndrome* focused more on guidelines for diagnosing PCOS, which are essential if short- and long-term intervention and follow-up outcome studies are to be undertaken. Finally, the guidelines of the *Turner Syndrome Study Group* provide more comprehensive statements about the care of children and adults with Turner syndrome. The main conclusions from this document are outlined above.

Self-esteem and social adjustment in young women with Turner syndrome – influence of pubertal management and sexuality: population-based cohort study

Carel JC, Elie C, Ecosse E, Tauber M, Leger J, Cabrol S, Nicolino M, Brauner R, Chaussain JL, Coste J
Pediatric Endocrinology, Hôpital Robert Debré, Paris, France
carel@paris5.inserm.fr
J Clin Endocrinol Metab 2006;91:2972–2979

Background: Girls with Turner syndrome often have induction of puberty delayed in an attempt to optimize height. However, the influence of different strategies of pubertal management on psychosocial adjustment and sex life has not been evaluated in detail.
Methods: Determinants of self-esteem, social adjustment, and initiation of sex life were assessed in relation to pubertal management in a prospective study of 566 women with Turner syndrome (aged 22.6 ± 2.6 years, range 18.3–31.2), from a population-based registry of GH-treated patients.
Results: Low self-esteem was found to be associated with otological problems and limited sexual experience, whereas low social adjustment was associated with lower paternal socioeconomic class and an absence of sexual experience. A delay in the age at first kiss or date was more prevalent in those girls with cardiac involvement or who had a lack of spontaneous pubertal development. Age at first sexual intercourse was related to age at puberty and paternal socioeconomic class. Thus, delayed induction of puberty had a long-lasting effect on sex life. In contrast, height and height gain due to GH treatment had no effect on outcomes.
Conclusions: Puberty should be induced at a physiologically appropriate age in girls with Turner syndrome to optimize self-esteem, social adjustment, and initiation of the patient's sex life.

Clinical significance of the parental origin of the X chromosome in Turner syndrome

Sagi L, Zuckerman-Levin N, Gawlik A, Ghizzoni L, Buyukgebiz A, Rakover Y, Bistritzer T, Admoni O, Vottero A, Baruch O, Fares F, Malecka-Tendera E, Hochberg Z

Division of Endocrinology, Meyer Children's Hospital, Haifa, Israel; Pediatric Endocrinology, Katowice University, Katowice, Poland; Pediatric Endocrinology, Parma University, Parma, Italy; Department of Pediatrics, Ismir University, Ismir, Turkey; 5 Pediatric Endocrinology, Haemek Hospital, Afula, Israel; Department of Pediatrics, Asaf Harofeh Hospital, Tzrifin, Israel; Department of Biochemistry and Molecular Genetics, Carmel Medical Center, Haifa, Israel; Faculty of Medicine, Technion-Israel Institute of Technology, Haifa, Israel
z_hochberg@rambam.health.gov.il

J Clin Endocrinol Metab 2006;92:846–852

Background: The phenotype in Turner syndrome (TS) is variable even in patients with a supposedly non-mosaic karyotype. Previous work has suggested that X-linked parent-of-origin effects might exist. Therefore, TS phenotype may be influenced by the parental origin of the missed X chromosome.

Methods: A multicenter prospective study of 83 TS patients (45,X or 46Xi[Xq]) and their parents was performed to determine parental origin of the X chromosome using highly polymorphic microsatellite markers on the X and Y chromosomes. Associations between the parental origin of the X chromosome and the unique phenotypic traits of TS (e.g., congenital malformations, anthropometry, skeletal defects, endocrine traits, education and vocation) were determined.

Results: Girls with a 45,X karyotype retained their maternal X(m) in 83% of cases, whereas 64% of those with a 46Xi(Xq) karyotype retained their paternal X(p) ($p < 0.001$). Kidney malformations were exclusively found in X(m) patients ($p = 0.030$). In addition, the X(m) group had lower total and LDL cholesterol ($p < 0.05$), and higher BMI SDS ($p = 0.03$) that was not maintained after hGH treatment. Ocular abnormalities were more common in the X(p) group ($p = 0.017$), who also had higher academic achievement. Response to GH therapy was comparable between both groups.

Conclusions: The parental origin of the missing short arm of the X chromosome has an impact on weight, renal development, ocular features and lipids. These findings suggest potential effects of as yet undetermined imprinted X chromosome genes.

In addition to the Turner Syndrome Study Group guidelines, several original articles have been published this year that report important findings for the management of TS in children and adults. Carel et al. provide data from 566 girls with TS to support the view that puberty should be induced at a physiologically appropriate age to optimize self-esteem, social adjustment, and initiation of sexual relationships. There has been a trend to delay puberty in some cases in an attempt to optimize any benefits of GH therapy before the pubertal growth spurt. However, this paper shows that delaying pubertal induction is not only associated with delayed onset of sexual relationships, but also with worse self-esteem and social adjustment. The sample size is impressively large, and the mean age of respondents was 22 years. Whether the effects of puberty timing will be perceived as less relevant with increasing age remains to be seen. However, in this formative period of life there are clearly issues. Furthermore, although the otological issues associated with TS have been appreciated for some time (e.g., sensorineuronal hearing loss), Carel et al. clearly show that such features can have an important negative impact on self-esteem. Differences in phenotypic features have been proposed to correlate with certain patterns of X-chromosomal loss but, in general, phenotypic variability can be quite great even in girls with monosomy (45,X). Another explanation for phenotypic differences is that the parent of origin effect of X-chromosomal inheritance is important, perhaps through a subset of imprinted genes [5]. By studying parental origin of the X chromosome in 83 girls with 45,X or 46XiXq, Sagi et al. have shown that inheritance of a maternal X chromosome was associated with renal abnormalities, lower LDL and cholesterol and higher pre-GH BMI, whereas a paternally-derived X chromosome was more frequently found with eye abnormalities and higher academic achievement. These studies add to the growing literature on potential imprinting effects of X-chromosomal genes. It remains to be determined whether long-term follow-up protocols should be modified depending on parental X-inheritance patterns.

Clomiphene, metformin, or both for infertility in the polycystic ovary syndrome

Legro RS, Barnhart HX, Schlaff WD, Carr BR, Diamond MP, Carson SA, Steinkampf MP, Coutifaris C, McGovern PG, Cataldo NA, Gosman GG, Nestler JE, Giudice LC, Leppert PC, Myers ER
Department of Obstetrics and Gynecology, Pennsylvania State University College of Medicine, M.S. Hershey Medical Center, Hershey, Pa., USA
rsl1@psu.edu
N Engl J Med 2007;356:551–566

Background: The polycystic ovary syndrome (PCOS) is a common cause of infertility. Clomiphene and insulin sensitizers are used alone and in combination to induce ovulation, but it is unknown whether one approach is superior to the other.
Methods: A total of 626 infertile women with the PCOS were randomly assigned to receive clomiphene citrate plus placebo, extended-release metformin plus placebo, or a combination of metformin and clomiphene for up to 6 months. Medication was discontinued when pregnancy was confirmed. All subjects were followed until delivery.
Results: The live-birth rate was 22.5% (47 of 209 subjects) in the clomiphene group, 7.2% (15 of 208) in the metformin group, and 26.8% (56 of 209) in the combination-therapy group. Among pregnancies, the rate of multiple pregnancy was 6.0% in the clomiphene group, 0% in the metformin group, and 3.1% in the combination-therapy group. The rates of first-trimester pregnancy loss did not differ significantly among the groups. However, the conception rate among subjects who ovulated was significantly lower in the metformin group (21.7%) than in either the clomiphene group (39.5%, p = 0.002) or the combination-therapy group (46.0%, p < 0.001). Adverse-event rates were similar in all groups, although gastrointestinal side effects were more frequent, and vasomotor and ovulatory symptoms less frequent, in the metformin group than in the clomiphene group.
Conclusions: Clomiphene is superior to metformin in achieving live birth in infertile women with the PCOS, although multiple births are a complication.

This study comparing clomiphene and metformin in the treatment of infertility in PCOS does not involve any new therapeutics or novel treatment strategies; rather, it compares two established treatments in a randomized-controlled fashion with sufficient numbers to address the question posed. Clomiphene was found to be superior to metformin in achieving live births in infertile women, but its use was associated with a higher risk of multiple births; thus, this study provides suitable data for the development of evidence-based guidelines, and allows for the appropriate counseling of patients in this regard. Similarly, in a multicenter, randomized trial that compared clomiphene plus metformin with clomiphene plus placebo in 225 infertile Dutch women with PCOS, the addition of metformin did not significantly improve rates of either ovulation or pregnancy [6]. These data contrast somewhat with the meta-analysis reported by Norman et al. discussed previously [7] but total numbers in this meta-analysis were less than those in the Legro study. All too often it is difficult or unethical to undertake a randomized controlled study once a treatment modality has become established, although data may be lacking on absolute benefits and risks. This problem can be particularly difficult in the study of rare conditions, as highlighted by the paucity of evidence-based data when recent consensus guidelines have been established (see *Important for clinical practice*). Sometimes taking one step backwards is necessary in order to take two steps forward.

A male contraceptive targeting germ cell adhesion

Mruk DD, Wong CH, Silvestrini B, Cheng CY
Population Council, Center for Biomedical Research, New York, N.Y., USA
d-mruk@popcbr.rockefeller.edu
Nat Med 2006;12:1323–1328

Background: Developing germ cells remain attached to Sertoli cells during spermatogenesis via testis-specific anchoring junctions. If the adhesion between these cell types is compromised, germ cells detach from the seminiferous epithelium, often resulting in infertility. Adjudin is capable of inducing germ cell loss from the epithelium, but serious side effects such as liver inflammation and muscle atrophy can occur in a subset of animals given this compound.

Methods: The effects of testis-specific targeting of Adjudin were studied by conjugating Adjudin to a recombinant follicle-stimulating hormone (FSH) mutant, which serves as its 'carrier'.

Results: Using this approach, infertility was induced in adult rats when 0.5 µg Adjudin/kg b.w. was administered intraperitoneally, which was similar to results when 50 mg/kg b.w. was given orally.

Conclusion: This targeted approach represents a substantial increase in Adjudin's selectivity and efficacy as a potential male contraceptive.

The quest for a simple, effective and reversible male contraceptive goes on. Current studies of testosterone alone or in combination with other factors are proving to be generally disappointing. Thus, other therapeutic strategies may be worth investigating. Potential approaches include non-steroidal factors such as 1-CDB-4022 that interfere with the process of spermatogenesis [8] or Adjudin, a compound that can cause germ cell loss from the epithelium by disrupting the adhesions between germ cells and Sertoli cells. Whilst Adjudin is effective in rats at high doses, its oral administration is associated with significant side effects such as liver damage in around one-third of animals. By linking the active compound to a recombinant mutant form of FSH, Mruk et al. have been able to target Adjudin to the Sertoli cells, thereby permitting the use of much smaller doses of the drug and avoiding unwanted systemic complications. This approach means that the compound would need to be given parentally or in depot form, unless an orally bioavailable FSH receptor binding compound could be developed. Also, it is not clear whether disrupting germ cell adhesion would have lasting effects on fertility in humans; fertility was restored in rats over a matter of weeks. Thus, it is likely that developing this approach for human use is some way off. Nevertheless, therapeutic targeting to endocrine systems is a useful strategy that could have applications to other areas of endocrine intervention.

New genes: responding to the desire to be an ovary

R-spondin1 is essential in sex determination, skin differentiation and malignancy

Parma P, Radi O, Vidal V, Chaboissier MC, Dellambra E, Valentini S, Guerra L, Schedl A, Camerino G
Dipartimento di Patologia Umana ed Ereditaria, Sezione di Biologia Generale e Genetica Medica, Università di Pavia, Pavia, Italy
camerino@unipv.it
Nat Genet 2006;38:1304–1309

Background: R-spondins are a recently characterized small family of growth factors, but their role in developmental endocrinology has not been elucidated.

Methods: Mapping and candidate gene analysis in kindred with a recessive syndrome characterized by XX sex reversal, palmoplantar hyperkeratosis and predisposition to squamous cell carcinoma of the skin.

Results: Disruption of the gene R-spondin1 (RSPO1) was found in patients with this condition.

Conclusion: This study shows for the first time that disruption of a single gene can lead to complete female-to-male sex reversal in the absence of the testis-determining gene, SRY.

For many years, ovarian development was viewed as a largely passive process, whereas testis development is an active process requiring the expression of genes such as SRY and SOX9, and followed by a distinct set of morphological changes. However, recent studies of gene expression profiles have started to reveal a distinct set of genes that are turned on in the developing ovary [9], and several morphological processes may have an effect on suppressing testis formation. Direct evidence for the existence of ovarian genes that oppose testis development comes from the identification of R-spondin1 as the gene responsible for the clinical syndrome of 'XX sex reversal' (testicular DSD), palmoplantar hyperkeratosis and predisposition to squamous cell carcinoma of the skin. Individuals (46,XX) with loss of function mutations in this gene develop testicular tissue in the absence of SRY. This finding provides strong evidence that ovarian development is an active process that involves repression of testis development as well as maintenance of ovarian commitment. Whether RSPO1 mutations might be found in individuals without an extended phenotype (e.g., SRY-negative 46,XX individuals with a male phenotype, or 46,XX ovotesticular DSD) remains to be seen. Similarly, overexpression or duplication of RSPO1 might be found in cases of testicular dysgenesis.

CXorf6 is a causative gene for hypospadias

Fukami M, Wada Y, Miyabayashi K, Nishino I, Hasegawa T, Nordenskjold A, Camerino G, Kretz C, Buj-Bello A, Laporte J, Yamada G, Morohashi K, Ogata T
Department of Endocrinology and Metabolism, National Research Institute for Child Health and Development, Tokyo, Japan
tomogata@nch.go.jp
Nat Genet 2006;38:1369–1371

Background: 46,XY disorders of sex development (DSD) refer to a wide range of abnormal genitalia, including hypospadias, which affects approximately 0.5% of male newborns.
Methods: Analysis of the gene CXorf6 in boys with hypospadias and investigation of CXorf6 expression during development in the mouse.
Results: Three different nonsense mutations of CXorf6 were found in individuals with hypospadias. The mouse homolog for CXorf6 was specifically expressed in fetal Sertoli and Leydig cells around the critical period for sex development.
Conclusions: These findings suggest that CXorf6 is a causative gene for hypospadias.

Hypospadias is one of the most frequent congenital anomalies in newborn males with minor degrees of hypospadias present in up to 1:200–500 live births, or even more [9]. The cause of hypospadias is unknown in the vast majority of cases. Defects in dihydrotestosterone synthesis and action can be found in rare cases, although in most of these situations the degree of hypospadias is relatively severe and associated with a small penis. Here, Fukami et al. describe mutations in an X-linked gene, Cxorf6, in 3 boys with penoscrotal hypospadias and a micropenis, out of a cohort of 166 patients. Postnatal hypothalamic-pituitary gonadal endocrine function was apparently normal. Cxorf6 encodes a hypothetical protein with poorly understood function, but which is expressed during a critical period of testis development in the mouse. In fact, Cxorf6 appears to be switched on in the developing testis from around e12, has weak expression soon after birth, and is not detected thereafter. This study raises the possibility that a number of other gene defects may account of cases of hypospadias, either through their actions at critical time periods of development or perhaps through an interaction with environmental modulators.

Kallmann syndrome: mutations in the genes encoding prokineticin-2 and prokineticin receptor-2

Dode C, Teixeira L, Levilliers J, Fouveaut C, Bouchard P, Kottler ML, Lespinasse J, Lienhardt-Roussie A, Mathieu M, Moerman A, Morgan G, Murat A, Toublanc JE, Wolczynski S, Delpech M, Petit C, Young J, Hardelin JP
Institut Cochin, INSERM U567, Université René Descartes, Paris, France
dode@cochin.inserm.fr
PLoS Genet 2006;2:e175

Background: Kallmann syndrome describes the association of anosmia (due to defective olfactory bulb morphogenesis) and hypogonadism (due to gonadotropin-releasing hormone deficiency). Loss-of-function mutations in KAL1 and FGFR1 underlie the X-chromosome-linked form and an autosomal dominant form of the disease, respectively. Mutations in these genes, however, only account for approximately 20% of all Kallmann syndrome cases.
Methods: Analysis of the candidate genes encoding the G-protein-coupled prokineticin receptor-2 (PROKR2) and one of its ligands, prokineticin-2 (PROK2), in a cohort of 192 patients with Kallmann syndrome.
Results: Ten heterozygous, homozygous, or compound heterozygous mutations were identified in PROKR2 and four heterozygous mutations were found in PROK2 in this cohort. In addition, 1 of the patients heterozygous for a PROKR2 mutation also harbored a missense mutation in KAL1, suggesting a possible digenic inheritance of the disease in this individual.

Conclusion: These findings reveal that insufficient prokineticin-signaling through PROKR2 leads to abnormal development of the olfactory system and reproductive axis in man. These findings also shed new light on the complex genetic transmission of Kallmann syndrome.

It is now 15 years since the description of KAL1 gene mutations in X-linked Kallmann syndrome. More recently, heterozygous mutations in FGFR1 have been reported in an autosomal dominant form of this condition. However, only a proportion of patients with Kallmann syndrome have been found to have changes in these genes, suggesting that additional candidate factors involved in olfaction and GnRH neuronal development are yet to be found. Using a candidate gene approach in part based on mouse data [10], Dode et al. report mutations in the G-protein-coupled prokineticin receptor-2 (PROK2) and one of its ligands (prokineticin-1, PROK2) in 14 patients with Kallmann syndrome out of a study cohort of 192 individuals. The mutations in PROKR2 were heterozygous, compound heterozygous or homozygous, whereas the PROK2 changes were all heterozygous changes that were either de novo or inherited in a dominant fashion. The description of a heterozygous PROKR2 mutation together with a heterozygous missense mutation in KAL1 in 1 patient with Kallmann syndrome further supports the concept that digenic or limited polygenic changes in a small subset of genes may contribute to anosmic or normosmic hypogonadotropic hypogonadism phenotypes (see *New paradigms*). Taken together, these findings substantially increase our insight into the genetic regulation of hypothalamic-pituitary reproductive axis development. It is likely that additional factors remain to be discovered and that combinatorial effects of several factors may be important for the expression of phenotype.

New hormones: seeking biomarkers of Leydig cell function

Changes in serum insulin-like factor 3 during normal male puberty

Ferlin A, Garolla A, Rigon F, Rasi Caldogno L, Lenzi A, Foresta C
University of Padova, Department of Histology, Microbiology and Medical Biotechnologies, Centre for Male Gamete Cryopreservation, Padova, Italy
carlo.foresta@unipd.it
J Clin Endocrinol Metab 2006;91:3426–3431

Background: Insulin-like factor 3 (INSL3) is produced by Leydig cells. In adults, INSL3 secretion is dependent on the state of differentiation of these cells, which is LH-dependent. However, the secretion and regulation of INSL3 during puberty is unknown.

Methods: INSL3 concentrations during normal male puberty were analyzed in relation to LH, FSH, testosterone, and testicular volume in 75 healthy male subjects aged 9.5–17.5 years, divided into five groups based on Tanner staging.

Results: INSL3 and LH levels increased from Tanner stage 2 to 4, whereas FSH increased from stage 2 to 3. Testosterone levels increased from stage 3 to 4. No differences were seen for all measured hormones between stages 4 and 5. However, INSL3 plasma concentrations at pubertal stages 4 and 5 are about one quarter of adult levels, whereas FSH, LH, and testosterone reached adult levels by stage 4. INSL3 and LH were significantly correlated during all stages of puberty.

Conclusion: This study describes the physiological dynamics of INSL3, showing that serum concentrations of this hormone increased progressively throughout puberty under the differentiating action of LH on Leydig cells, and preceding the rise in testosterone. INSL3 may therefore represent a marker of Leydig cell differentiation and function. However, a prolonged exposure to LH seems to be necessary to reach INSL3 concentrations of adults.

Serum insulin-like factor 3 levels during puberty in healthy boys and boys with Klinefelter syndrome

Wikstrom AM, Bay K, Hero M, Andersson AM, Dunkel L
Hospital for Children and Adolescents, Helsinki University Central Hospital, Helsinki, Finland
anne.wikstrom@fimnet.fi

J Clin Endocrinol Metab 2006;91:4705–4708

Background: Levels of the Leydig cell-specific hormone insulin-like factor 3 (INSL3) are incompletely characterized in boys during pubertal development.

Methods: INSL3 levels during spontaneous puberty were measured in 30 healthy boys with idiopathic short-stature (ISS) (aged 9.0–14.5 years), half of whom received aromatase inhibitors for 24 months, and 14 boys with Klinefelter syndrome (KS) and Leydig cell dysfunction (aged 10–13.9 years). Serum INSL3 levels were correlated with in bone age, Tanner pubertal stages, and LH and testosterone concentrations.

Results: Onset of puberty was associated with a significant increase in INSL3 levels from Tanner G1 to Tanner G2. Adult INSL3 levels were attained at bone age 13–14 years. ISS boys with letrozole-induced hypergonadotropic hyperandrogenism had, after 12 months of therapy, higher INSL3 levels than did placebo-treated boys. KS boys had an initial increase in INSL3 similar to that in healthy boys, but INSL3 concentrations leveled off despite LH hyperstimulation. Positive correlations occurred between serum INSL3 and LH and between INSL3 and testosterone levels in all three groups ($p < 0.0001$).

Conclusions: The Leydig cell-specific hormone INSL3 may serve as a new marker for onset and progression of puberty in boys. The increase in INSL3 levels seen during puberty seems to be dependent on LH stimulation. INSL3 concentrations may indicate Leydig cell dysfunction from midpuberty onward in boys with KS.

Position statement: utility, limitations, and pitfalls in measuring testosterone – an Endocrine Society position statement

Rosner W, Auchus RJ, Azziz R, Sluss PM, Raff H
St. Luke's/Roosevelt Hospital Center, New York, N.Y., USA
wr7@columbia.edu

J Clin Endocrinol Metab 2007;92:405–413

Background: The objective of the study was to evaluate the current state of clinical assays for total and free testosterone.

Methods: Five participants were appointed by The Endocrine Society to undertake this task using published data from search engines and the College of American Pathologists, as well as expert opinion.

Results and Conclusion: Laboratory proficiency testing should be based on the ability to measure accurately and precisely samples containing known concentrations of testosterone, not only on agreement with others using the same method. Normative values for total and free testosterone should be established for both genders and children when such standardization is in place, taking into account the many variables that influence serum testosterone concentration.

Initial studies of INSL3 focused on its role in testis descent, as mutations in INSL3 (or its G-protein-coupled receptor, GREAT) have been found in boys with congenital cryptorchidism. However, the development of assays for this peptide has raised the possibility that INSL3 may be a useful marker of testicular Leydig cell function during development and in certain endocrine conditions [11]. Testosterone and INSL3 provide different information on the status of the Leydig cell. Testosterone better reflects the steroidogenic activity, whereas INSL3 might better reflect the differentiation status of the Leydig cell or long-term tropic effects of LH action. The two studies presented here show that INSL3 levels rise during the early stages of puberty in boys, mimicking the rise in LH at this time, and preceding the elevation in testosterone seen typically between Tanner stages III-IV. Furthermore, INSL3 levels were lower from midpuberty in boys with Klinefelter syndrome. Thus, INSL3 may become a useful marker for impending Leydig cell dysfunction in the future, or as a marker of Leydig cell reserve. Whether measurement of this hormone would be useful for assessing Leydig cell function in infants with disorders of sex development, or as a marker to help differentiate constitutionally delayed puberty from hypogonadotropic hypogonadism, remains to be seen. Increasing issues are arising about the standardization of measurement of testosterone and lack of appropriate normative data, which precipitated publication of a position statement on this subject by The Endocrine Society this year. Thus, additional markers of Leydig cell function, such as INSL3, could be very valuable.

Reviews

Germ cell tumors in the intersex gonad: old paths, new directions, moving frontiers

Cools M, Drop SL, Wolffenbuttel KP, Oosterhuis JW, Looijenga LH
Department of Pathology, Erasmus MC-University Medical Center Rotterdam, Josephine Nefkens Institute, The Netherlands
l.looijenga@erasmusmc.nl
Endocr Rev 2006;27:468–484

Background: The risk of developing germ cell tumors is an important factor to consider in the management of patients with disorders of sex development (DSD). However, this risk is often hard to predict. Recently, major progress has been made in identifying gene products related to germ cell tumor development (e.g., testis-specific protein-Y encoded and OCT3/4), in recognizing early changes of germ cells (maturation delay, preneoplastic lesions, and in situ neoplasia), and in appreciating the role of 'undifferentiated gonadal tissue' in the development of gonadoblastoma. It is expected that the combination of these findings will allow for estimation of the risk for tumor development in the individual patient. *Method:* This article reviews recent literature regarding the prevalence of germ cell tumors in patients with DSD. *Results and Conclusion:* A clear perspective on the literature is hindered by confusing terminology regarding different forms of intersex disorders and unclear criteria for the diagnosis of malignant germ cells at an early age (maturation delay vs. early steps in malignant transformation). It is hoped that a better understanding of germ cell tumor development and a new classification system for patients with DSD (see *Important for clinical practice*) will help to refine our insight in the prevalence and progression of germ cell tumors in specific diagnostic groups.

Food for thought: tea tree oil?

Prepubertal gynecomastia linked to lavender and tea tree oils

Henley DV, Lipson N, Korach KS, Bloch CA
Receptor Biology Section, Laboratory of Reproductive and Developmental Toxicology, National Institute of Environmental Health Sciences, Research Triangle Park, N.C., USA
korach@niehs.nih.gov
N Engl J Med 2007;356:479–485

Background: Most cases of male prepubertal gynecomastia are classified as idiopathic. *Methods:* Possible causes of gynecomastia were investigated in 3 prepubertal boys who were otherwise healthy and had normal serum concentrations of endogenous steroids. *Results:* In all 3 boys, the development of gynecomastia coincided with the topical application of products that contained lavender and tea tree oils, and regressed when use of these products was stopped. Studies in human cell lines indicated that the two oils have estrogenic and anti-androgenic activities. *Conclusion:* Repeated topical exposure to lavender and tea tree oils probably caused prepubertal gynecomastia in these boys.

Although this report contains only a small number of effectively anecdotal cases, it does provide important direct evidence for the potentially estrogenic effects of certain 'environmental' compounds in humans, and is backed up by detailed in vitro studies of estrogenic and anti-androgenic activity. Whether all boys would respond to such oils similarly is unclear – although randomized controlled trials are unlikely to be possible. Furthermore, larger population studies are needed to assess how frequent this association with prepubertal gynecomastia really is. Nevertheless, these cases do show the great importance of taking a detailed history of exposure to 'unusual' environmental agents when children present with atypical or precocious development. As the gynecomastia in these cases was reversible following withdrawal of the agent, unnecessary surgery could be avoided.

Acknowledgment
J.C.A. is a Wellcome Trust Senior Research Fellow in Clinical Science (079666).

References

1. Savage DB, Agostini M, Barroso I, Gurnell M, Luan J, Meirhaeghe A, et al: Digenic inheritance of severe insulin resistance in a human pedigree. Nat Genet 2002;31:379–384.
2. Pitteloud N, Meysing A, Quinton R, Acierno JS Jr, Dwyer AA, Plummer L, et al: Mutations in fibroblast growth factor receptor 1 cause Kallmann syndrome with a wide spectrum of reproductive phenotypes. Mol Cell Endocrinol 2006; 254–255:60–69.
3. Trarbach EB, Costa EM, Versiani B, de Castro M, Baptista MT, Garmes HM, et al: Novel fibroblast growth factor receptor 1 mutations in patients with congenital hypogonadotropic hypogonadism with and without anosmia. J Clin Endocrinol Metab 2006;91:4006–4012.
4. Xu N, Qin Y, Reindollar RH, Tho SP, McDonough PG, Layman LC: A mutation in the fibroblast growth factor receptor 1 gene causes fully penetrant normosmic isolated hypogonadotropic hypogonadism. J Clin Endocrinol Metab 2007;92:1155–1158.
5. Skuse DH, James RS, Bishop DV, Coppin B, Dalton P, Aamodt-Leeper G, et al: Evidence from Turner's syndrome of an imprinted X-linked locus affecting cognitive function. Nature 1997;387:705–708.
6. Moll E, Bossuyt PM, Korevaar JC, Lambalk CB, van der Veen F: Effect of clomifene citrate plus metformin and clomifene citrate plus placebo on induction of ovulation in women with newly diagnosed polycystic ovary syndrome: randomised double-blind clinical trial. BMJ 2006;332:1485.
7. Lin L, Woodruff TK, Achermann JC: Reproductive endocrinology; in Carel JC, Hochberg Z (eds): Yearbook of Pediatric Endocrinology 2004. Basel, Karger, 2004, pp 143–156.
8. Hild SA, Marshall GR, Attardi BJ, Hess RA, Schlatt S, Simorangkir DR, et al: Development of l-CDB-4022 as a non-steroidal male oral contraceptive: induction and recovery from severe oligospermia in the adult male cynomolgus monkey (Macaca fascicularis). Endocrinology 2007;148:1784–1796.
9. Ferraz-de-Souza B, Lin L, Woodruff TK, Achermann JC: Reproductive endocrinology; in Carel JC, Hochberg Z (eds): Yearbook of Pediatric Endocrinology 2006. Basel, Karger, 2006, pp 87–101.
10. Matsumoto S, Yamazaki C, Masumoto KH, Nagano M, Naito M, Soga T, et al: Abnormal development of the olfactory bulb and reproductive system in mice lacking prokineticin receptor PKR2. Proc Natl Acad Sci USA 2006;103: 4140–4145.
11. Lin L, Woodruff TK, Achermann JC: Reproductive endocrinology; in Carel JC, Hochberg Z (eds): Yearbook of Pediatric Endocrinology 2005. Basel, Karger, 2005, pp 89–106.

Adrenals

Stefan A Wudy and Michaela F Hartmann

Steroid Research and Mass Spectrometry Unit, Division of Pediatric Endocrinology and Diabetology, Center of Child and Adolescent Medicine, Justus Liebig University, Giessen, Germany

Preface

Recent years have seen a tremendous growth in international communication. The technical means of communication have undergone a major revolution. Scholars and scientists can communicate almost instantly via phone, fax and particularly by e-mail. Some of them have already chosen to post their scientific results on their websites instead of having to wait for months and sometimes years to have them published.

One unspoken or spoken motive of all of these developments is the expectation that the new technical improvements in communication should facilitate research and should bring international discussion of important issues in one's home country. Indeed, such an undertaking as the *Yearbook of Pediatric Endocrinology* would have been hardly possible without the instruments of modern communication. Without the 'net' we authors would have never achieved retrieving and selecting specific literature as well as communicating with each other over large distances in such a small amount of time.

This year's selection directs the readers' attention to new actions of old hormones such as DHEA and its sulfate or cortisol. Furthermore, the response of the adrenals to ACTH will be a major topic. Again, amongst important enzymes to be discussed, the enzyme 11β-hydroxysteroid dehydrogenase – hope of many fighters of the global epidemic obesity – will be one of the main focuses within our chapter. More than in any other chapter before, we will learn from the steroid metabolism in animals: zebrafish, zebra finches and horses will cross our way. And last but not least, the readers will get a short update on the current role of stem cells in the prospective cure of adrenal disease.

This year's annual meeting of ESPE will be held in Helsinki, Finland's capital. In this context and in the light of the above-mentioned rapid developments of modern communication, it seems to be worthwhile remembering Tekla Hultin (1864–1943), the first female PhD in Finland who on November 11 1889 spoke on the question 'Does the growth of culture bring about happiness for humanity?'. Could she have known of the meanwhile established tradition of the *Yearbook of Pediatric Endocrinology*, I am pretty sure that she would doubtlessly have answered this question with 'yes'.

New concepts: unraveling the mechanisms of septic shock

Dissociation of serum dehydroepiandrosterone and dehydroepiandrosterone sulfate in septic shock

Arlt W, Hammer F, Sanning P, Butcher SK, Lord JM, Allolio B, Annane D, Stewart PM
Division of Medical Sciences, University of Birmingham, Institute of Biomedical Research, Birmingham, UK
w.arlt@bham.ac.uk
J Clin Endocrinol Metab 2006;91:2548–2554

Background: Dehydroepiandrosterone (DHEA) substitution in sepsis has been advocated because DHEA sulfate (DHEAS) decreases in sepsis. Experimental sepsis in rodents leads to downregulation of DHEA sulfotransferase, which inactivates DHEA to DHEAS, thus causing higher DHEA levels. This study was conducted to test whether serum DHEA and DHEAS are dissociated in septic shock.
Method: The study had a cross-sectional design with 181 patients with septic shock, 31 patients with acute trauma, and 60 healthy controls. Serum cortisol, DHEA, and DHEAS were measured before and 60 min after ACTH stimulation.

Results: Serum cortisol significantly increased and DHEAS significantly decreased in both septic shock and trauma patients. Compared with healthy controls, DHEA significantly increased in sepsis but decreased after trauma. In sepsis, neither cortisol nor DHEA increased significantly after ACTH. The cortisol to DHEA ratio was significantly increased in non-survivors of septic shock ($p = 0.026$).

Conclusion: The observed dissociation of DHEA and DHEAS in septic shock is not in accordance with the previous concept of sepsis-associated DHEA deficiency. Increased DHEA levels may maintain the balance between glucocorticoid- and DHEA-mediated immune and vascular effects. Most severe disease and mortality was found to be associated with an increased cortisol to DHEA ratio, which the authors suggest as a novel prognostic marker in septic shock.

Sepsis presents the most common cause of death in non-coronary intensive care unit patients. Adrenal insufficiency might play an important role within this context. The authors examined a large sample of septic shock patients and hypothesized that low circulating DHEAS in septic shock may not indicate true DHEA deficiency. Their results confirmed earlier findings of significantly lower serum DHEAS in septic shock patients. However, the authors found increased DHEA levels in septic patients, thus shattering the previous concept of DHEA deficiency. The upregulation of DHEA might be a sepsis-typical phenomenon which may aim at maintenance of the balance between glucocorticoid- and DHEA-mediated effects on the immune and vascular system. Furthermore, the authors suggest that the ratio cortisol/DHEA is a novel prognostic marker in septic shock, indicating an exhausted counterregulatory mechanism in the most critical patients. More studies are needed, in particular those investigating whether a combined treatment with hydrocortisone and DHEA would be superior to administration of hydrocortisone alone.

New hopes: obesity – a treatable disorder of steroid metabolism? Part I

Depot-specific modulation of rat intra-abdominal adipose tissue lipid metabolism by pharmacologic inhibition of 11β-hydroxysteroid dehydrogenase type 1

Berthiaume M, Laplante M, Festuccia W, Gelinas Y, Poulin S, Lalonde J, Joanisse DR, Thieringer R, Deshaies Y
Laval Hospital Research Center and Department of Anatomy and Physiology, Faculty of Medicine, Laval University, Quebec, QC, Canada; Division of Kinesiology, Department of Social and Preventive Medicine, Faculty of Medicine, Laval University, Quebec, QC, Canada, and Department of External Scientific Affairs, Merck Research Laboratories, Rahway, N.J., USA
Endocrinology 2007;148:2391–2397 [Epub ahead of print]

Background: The metabolic consequences of visceral obesity have been correlated with amplification of glucocorticoid action by 11β-hydroxysteroid dehydrogenase type 1 (11β-HSD1) in adipose tissue. The authors assessed in a rat model of diet-induced obesity the effects of pharmacologic 11β-HSD1 inhibition on the morphology and expression of key genes of lipid metabolism in intra-abdominal adipose depots.

Method: Rats fed a high-sucrose, high-fat diet were treated or not with a specific 11β-HSD1 inhibitor (Compound A) for 3 weeks.

Results: Compound A did not alter food intake or body weight gain, but specifically reduced mesenteric adipose weight and adipocyte size. In mesenteric fat, the inhibitor decreased mRNA levels of genes involved in lipid synthesis and fatty acid cycling, and increased the activity of the fatty acid oxidation-promoting enzyme CPT1. In striking contrast, in the epididymal depot, 11β-HSD1 inhibition increased mRNA levels of those genes related to lipid synthesis/cycling and slightly decreased CPT1 activity, whereas gene expression remained unaffected in the retroperitoneal depot.

Conclusion: The authors found that pharmacologic inhibition of 11β-HSD1, at a dose that does not alter food intake, fat accretion specifically in the mesenteric adipose depot was reduced and that divergent intra-abdominal depot-specific effects on genes of lipid metabolism were exerted reducing steatosis and lipemia.

The concept of 'a mini-Cushing's syndrome' has been suggested in the genesis of visceral obesity and metabolic syndrome [1]. Within this context the enzyme 11β-HSD1 in adipose tissue seems to play a major role amplifying glucocorticoid action. Therefore, pharmacologic inhibition of 11β-HSD1 seems to be a highly attractive therapeutic approach for the metabolic effects of visceral obesity. This study assesses the effects of a 3-week course of pharmacological inhibition of this key enzyme of cortisol metabolism on intra-abdominal adipose depot distribution as well as on the metabolic profile of rats. The authors found reduced fat accretion, decreased lipogenic gene expression, and increased oxidative enzyme activity in the mesenteric fat depot. This study in rats suggests pharmacologic 11β-HSD1 inhibition an attractive approach in metabolic syndrome. However, we need more studies with respect to correct dosage as well as duration of such therapeutic agents. In particular, proper caution should be exerted because these drugs might also affect the brain and the central regulation of energy balance!

The adrenocorticotropin stimulation test: contribution of a physiologically based model developed in horse for its interpretation in different pathophysiological situations encountered in man

Bousquet-Melou A, Formentini E, Picard-Hagen N, Delage L, Laroute V, Toutain PL
Unité Mixte de Recherche 181 de Physiopathologie et Toxicologie Expérimentales, Institut National de la Recherche Agronomique et Ecole Nationale Vétérinaire de Toulouse, Ecole Nationale Vétérinaire de Toulouse, Toulouse, France
a.bousquet-melou@envt.fr
Endocrinology 2006;147:4281–4291

Background: The authors characterized the adrenal response to ACTH in horses. They developed a model coupling the non-linear disposition of cortisol with a physiologically based model for cortisol secretion by the adrenals. They assumed that the response to ACTH resulted from two mechanisms: a stimulation of the cortisol secretion rate and control of the duration of the secretion.

Method: Seven doses of ACTH were tested in horses, a species similar to man with respect to adrenal function.

Results: The main finding was that the secretion rate of the adrenal gland could be described by a zero-order process that was maximal for a relatively low dose of ACTH (0.1 μg/kg). At higher doses, the increasing adrenal gland response was only due to the prolongation of the time of its secretion.

Conclusion: The authors were able to reproduce and explain many adrenal gland responses that were dimmed by the different non-linearities of the system.

Did you know that horses are similar to humans? At least when it comes to comparing adrenal function this seems to be true. I do not know whether horses like maths, but the inclined reader of this paper should not be repelled by mathematical models. For all those not indulging in mathematical formulas since school any more, the essentials of this remarkable paper are that ACTH tests seem to be only able to explore concentration-dependent mechanisms of the adrenal response at very low ACTH doses. As soon as the dose exceeds 0.1 μg/kg, the response reflects different time-dependent mechanisms. These results are in agreement with the fact that the adrenal glands do not accumulate a pool of releasable cortisol but instead only increase cortisol synthesis. I still suggest to carry out experiments transferring these findings to the human being and then to draw consequences for reasonable ACTH testing.

Mechanisms of disease: the adrenocorticotropin receptor and disease

Clark AJ, Metherell LA
Centre for Endocrinology, William Harvey Research Institute at Barts, London, UK
a.j.clark@qmul.ac.uk
Nat Clin Pract Endocrinol Metab 2006;2:282–290

Background: The action of ACTH to stimulate glucocorticoid production by the adrenals is an essential physiologic process. It depends on a single unique genetic component – the ACTH receptor or melanocortin-2 receptor. Genetic defects causing abnormalities in this receptor or in a protein required for its expression at the cell surface result in a potentially fatal disease (familial glucocorticoid deficiency). Overexpression of this receptor or inability to desensitize it can be seen in adrenal adenomas or hyperplasia associated with glucocorticoid overproduction (Cushing syndrome). Regarding depressive illness and septic shock, the origin of these latter disturbances is undoubtedly complex and multifactorial, but there is strong evidence that a component of this phenomenon is an altered responsiveness of the ACTH receptor to ACTH.

Please consider that (1) ACTH plays a key role in mediating the stress response, (2) inactivating mutations in the ACTH receptor cause the inherited syndrome of ACTH insensitivity, (3) benign and malignant adrenal neoplasms often bear disturbances of ACTH receptor expression, and (4) in common disorders such as depression or septic shock an altered responsiveness to ACTH is often present. This excellent review does not deserve to be further commented, no – to read this article is a must for every serious endocrinologist.

Cortisol stimulates cell cycle activity in the cardiomyocyte of the sheep fetus

Giraud GD, Louey S, Jonker S, Schultz J, Thornburg KL
Heart Research Center, Oregon Health and Science University, Portland, Oreg., USA
Endocrinology 2006;147:3643–3649

Background: The authors hypothesized that cortisol would suppress cardiomyocyte proliferation and stimulate cardiomyocyte binucleation and enlargement, which are signs of terminal differentiation.
Method: Cardiomyocyte dimensions and percent binucleation were determined in isolated cardiac myocytes from 7 cortisol-treated and 7 control fetuses. Cortisol was infused into the circumflex coronary artery at subpressor rates.
Results: Cortisol infusion had no hemodynamic effects. It increased heart weight significantly. Heart to body weight ratio was greater in treated hearts. Ventricular myocyte length, width, and percent binucleation were not different between groups.
Conclusion: Increases in fetal heart mass associated with subpressor doses of cortisol are due to cardiomyocyte proliferation and not hypertrophic growth.

The authors present a somewhat unexpected and exciting finding that cortisol acts as a growth hormone in the ovine fetal heart, stimulating cardiac myocyte hyperplasia and not maturation. On the one hand, this paper presents a valuable contribution to understand the role of corticosteroids in cardiomyocyte maturation. On the other hand, this observation raises at least two major issues. First, it is still unknown by which receptor these effects are mediated. Second, we have to investigate more intensively possible implications for premature human neonates receiving exogenous glucocorticoids before birth! [2]

In humans, early cortisol biosynthesis provides a mechanism to safeguard female sexual development

Goto M, Piper Hanley K, Marcos J, Wood PJ, Wright S, Postle AD, Cameron IT, Mason JI, Wilson DI, Hanley NA
Human Genetics Division and Early Human Development and Stem Cells Group, University of Southampton, Southampton, UK
J Clin Invest 2006;116:953–960

Background: Differentiation of the human external genitalia is established at 7–12 weeks post-conception. During this period, maintaining the appropriate intrauterine hormone environment is critical. This regulation extends to the human fetal adrenal cortex, as evidenced by the virilization that is associated with various forms of congenital adrenal hyperplasia. The mechanism underlying these clinical findings has remained unknown.
Method: The authors investigated the expression of the orphan nuclear receptor nerve growth factor IB-like (NGFI-B) and its regulatory target, the steroidogenic enzyme 3β-hydroxysteroid dehydrogenase type 2 (HSD3B2).
Results: Cortisol biosynthesis was maximal at 8–9 weeks post-conception under the regulation of ACTH. Negative feedback was apparent at the anterior pituitary corticotrophs. ACTH also stimulated the adrenal gland to secrete androstenedione and testosterone.
Conclusion: These data show a distinctive mechanism for normal human development whereby cortisol production, determined by transient NGFI-B and HSD3B2 expression, provides feedback at the anterior pituitary to modulate androgen biosynthesis and safeguard normal female sexual differentiation.

This is a very interesting contribution to understand the role of the fetal adrenal cortex and its capacity of cortisol and androgen biosynthesis during the first trimester of human development. The authors suggest a delicate balance during early female differentiation which is vulnerable to androgen before the protective appearance of placental aromatase. A transient expression of adrenocortical nerve growth factor IB-like inducing 3β-hydroxysteroid dehydrogenase type 2 would cause early cortisol biosynthesis and thus inhibit ACTH production by the anterior pituitary. This would minimize ACTH-induced androgen secretion and thus cause a transient mechanism safeguarding the most sensitive period of female sexual development. To conclude, becoming a female seems by no means to be as passive a process than has previously been thought.

Dehydroepiandrosterone is an anabolic steroid like dihydrotestosterone, the most potent natural androgen, and tetrahydrogestrinone

Labrie F, Luu-The V, Martel C, Chernomoretz A, Calvo E, Morissette J, Labrie C
Molecular Endocrinology and Oncology Laboratory, Laval University Hospital Research Center (CRCHUL) and Laval University, Quebec City, Que., Canada
fernand.labrie@crchul.ulaval.ca
J Steroid Biochem Mol Biol 2006;100:52–58

Background: In 2004, the US Controlled Substances Act was modified to include androstenedione (4-dione) as an anabolic steroid. However, despite the common knowledge that dehydroepiandrosterone (DHEA) is the precursor of testosterone, DHEA was excluded from the list of anabolic steroids.
Method: The authors used DNA microarray technology to analyze the expression profile of practically all the 30,000 genes of the mouse genome modulated by DHEA and dihydrotestosterone (DHT) in classical androgen-sensitive tissues.
Results: Daily subcutaneous injections of DHT or DHEA for 1 month in gonadectomized mice increased ventral prostate, dorsal prostate, seminal vesicle and preputial gland weight. As early as 24 h after a single

injection of the two steroids, 878, 2,681 and 14 probe sets were commonly stimulated or inhibited in the prostate, seminal vesicles and preputial glands, respectively, compared to tissues from gonadectomized control animals.

Conclusion: The present microarray data show proof of the androgenic/anabolic activity of DHEA. The data reveal that DHEA is transformed into androgens in the human peripheral tissues as well as in laboratory animal species exerting potent androgenic/anabolic activity.

DHEA [3] has so far not been listed by the World Anti-Doping Agency as an anabolic steroid. In many countries the substance is regarded as an anti-aging drug and is available over the counter. Using gene expression profiling, the authors have convincingly shown that DHEA is an anabolic steroid like DHT. Another interesting aspect of this paper is that of 'intracrinology'. While ovaries and testes are the exclusive sources of androgens and estrogens in lower mammals, in man and higher primates, sex steroids are largely synthesized locally in peripheral tissues. DHEA, at physiological concentrations, induces high levels of intraprostatic DHT resulting in marked stimulation of ventral prostate weight and increased expression of androgen-sensitive genes. Therefore the question arises whether the measurement of serum androgens reliably reflects biological and clinical phenomena!

New mechanisms: singing – a function of steroids?
Music lessons by the zebra finch

Widespread capacity for steroid synthesis in the avian brain and song system

London SE, Monks DA, Wade J, Schlinger BA
University of California, Los Angeles, Los Angeles, Calif., USA
slondon@igb.uiuc.edu
Endocrinology 2006;147:5975–5987

Background: The zebra finch song system presents a sensorimotor neural circuit sensitive to steroids throughout life. It organizes and functions largely independent of gonadally derived steroids.

Method and Results: The authors demonstrated that the steroidogenic acute regulatory protein (StAR), cytochrome P_{450} side-chain cleavage (CYP11A1), and 3β-hydroxysteroid dehydrogenase/Δ5-Δ4 isomerase are expressed in both developing and adult zebra finch brain.

Conclusion: The data suggest neurosteroids may modulate multiple brain functions, including sensory and motor systems. Notably, whereas expression of other steroidogenic genes such as aromatase has been essentially absent from the song system, each of the major song nuclei express at least a subset of steroidogenic genes described here, establishing the song system as a potential steroidogenic circuit.

The zebra finch song system is steroid-sensitive at all ages, but its incomplete dependence on gonadally derived steroids suggests that the brain may provide steroids essential to its organization and function. Thus, neurosteroidogenesis may broaden the role of steroids in the brain [4]. By uncoupling the synthesis of sex steroids from gonads, the role of sex steroids may be expanded in the brains beyond those primarily useful for reproductive behaviors. From the example of the zebra finch, we learn that neurosteroidogenesis may be a crucial factor by which the brain regulates sensory and motor functions.

Gender development in women with congenital adrenal hyperplasia as a function of disorder severity

Meyer-Bahlburg HF, Dolezal C, Baker SW, Ehrhardt AA, New MI
NYS Psychiatric Institute/Department of Psychiatry, Columbia University, NYSPI Unit 15, New York, N.Y., USA
meyerb@childpsych.columbia.edu
Arch Sex Behav 2006;35:667–684

Background: Prenatal-onset CAH in 46,XX individuals is associated with variable masculinization/defeminization of the genitalia and of behavior. This is presumably both due to excess prenatal androgen production. The purpose of this study was (1) to extend the gender-behavioral investigation to the mildest subtype of 46,XX CAH, the non-classical variant, (2) to replicate previous findings on moderate and severe variants of 46,XX CAH using a battery of diversely constructed assessment instruments, and (3) to evaluate the utility of the chosen assessment instruments for this area of work.
Method: 63 women with classical CAH were studied (42 had salt wasting and 21 were simple virilizers), 82 women had the non-classical type, and 24 related non-CAH sisters and female cousins served as controls.
Results: Non-classical women showed a few signs of gender shifts in the expected direction, simple virilizing women were intermediate, and salt wasting women were found to be most severely affected. Regarding gender identity, two salt wasting women were gender-dysphoric, and a third had changed to male in adulthood. All others identified as women.
Conclusion: Behavioral masculinization/defeminization was pronounced in salt wasting-CAH women, slight but still clearly present in simple virilizing women, and probable, but still in need of replication in non-classical women.

The clinical spectrum of patients with 21-hydroxylase deficiency extends from the mildest 'non-classical' forms to the severer classical forms (simple virilizers, salt wasters). This study for the first time investigates gender outcome in a relatively large sample of women with non-classical 21-hydroxylase deficiency in comparison to the classical forms of 21-hydroxylase deficiency and normal controls. Behavioral masculinization/defeminization correlated with the severity of 21-hydroxylase deficiency: it was pronounced in women with a salt wasting form, slight but clearly demonstrable in simple virilizing women, but questionable in non-classical women. This study is a valuable contribution to a neglected field of research. However, the assessment instruments in this study clearly had their limitations: they were not well suited as measures of discrete behaviors that could be compared to those behavioral units used by animal researches in the investigation of hormone-, dose-, and timing-specific hormone behavior relationships. The authors furthermore point out further hindrances of such a study such as a relatively small sample size, high rates of non-participation and a cross-sectional design. This reviewer wonders whether a further study could be conducted on an ESPE-wide basis?

Mechanism of StAR's regulation of mitochondrial cholesterol import

Miller WL
Department of Pediatrics, University of California, San Francisco, Calif., USA
Mol Cell Endocrinol 2007;265–266:46–50

The steroidogenic acute regulatory protein (StAR) regulates the acute steroidogenic response by moving cholesterol from the outer to inner mitochondrial membrane. However, the mechanism of StAR's action has remained enigmatic. The authors showed that StAR acts on the outer membrane, needs cholesterol binding, and requires the structural change previously described as a pH-dependent molten globule.

The current concept is that StAR's interaction with protonated phospholipid head groups on the outer mitochondrial membrane leads to a molten globule transition needed for StAR to take up cholesterol. A functional interaction between StAR and the peripheral benzodiazepine receptor is suggested. Whereas many models have revealed that StAR delivers cholesterol to peripheral benzodiazepine receptor, the authors suggest that StAR removes cholesterol from the cholesterol-binding domain of peripheral benzodiazepine receptor and delivers it to the inner mitochondrial membrane.

This excellent review is not only for all of those indulging in endocrine mechanisms! It should be a pleasure for all real endocrinologists to read this excellent update on the molecular mechanisms concerning steroidogenic acute regulatory protein (StAR). May the authors remind our readers of last year's *Yearbook of Pediatric Endocrinology*, where we have already dwelled on this highly interesting 'two-hit' disease [5]?

Important for clinical practice: pheochromocytoma update

Pheochromocytoma: recommendations for clinical practice from the First International Symposium

Pacak K, Eisenhofer G, Ahlman H, Bornstein SR, Gimenez-Roqueplo AP, Grossman AB, Kimura N, Mannelli M, McNicol AM, Tischler AS
National Institute of Child Health and Development, NIH, Bethesda, Md., USA
Nat Clin Pract Endocrinol Metab 2007;3:92–102

The First International Symposium on Pheochromocytoma was held in October 2005. Recommendations were made concerning biochemical diagnosis, localization, genetics, and treatment. Measurement of plasma or urinary fractionated metanephrines, the most accurate screening approach, was recommended as the first-line test for diagnosis. Localization studies should only follow reasonable clinical evidence of a tumor. Preoperative pharmacologic blockade of circulatory responses to catecholamines is mandatory. Mutation testing should be considered; however, it is not currently cost-effective to test every gene in every patient. Inadequate methods to distinguish malignant from benign tumors and a lack of effective treatments for malignancy are important problems requiring further studies.

This article reminds us of the fact that the adrenals are not exclusively composed of steroidogenic tissue. The paper is devoted to the adrenal medulla and summarizes the latest recommendations of the First International Symposium on Pheochromocytoma held in 2005. It is an excellent clinical help regarding the latest updates on diagnosis, localization, genetics and treatment of pheochromocytomas – a 'must' for the clinical endocrinologist's library!

Food for thought: diabetes – a disease not only affecting insulin!

Exaggerated adrenarche and altered cortisol metabolism in type 1 diabetic children

Remer T, Maser-Gluth C, Boye KR, Hartmann MF, Heinze E, Wudy SA
Department of Nutrition and Health, Research Institute of Child Nutrition, Dortmund, Germany
remer@fke-do.de
Steroids 2006;71:591–598

Background: A few data from the literature suggest altered steroid metabolism in type 1 diabetes. The aim of this study was to test the hypothesis that adrenarche is affected under conventional intensive insulin therapy.

Method: In 24-hour urine samples of 109 patients aged 4–18 years with type 1 diabetes of more than 1 year, steroids were profiled using gas chromatography-mass spectrometry. Additionally, urinary free cortisol and cortisone were quantified by RIA after extraction and chromatographic purification. Data on urinary steroids from 400 healthy controls served as reference values. Enzyme activities were assessed by established steroid metabolite ratios, e.g. 5α-reductase and 11β-hydroxysteroid dehydrogenase type 2 (11β-HSD2) by 5α-tetrahydrocortisol/tetrahydrocortisol and urinary free cortisol/cortisone, respectively. Urinary markers of adrenarche, especially dehydroepiandrosterone and its direct metabolites, were elevated in patients, as were urinary 6β-hydroxycortisol, urinary free cortisol, and 11β-HSD2 activity.

Results: Overall cortisol secretion, reflected by the sum of major urinary cortisol metabolites, was mostly normal and activity of 5α-reductase clearly reduced.

Conclusion: The authors found evidence for an exaggerated adrenarche in type 1 diabetes children, which may account for hyperandrogenic symptoms in diabetic females. Furthermore, a reduced cortisol inactivation via 5α-reductase that was not compensated by a fall in cortisol secretion was found.

This paper draws our attention on the consequences of chronic hyperglycemia on steroid metabolism, a topic rarely touched upon. The authors provide evidence for a potentially clinically relevant alteration in cortisol metabolism with a markedly increased 11β-HSD2 activity and an exaggerated adrenarche [6] in type 1 diabetic children and adolescents. Obviously, insulin can increase the metabolic clearance of DHEA and its sulfate while DHEA-S secretion is likely to be increased. Elevated excretion rates of 6β-hydroxylcortisol and cortisone might point to a mild form of hypercortisolism and to a potential role of steroids in the induction of insulin resistance.

New mechanisms: development of pituitary-interrenal interaction – lessons from the zebrafish

Pituitary-interrenal interaction in zebrafish interrenal organ development

To TT, Hahner S, Nica G, Rohr KB, Hammerschmidt M, Winkler C, Allolio B
Endocrinology and Diabetes Unit, Department of Medicine, University of Wuerzburg, Wuerzburg, Germany
Allolio_b@medizin.uni-wuerzburg.de
Mol Endocrinol 2007;21:472–485

Background: The authors elucidated pituitary adrenal interactions during development by studying the organogenesis of the interrenal organ, which is the teleost homolog of the mammalian adrenal gland in zebrafish.

Method: Wild-type zebrafish interrenal development was compared with that of mutants lacking pituitary cell types including corticotrophs.

Results: Until 2 days post-fertilization (2 dpf), interrenal development assessed by transcripts of key steroidogenic genes (cyp11a1, mc2r, star) was found to be independent of proopiomelanocortin. However, at 5 dpf, lack of pituitary cells leads to reduced expression of steroidogenic genes at both the transcriptional and the protein level.

Conclusion: The authors demonstrated a gradual transition from early pituitary-independent interrenal organogenesis to developmental control by the anterior domain of pituitary corticotrophs acting via Mc2 receptors.

The inclined reader will again note the importance of animal models in steroid research. It actually seems that this year's selection of papers is more or less devoted to animals helping to understand steroid metabolism and its regulation. While the zebra finch has nicely demonstrated the importance of – gonadally indifferent – neurosteroids, the zebrafish interrenal glands seem to be a suitable model for studying adrenal development. Indeed the authors demonstrate that interrenal development in the zebrafish shares many conserved molecular and developmental mechanisms with higher vertebrates, in particular when it comes to studying transcription factors involved in adrenal development. In this paper we learn that it is the Mc2 receptor which after an early phase of pituitary independent development and steroidogenic enzyme activity is needed for further functional differentiation of the interrenal organ.

Inhibition of 11β-HSD1 activity in vivo limits glucocorticoid exposure to human adipose tissue and decreases lipolysis

Tomlinson JW, Sherlock M, Hughes B, Hughes SV, Kilvington F, Bartlett W, Courtney R, Rejto P, Carley W, Stewart PM
Division of Medical Sciences, Institute of Biomedical Research, University of Birmingham, Queen Elizabeth Hospital, Edgbaston, Birmingham, UK; Department of Clinical Chemistry and Immunology, Heart of England NHS Foundation Trust, Birmingham, UK, and Pfizer Global R&D, La Jolla Laboratories, San Diego, Calif., USA
J Clin Endocrinol Metab 2007;92:857–864

Background: The authors aimed at comparing markers of 11β-HSD1 activity and demonstrating that inhibition of 11β-HSD1 activity limits glucocorticoid availability to adipose tissue.
Methods: Seven healthy male volunteers participated in this clinical study. Carbenoxolone was used in a single dose (100 mg) and the probands received 72 h of continuous treatment (300 mg/day). Inhibition of 11β-HSD1 was examined using five different mechanistic biomarkers (serum cortisol and prednisolone generation, urinary corticosteroid metabolite analysis by gas chromatography/mass spectrometry, and adipose tissue microdialysis examining cortisol generation and glucocorticoid-mediated glycerol release).
Results: Each biomarker demonstrated reduced 11β-HSD1 activity after CBX administration.
Conclusion: Carbenoxolone is able to inhibit rapidly the generation of active GC in human adipose tissue. Limiting glucocorticoid availability in vivo has functional consequences including decreased glycerol release.

Carbenoxolone – a derivative of glycyrrhetinic acid, the active principal of licorice – is an inhibitor of 11β-hydroxysteroid dehydrogenase type 1 and type 2. Clinical studies in patients with type 2 diabetes have shown improvement of insulin sensitivity and decreased glucose production rates. In this paper the authors show in healthy adult males that carbenoxolone is able to access adipose tissue and to inhibit the generation of bioactive cortisol and prednisolone through inhibition of 11β-hydroxysteroid dehydrogenase type 1. This observation has important implications for selective inhibition of 11β-hydroxysteroid dehydrogenase type 1 as a therapeutic strategy in humans. However, carbenoxolone is not a selective inhibitor of both type 1 and type 2 11β-hydroxysteroid dehydrogenases and therefore bears the risk of inducing apparent mineralocorticoid excess, as all chronic users of licorice will know. Consequently, this substance will not be suited as a future therapeutic drug.

Differentiation of adult stem cells derived from bone marrow stroma into Leydig or adrenocortical cells

Yazawa T, Mizutani T, Yamada K, Kawata H, Sekiguchi T, Yoshino M, Kajitani T, Shou Z, Umezawa A, Miyamoto K
Department of Biochemistry, Faculty of Medical Sciences, University of Fukui, Fukui, Japan
Endocrinology 2006;147:4104–4111

Background: The authors investigated whether MSCs from rat, mouse, and human are able to differentiate into steroidogenic cells.
Method and Results: It was found that when transplanted into immature rat testes, adherent marrow-derived cells were found to be engrafted and differentiated into steroidogenic cells that were indistinguishable from Leydig cells. Isolated murine marrow-derived cells transfected with green fluorescence protein driven by the promoter of P_{450} side-chain cleaving enzyme gene (CYP11A), a steroidogenic cell-specific gene, were used to examine steroidogenic cell production in vitro. During in vitro differentiation, green fluorescence protein-positive cells similar to Leydig cells, were found. Stable transfection of murine marrow-derived cells with a transcription factor, steroidogenic factor-1, followed by treatment with cAMP almost recapitulated the properties of Leydig cells. Transfection of human marrow-derived cells

with steroidogenic factor-1 also led to their conversion to steroidogenic cells, but they appeared to be glucocorticoid rather than testosterone-producing cells.

Conclusion: These results indicate that marrow-derived cells represent a useful source of stem cells for producing steroidogenic cells that may provide basis for their use in cell and gene therapy.

Stem cells are self-renewing elements. They have the capacity to generate multiple distinct cell lineages. Even in adults they exist in various tissues and have been isolated from a variety of differentiated tissues such as bone marrow, umbilical blood, brain and fat, while bone marrow-derived mesenchymal stem cells have been shown to differentiate into adipocytes chondrocytes and osteoblasts both in vivo and ex vivo. The authors in this paper show that rodent mesenchymal stem cells have the potential to differentiate into steroidogenic cells in vivo and in vitro. Thus, mesenchymal stem cells represent a powerful tool not only for studying the differentiation of the steroidogenic lineage but also for future therapeutic approaches concerning steroidogenic organs. Let's look forward to the future!

Closing remark

Of course, phone, fax and e-mail have tremendously helped in writing another yearbook chapter. But do we only profit from these developments in communication or is there a slight danger that one day there will be no more 'real' ESPE meetings but only 'virtual' ESPE conferences? Indeed the unresolved question seems to be whether technical means can serve the same function as face-to-face personal interaction? Therefore we will have to show – more than ever before – that personal relationships and personal contacts within ESPE are of continued importance. Let's all look forward to meeting personally in Helsinki again!

It has now been for 4 years that these 'first-generation' authors (S.A.W. and M.H.) have had the privilege of compiling the Adrenals' chapter in the *Yearbook of Pediatric Endocrinology*. Despite this huge workload, the authors have always enjoyed this task because it permitted them the opportunity to get an excellent overview over current research and developments in the field of steroidology. We hope that our readers have enjoyed and profited from the selections as well. To maintain a balance in selecting and commenting the literature it is now time for a change, and we wish our successors all the best with this highly challenging and interesting task.

References
1. Wolf G: Glucocorticoids in adipocytes stimulate visceral obesity. Nutr Rev 2002;60:148–151.
2. Newnham JP: Is prenatal glucocorticoid administration another origin of adult disease? Clin Exp Pharmacol Physiol 2001;28:957–961.
3. Labrie F, Luu-The V, Belanger A, Lin SX, Simard J, Labrie C: Is DHEA a hormone? Starling review. J Endocrinol 2005;187:169–196.
4. Mellon SH, Griffin LD: Neurosteroids: biochemistry and clinical significance. Trends Endocrinol Metab 2002;13:35–43.
5. Wudy SA, Hartmann MF: Adrenals; in Carel JC, Hochberg Z (eds): Yearbook of Pediatric Endocrinology 2006. Basel, Karger, 2006, pp 103–115.
6. Remer T, Boye KR, Hartmann MF, Wudy SA: Urinary markers of adrenarche: reference values in healthy subjects aged 3–18 years. J Clin Endocrinol Metab 2005;90:2015–2021.

Type 1 Diabetes

Francesco Chiarelli and Cosimo Giannini

Department of Pediatrics, University of Chieti, Chieti, Italy

It is well known that type 1 diabetes is a chronic autoimmune disease in which the breakdown of normal tolerance to the β cell allows the activation of T cell to multiple antigens. This induces a progressive destruction of β cells and a state of chronic insulin deficiency. Multiple genetic and environmental risk factors have been evaluated for better understanding the mechanisms causing type 1 diabetes with the aim of improving prediction and possibly prevention of β cell impairment and failure. Meanwhile, it remains of paramount importance to reach the best metabolic and glycemic control from the very beginning of diabetes in children and adolescents; new technologies have improved the day-to-day diabetes care and there is hope that a closed-loop device will allow a more physiological insulin delivery. There is also hope for finding a cure for diabetes by teaching stem cells to produce insulin, by implementing β cell and pancreas transplantation and by applying gene therapy.

Mechanism of the year

Kv1.3 channels are a therapeutic target for T-cell-mediated autoimmune diseases

Beeton C, Wulff H, Standifer NE, Azam P, Mullen KM, Pennington MW, Kolski-Andreaco A, Wei E, Grino A, Counts DR, Wang PH, LeeHealey CJ, Andrews BS, Sankaranarayanan A, Homerick D, Roeck WW, Tehranzadeh J, Stanhope KL, Zimin P, Havel PJ, Griffey S, Knaus HG, Nepom GT, Gutman GA, Calabresi PA, Chandy KG
Department of Physiology and Biophysics, University of California, Irvine, Calif., USA
gchandy@uci.edu
Proc Natl Acad Sci USA 2006;103:17414–17419

Background: Autoreactive memory T lymphocytes are implicated in the pathogenesis of autoimmune diseases.

Methods and Results: Here the authors demonstrate that disease-associated autoreactive T cells from patients with type 1 diabetes mellitus or rheumatoid arthritis are mainly CD4+ CCR7-CD45RA-effector memory T cells with elevated Kv1.3 potassium channel expression. In contrast, T cells with other antigen specificities from these patients, or autoreactive T cells from healthy individuals and disease controls, express low levels of Kv1.3 and are predominantly naive or central-memory cells. In effector memory T cells, Kv1.3 traffics to the immunological synapse during antigen presentation where it colocalizes with Kvβ2, SAP97, ZIP, p56(lck), and CD4. Although Kv1.3 inhibitors do not prevent immunological synapse formation, they suppress CA^{2+} signaling, cytokine production, and proliferation of autoantigen-specific effector memory T cells at pharmacologically relevant concentrations while sparing other classes of T cells. Kv1.3 inhibitors ameliorate pristane-induced arthritis in rats and reduce the incidence of experimental autoimmune diabetes in diabetes-prone BB rats. Repeated dosing with Kv1.3 inhibitors in rats has not revealed systemic toxicity.

Conclusions: Further development of Kv1.3 blockers for autoimmune disease therapy is warranted.

Type 1 diabetes is an autoimmune disease characterized by a permissive immune system that fails to impose tolerance to arrays of self-antigens [1]. Therefore, disease-modifying immunotherapies capable of selectively suppressing autoantigens reaction are under investigation. Because the disease-associated autoreactive T cells are mainly costimulation-independent by CCR7-effector memory T cells, immunomodulators able to selectively suppress effector memory T cells without affecting other lymphoid subsets would be relevant [2]. This study evaluated disease-associated autoreactive T cells from patients with type 1 diabetes or rheumatoid arthritis and tested whether a selective blockers of Kv1.3 (a homotetrameric human K^+ channel which regulates membrane potential and Ca^{2+} signalling in human T cells, overexpressed in activated CD4+ and CD8+ effector memory T/effector memory$_{CD45RA+}$ T cells) could reduce autoimmune-mediated disease in rat models of type 1 diabetes or rheumatoid arthritis, without causing toxicity. It was shown that disease-associated autoreactive T cells in type 1 diabetes, multiple sclerosis and rheumatoid arthritis are mainly CCR7-Kv1.3^{high} effector memory T cells. Furthermore, utilizing a selective Kv1.3 blocker to discern whether effector memory T-cell function can be preferentially suppressed without impacting naive/T central memory cells in rheumatoid arthritis and type 1 diabetes patients, it was observed that Kv1.3 blockers might globally suppress effector memory T/effector memory$_{CD45RA+}$ T cells and compromise the ability to respond to pathogens. Nonetheless, conducting a prevention trial of PAP1 (a small-molecule Kv1.3 inhibitor) in BB rats (a standard model for type 1 diabetes), it was also demonstrated that Kv1.3 inhibitors reduce the incidence of autoimmune diabetes without relevant side effects. These encouraging data provide a rationale for evaluating Kv1.3 inhibitors as a therapy for type 1 diabetes and for preventing autoimmune destruction of HLA-matched grafted islets. Highly selective immune system modulation represents an innovating and promising therapeutic opportunity which would be ideal in prevention of type 1 diabetes.

New paradigms

Intrahepatic transplanted islets in humans secrete insulin in a coordinate pulsatile manner directly into the liver

Meier JJ, Hong-McAtee I, Galasso R, Veldhuis JD, Moran A, Hering BJ, Butler PC
Larry Hillblom Islet Research Center, University of California, Los Angeles David Geffen School of Medicine, Los Angeles, Calif., USA
pbutler@mednet.ucla.edu
Diabetes 2006;55:2324–2332

Background: Intrahepatic islet transplantation is an experimental therapy for type 1 diabetes.
Methods: In the present studies, the authors sought to address the following questions: (1) in humans, do intrahepatic transplanted islets re-establish coordinated pulsatile insulin secretion? and (2) to what extent is insulin secreted by intrahepatic transplanted islets delivered to the hepatic sinusoids (therefore effectively restoring a portal mode of insulin delivery) versus delivered to the hepatic central vein (therefore effectively providing a systemic form of insulin delivery)? To address the first question, the authors examined insulin concentration profiles in the overnight fasting state and during a hyperglycemic clamp (ca. 150 mg/dl) in 10 recipients of islet transplants and 10 control subjects. To address the second question, the authors measured first-pass hepatic insulin clearance in two recipients of islet autografts after pancreatectomy for pancreatitis versus 5 control subjects by direct catheterization of the hepatic vein.
Results: The authors report that coordinate pulsatile insulin secretion is re-established in islet transplant recipients and that glucose-mediated stimulation of insulin secretion is accomplished by amplification of insulin pulse mass. Direct hepatic catheterization studies revealed that intrahepatic islets in humans do deliver insulin directly to the hepatic sinusoid because approximately 80% of the insulin is extracted during first pass.
Conclusions: In conclusion, intrahepatic islet transplantation effectively restores the liver to pulsatile insulin delivery.

β-Cell replacement is an attractive potential treatment in order to mimic as close as possible the insulin variation in all physiological and pathological conditions and to avoid any disadvantage related to insulin replacement. Performed in conjunction with kidney transplants or as solitary grafts, β-cell transplantation can be either a whole organ pancreas transplant or an islet cell transplant [3]. However, due to the related surgical morbidities and long-term mortality, islet cell transplantation represents a suitable procedure which offers several advantages. In particular, by secreting insulin directly into the portal-venous circulation to the liver, intrahepatic transplanted cells might reproduce the physiological variations of insulin secretion. In general, whole organ transplants have a more sustained and durable function and are more widely available than their counterparts, but entail a much more invasive procedure. In this study, 10 patients with type 1 diabetes were studied after islet transplantation in order to evaluate whether intrahepatic transplanted islets in humans may serve as a reliable pacemaker for pulsatile insulin secretion in a coordinated pulsatile manner. Thus, pulsatile insulin secretion, determined by deconvolution analysis of 1-minute insulin concentrations, was measured in the basal fasting state and during a hyperglycemic clamp followed by an acute intravenous arginine (5 g) bolus. It was shown that insulin secretion in islet transplant recipients is pulsatile and glucose-induced insulin secretion is accomplished through amplification of pulse size. Furthermore, by studying insulin concentrations in samples obtained simultaneously from the hepatic vein and the arterialized hand vein in 1-minute intervals over 40 min, it was shown a similar hepatic first-pass insulin extraction in intraportal islet autotransplanted patients compared with healthy control subjects. These results imply a direct insulin delivery into hepatic sinusoids rather than into the hepatic central vein. This appears to be an interesting approach which should re-establish a pulsatile pattern of insulin release in patients with type 1 diabetes through intraportal islet transplantation which is able mimic both the physiological 80% first passage insulin clearance and the balance between hepatic and extrahepatic insulin exposure. However, no long-term related effect can be drawn by this study in order to evaluate the lifelong efficacy of the intraportal islet transplantation. Although promising, the surgical- and method-related consequences such as thrombosis, bleeding, and exposure of the islets to high gut-derived environmental toxins and immunosuppressive drugs used to prevent rejection, reduce drastically the utility of this procedure in the short-term. However, the well-reproduced physiological route of intraportal insulin delivery stimulates further studies as well as new pharmacological approaches in this field.

New hope

Production of pancreatic hormone-expressing endocrine cells from human embryonic stem cells

D'Amour KA, Bang AG, Eliazer S, Kelly OG, Agulnick AD, Smart NG, Moorman MA, Kroon E, Carpenter MK, Baetge EE
Novocell Inc., San Diego, Calif., USA
gage@salk.edu
Nat Biotechnol 2006;24:1392–1401

Background: Of paramount importance for the development of cell therapies to treat diabetes is the production of sufficient numbers of pancreatic endocrine cells that function similarly to primary islets.
Methods and Results: the authors have developed a differentiation process that converts human embryonic stem cells to endocrine cells capable of synthesizing the pancreatic hormones insulin, glucagon, somatostatin, pancreatic polypeptide and ghrelin. This process mimics in vivo pancreatic organogenesis by directing cells through stages resembling definitive endoderm, gut-tube endoderm, pancreatic endoderm and endocrine precursor – en route to cells that express endocrine hormones. The human embryonic stem cell-derived insulin-expressing cells have an insulin content approaching that of adult islets. Similar to fetal β cells, they release C-peptide in response to multiple secretory stimuli, but only minimally to glucose.
Conclusions: Production of these human embryonic stem cell-derived endocrine cells may represent a critical step in the development of a renewable source of cells for diabetes cell therapy.

During the gastrulation stage of embryogenesis the definitive endoderm germ layer, which is generated in an area termed the primitive streak, progressively proliferates and differentiates into different gastrointestinal cells including the endocrine pancreatic cells. A complex and strict step-by-step activation of several transcription factor genes and signals from the adjacent growing tissue are necessary to allow a complete and precise production of the different insular cells [4]. The unlimited replicative capacity and the ability to produce most, if not all, differentiated cell types allow to retain the human embryonic stem cells, a potential and interesting approach in type 1 diabetes [5]. In this study characterizing the differentiation process at the RNA and protein levels using real-time PCR,

Western blotting, immunofluorescence and flow cytometry, it was shown that definitive endoderm derived from human embryonic stem cells can be efficiently differentiated to hormone-expressing endocrine cells. The authors reproduced a five-stage protocol for differentiating human embryonic stem cells to endocrine hormone-expressing cells through a series of endodermal intermediates resembling those that occur during pancreatic development in vivo. Furthermore, insulin content of the insulin-expressing cells approached that of adult islets. In addition, C-peptide release occurred in response to multiple secretory stimuli. However, the insulin-expressing cells' response to glucose was less effective than to what occurs in the fetal β-cell. Although endocrine hormone-expressing cells were well reproduced, it was not defined whether a differentiation process occurs via an inductive or a selective mechanism. These interesting issues need to be addressed in future studies in order to completely explore the β-cell organogenesis. This model might represent a promising way to restore a renewable source of pancreatic β cells.

Preparation and in vitro and in vivo characterization of composite microcapsules for cell encapsulation

Blasi P, Giovagnoli S, Schoubben A, Ricci M, Rossi C, Luca G, Basta G, Calafiore R
Department of Chemistry and Technology of Drugs, School of Pharmacy, University of Perugia, Perugia, Italy
kaolino@unipg.it
Int J Pharm 2006;324:27–36

Background: Cell encapsulation technology raises great hopes in medicine and biotechnology. Transplantation of encapsulated pancreatic islets represents a promising approach to the final cure of type 1 diabetes mellitus. Unfortunately, long-term graft survival and functional competence remain only partially fulfilled. Failure was often ascribed to the lack of biocompatibility generating inflammatory response, limited immunobarrier competence, hypoxia, and low β-cell replication.

Methods: In the present work, ketoprofen-loaded biodegradable microspheres, embedded into alginate/poly-L-ornithine/alginate microcapsules, were prepared in order to release ketoprofen at early stages after implantation. Morphology, size, in vitro release behavior, and in vivo biocompatibility were assessed. The effect of some preparation parameters was also evaluated. Polymeric microspheres were spherical and smooth, two populations of about 5 and 20 μm of mean diameter characterized the particle size distribution.

Results: A high burst effect was observed for all preparations during in vitro release studies. Ketoprofen, plasticizing the polymeric matrix, could be responsible of this release behavior. Alginate/poly-L-ornithine/alginate microcapsules were not modified upon ketoprofen-loaded microsphere encapsulation and an optimal dispersion was obtained. The composite system showed good biocompatibility when a high molecular weight polymer was employed. Therefore, a potentially suitable composite system for cell encapsulation was obtained.

Conclusions: This system may be successfully used to release non-steroidal anti-inflammatory drugs and other active molecules capable of improving cell system functional performance and lifespan.

During the past decades several encouraging advances have been achieved in pancreas transplantation for the treatment of patients with type 1 diabetes. Although pancreatic cell transplantation represents the most suitable treatment in selected patients, several side effects and problems limit the applicability of this procedure in a large number of patients. In fact, insulin independence in most patients is of relatively short duration, persisting on average for only 3–5 years [6]. Thus, new experimental approaches to significantly improve the lifespan of transplanted pancreatic endocrine cells are under investigation [7]. In the present study, composite microcapsules capable of releasing ketoprofen (a non-steroid anti-inflammatory drug) were used to encapsulate pancreatic endocrine cells. For this purpose, ketoprofen-loaded polylactic acid and polylactic-co-glycolic acid microspheres were prepared. This system may represent a potentially suitable composite system for transplantation of pancreatic islets that could improve the islet lifespan (minimizing the immunoreactivity to the graft). Further studies are obviously needed to evaluate the effectiveness of the composite system in human islet transplantation.

The effect of glucose variability on the risk of microvascular complications in type 1 diabetes

Kilpatrick ES, Rigby AS, Atkin SL
Department of Clinical Biochemistry, Hull Royal Infirmary, Hull, UK
eric.kilpatrick@hey.nhs.uk
Diabetes Care 2006;29:1486–1490

Background: It is not known whether glycemic instability may confer a risk of microvascular complications that is in addition to that predicted by the mean blood glucose value alone. This study has analyzed data from the Diabetes Control and Complications Trial (DCCT) to assess the effect of glucose variability on the risk of retinopathy and nephropathy in patients with type 1 diabetes.

Methods: Pre- and postprandial 7-point glucose profiles were collected quarterly during the DCCT in 1,441 individuals. The mean area under the curve glucose and the SD of glucose variability within 24 h and between visits were compared with the risk of retinopathy and nephropathy, having adjusted for age, sex, disease duration, treatment group, prevention cohort, and phase of treatment.

Results: Multivariate Cox regression showed that within-day and between-day variability in blood glucose around a patient's mean value has no influence on the development or progression of either retinopathy (p = 0.18 and p = 0.72, respectively) or nephropathy (p = 0.32 and p = 0.57). Neither preprandial (p = 0.18) nor postprandial (p = 0.31) glucose concentrations preferentially contribute to the probability of retinopathy.

Conclusions: This study has shown that blood glucose variability does not appear to be an additional factor in the development of microvascular complications. Also, pre- and postprandial glucose values are equally predictive of the small-vessel complications of type 1 diabetes.

The association between glycemic control defined as HbA1c values and the risk of microvascular complications has clearly been defined in previous clinical trials (Stockholm Study, Oslo Study, Kroc Study and, finally, the DCCT) [8–11]. In fact, the higher the HbA1c values, the greater is the risk of either developing or worsening retinopathy, nephropathy and neuropathy. However, although HbA1c values have been shown to reflect the glycemic trend within the previous 3 months, this surrogate marker does not take into account the day-by-day and especially the 24-hour variability or to reveal hyperglycemic episodes [12]. Thus, despite low HbA1c levels, well-controlled patients may experience acute hyperglycemia which should increase the risk of diabetes-related complications [13]. Analyzing data from the 1,441 patients with type 1 diabetes recruited for the DCCT, this study evaluated the relationship between pre- or postprandial glycemia and the development of microvascular complications. It was shown that the development or progression of either retinopathy or nephropathy in patients with type 1 diabetes is not influenced by the variability in blood glucose. In fact, the risk of developing microvascular complications was not statistically different between patients with wide blood glucose fluctuations compared with those with little glycemic fluctuations throughout the day. Furthermore, the risk of developing microvascular complications was not related either to the pre- or to the postprandial glucose concentrations. Although these results should reassure patients and their caring physicians that no additional risk factors are added to glucose fluctuations, it appears of foremost importance to remark the clear relationship between glycemic control and microvascular complications. The current American Diabetes Association recommendations do not suggest a need to measure postprandial blood glucose in preference to basal values; this study confirms that there is no specific need for this to change in order to reduce the likelihood of microvascular complications.

Responses against islet antigens in NOD mice are prevented by tolerance to proinsulin but not IGRP

Krishnamurthy B, Dudek NL, McKenzie MD, Purcell AW, Brooks AG, Gellert S, Colman PG, Harrison LC, Lew AM, Thomas HE, Kay TW
St Vincent's Institute, Fitzroy, Vic., Australia
eric.kilpatrick@hey.nhs.uk

J Clin Invest 2006;116:3258–3265

Background: Type 1 diabetes (T1D) is characterized by immune responses against several autoantigens expressed in pancreatic β cells. T cells specific for proinsulin and islet-specific glucose-6-phosphatase catalytic subunit-related protein (IGRP) can induce T1D in NOD mice. However, whether immune responses to multiple autoantigens are caused by spreading from one to another or whether they develop independently of each other is unknown.

Methods and Results: As cytotoxic T cells specific for IGRP were not detected in transgenic NOD mice tolerant to proinsulin, the authors determined that immune responses against proinsulin are necessary for IGRP-specific T cells to develop. On the other hand, transgenic overexpression of IGRP resulted in loss of intra-islet IGRP-specific T cells but did not protect NOD mice from insulitis or T1D, providing direct evidence that the response against IGRP is downstream of the response to proinsulin.

Conclusions: These results suggest that pathogenic proinsulin-specific immunity in NOD mice subsequently spreads to other antigens such as IGRP.

Autoimmune response to a number of antigens represents the evolution of the course of type 1 diabetes in humans and NOD mice. The breakdown of normal tolerance to the β-cell allows the activation of T cells to multiple specificities that results in a continuously increasing production of antibodies against the insulin-producing cells [1]. Although different antigens have been shown to be involved in the autoimmune destruction of β cells, so far no convincing evidence has been reported to determine whether the disease is initiated by polyclonal activation of T cells specific of single vs. multiple antigens. The present study investigated the relationship between immune response to proinsulin and other significant autoantigens. Evaluating the fate of $IGRP_{206-214}$-specific T cells transgenic NOD mice overexpressing proinsulin 2 in APCs (NOD-PI mice), it was demonstrated that immune response to $IGRP_{206-214}$ does not develop in NOD-PI mice. Furthermore, using a NOD mice model overexpressing IGRP under the control of MHC class II promoter, it was shown that IGRP response occurs only when proinsulin responses have been established and that the immune response 'spreads' from proinsulin to IGRP. Although IGRP itself has not been shown to be a significant antigen in human type 1 diabetes, the concept of initiating and effector antigens may apply to it. These data suggest that the development of immune responses against multiple autoantigens is a necessary step. This is reminiscent of the clinical situation where individuals who are positive for a single autoantibody have a low risk of the disease, probably reflecting the lack of spreading of the immune response. This is an important distinction, because the effect of tolerance to proinsulin on immune responses to other antigens is a relevant issue in clinical trials for prevention of type 1 diabetes in humans. The findings of this study suggest that primary prevention should be most effective if targeted at the initiating antigen such as proinsulin. Once insulitis is established, tolerance induction to other β-cell antigens needs to be considered as well. Further investigations on how the response to autoantigens develops will help to fully understand how antigen-specific tolerance induction could prevent type 1 diabetes.

Francesco Chiarelli/Cosimo Giannini

The relation of ambulatory blood pressure and pulse rate to retinopathy in type 1 diabetes mellitus: the renin-angiotensin system study

Klein R, Moss SE, Sinaiko AR, Zinman B, Gardiner R, Suissa S, Donnelly SM, Kramer MS, Goodyer P, Strand T, Mauer M
Department of Ophthalmology and Visual Sciences, University of Wisconsin School of Medicine and Public Health, Madison, Wisc., USA
kleinr@epi.ophth.wisc.edu
Ophthalmology 2006;113:2231–2236

Background: To examine the association of ambulatory blood pressure (ABP) and ambulatory pulse rate (APR) with diabetic retinopathy in persons with type 1 diabetes in the Renin-Angiotensin System Study (RASS), a multicenter primary diabetic nephropathy prevention trial.

Methods: Cross-sectional study of 194 normotensive RASS participants in three centers who are 16 years of age or older with type 1 diabetes mellitus of 2–20 years' duration. ABP and APR were monitored using standardized protocols. Patients were defined as non-dippers if the night-to-day ratios for both systolic and diastolic blood pressures were >0.9. Diabetic retinopathy was determined by masked grading of 30° color stereoscopic fundus photographs of seven standard fields using the Early Treatment Diabetic Retinopathy Study severity scale.

Results: No diabetic retinopathy was present in 32%, mild non-proliferative diabetic retinopathy (NPDR) was present in 55%, and moderate to severe NPDR or proliferative diabetic retinopathy was present in 13% of the cohort. Neither 24-hour systolic ABP or diastolic ABP, daytime systolic or diastolic ABP, nor nighttime diastolic ABP were related to severity of diabetic retinopathy. Statistically significant associations were found between nighttime systolic ABP and mean ABP and diabetic retinopathy. Among those with no diabetic retinopathy, 19% were non-dippers; for those with mild NPDR, 28% were non-dippers, and for those with severe NPDR or proliferative diabetic retinopathy, 36% were non-dippers (p = 0.08). The ratio of nighttime to daytime APR, but not the 24-hour APR or daytime or nighttime APR, was related positively to the severity of DR. In multivariable analyses, only the nighttime systolic ABP was related to severity of diabetic retinopathy (p < 0.05).

Conclusions: These data suggest that ABP, especially during the night, may provide a better measure than clinical BP regarding the relationship of BP to the severity of retinopathy in normotensive persons with type 1 diabetes without clinical diabetic nephropathy.

Diabetes retinopathy remains the major cause of acquired blindness in youngsters and adults of developed countries. Adequate screening programs allow to detect early diabetic retinopathy in a large proportion of young people with a disease duration of more than 11 years. Several studies evaluated the mechanisms involved in the onset and progression of early retinal alterations [11]. Although chronic hyperglycemia has been proven to be one of the foremost factors affecting retinal damage, other factors such us blood pressure have been supposed to play a role in diabetic retinopathy. By using data from the Renin-Angiotensin System Study, a parallel, double-blind, placebo-controlled, multicenter, primary prevention clinical trial of diabetic nephropathy [14], this study evaluated whether ABP and APR may be associated with the severity of diabetic retinopathy in normotensive patients with type 1 diabetes who have clinically normal renal function. It was clearly shown that nighttime systolic ABP is associated with the severity of diabetic retinopathy, while no association was detected between clinical blood pressure and clinical and APR. These results suggest that in normotensive patients with type 1 diabetes, the 24-hour continuous monitoring blood pressure could represent a marker of risk for diabetic retinopathy. Longitudinal studies are now needed to confirm the predictive role of ABP monitoring on later development of diabetic retinopathy.

Persistent renal hypertrophy and faster decline of glomerular filtration rate precede the development of microalbuminuria in type 1 diabetes

Zerbini G, Bonfanti R, Meschi F, Bognetti E, Paesano PL, Gianolli L, Querques M, Maestroni A, Calori G, Del Maschio A, Fazio F, Luzi L, Chiumello G
Department of Medicine, San Raffaele Scientific Institute, Milan, Italy
g.zerbini@hsr.it
Diabetes 2006;55:2620–2625

Background: Soon after the onset of type 1 diabetes, renal hypertrophy and hyperfiltration become manifest, particularly among patients who will subsequently develop diabetic nephropathy. Whether these early renal dysfunctions are involved in the pathogenesis of diabetic nephropathy is currently unclear.
Methods: The authors evaluated, during the same day, kidney volume and glomerular filtration rate (GFR) in 146 patients with type 1 diabetes and normal renal function. All the individuals were then monitored for a mean of 9.5 ± 4.4 years for the development of microalbuminuria. Kidney volume and GFR were re-evaluated in a subset of 68 patients 4 years after baseline.
Results: During follow-up, microalbuminuria developed in 27 of 146 diabetic patients. At baseline, kidney volume (312.8 ± 52.6 vs. 281.4 ± 46.1 vs. $236.8 \pm 41.6 \,\mathrm{ml/1.73\,m^2}$, $p < 0.05$) but not GFR was increased in patients predisposed to microalbuminuria. The risk of progression was higher in patients with increased kidney volume ($p = 0.0058$). Patients predisposed to microalbuminuria showed a stable increase in kidney volume ($p = 0.003$), along with a faster decline of GFR ($p = 0.01$). Persistent renal hypertrophy and faster decline of GFR precede the development of microalbuminuria in type 1 diabetes.
Conclusions: These findings support the hypothesis that renal hypertrophy precedes hyperfiltration during the development of diabetic nephropathy.

Despite the development of microalbuminuria a few years after clinical onset of diabetes, it is well established that increased kidney volume and higher GFR may be detected as early as at onset of diabetes, especially in patients who will later develop nephropathy [15]. Although these abnormalities become evident quite simultaneously, the 'vascular hypothesis' retains that glomerular hyperfiltration due to defects of vascular control represents the primary event followed by hypertrophy [16]. On the other hand, the 'tubular hypothesis' suggests that the first event in diabetic nephropathy is increased kidney volume (due to hyperglycemia) followed by hyperfiltration [17]. This prospective study evaluated whether kidney volume and GFR are increased in subjects with type 1 diabetes mellitus and their relation to later development of microalbuminuria. In patients who developed microalbuminuria during the follow-up period, increased kidney volume was detected earlier than impaired GFR and both progressed during the course of diabetes. Furthermore, the rate of progression to microalbuminuria was significantly higher in patients with increased kidney volume. This study represents an important progress in the knowledge of diabetes-related kidney disease. A thorough understanding of the mechanisms involved in the development of renal hypertrophy is needed in order to evaluate approaches for the primary prevention of diabetic nephropathy.

Lower bone mineral content in children with type 1 diabetes mellitus is linked to female sex, low insulin-like growth factor type I levels, and high insulin requirement

Leger J, Marinovic D, Alberti C, Dorgeret S, Chevenne D, Marchal CL, Tubiana-Rufi N, Sebag G, Czernichow P
Pediatric Endocrinology Unit and INSERM U 690, Hôpital Robert Debré, Paris, France
juliane.leger@rdb.ap-hop-paris.fr
J Clin Endocrinol Metab 2006;91:3947–3953

Background: Studies on bone mineral characteristics in children with type 1 diabetes have generated conflicting results. Our objective was to investigate bone mineral characteristics in children with type 1 diabetes and to analyze their associations with bone metabolism and the IGF-1 system.
Methods: A cohort of Caucasian patients with type 1 diabetes for at least 3 years and healthy children was recruited between January 2003 and June 2004. This was a university hospital-based study. A total of

Francesco Chiarelli/Cosimo Giannini

127 patients and 319 controls aged 6–20 years participated. Dual-energy x-ray absorptiometry was performed in patients and controls. Serum bone alkaline phosphatase, cross-laps, IGF-1, and IGF-binding protein 3 levels were determined in patients with values analyzed using normative data from 1,150 healthy children.

Results: After adjustment for age, sex, pubertal stage, and body mass index SD score, total body bone mineral content/lean body mass was significantly lower in patients than in controls ($p < 0.04$). This difference was a result of the differences between the girls of the two groups. Girls with T1DM had significantly lower lumbar spine and total body bone mineral content than control girls ($p = 0.002$), whereas no such difference was observed in boys. Serum bone alkaline phosphatase level was significantly lower in girls than in boys ($p = 0.04$). Low serum IGF-1 levels and the administration of large amounts of insulin were found to have independent deleterious effects on bone mineral content for children of all ages and both sexes, whereas disease duration and glycosylated hemoglobin levels did not.

Conclusions: A sex-related difference in the impairment of bone mineral characteristics was identified in children with T1DM. Longitudinal studies are required to investigate whether boys may gain slightly less bone mass during skeletal growth.

Due to systemic rather than portal injections of insulin, serum insulin concentrations are not physiological in patients with diabetes, leading to abnormalities of the GH-IGF-1 axis. Low hepatic insulin concentrations results in lower IGF-1 and IGFBP-3 levels that have been widely reported in patients with type 1 diabetes, particularly in those with poor metabolic control. The impaired GH-IGF-1 axis results in blunted growth and appears to influence bone mineralization [18]. Performing a dual-energy X-ray absorption, this cross-sectional study evaluated bone turnover, bone mineral content and body composition in a group of 127 young patients with type 1 diabetes at different pubertal stages. Similar values were observed in boys with type 1 diabetes and controls, whereas girls with type 1 diabetes had lower lumbar spine and total body bone mineral content and lower lean body mass. Furthermore, total body bone mineral content for lean body mass was lower in patients than controls. The observed differences resulted primarily from girls. There was a significant relation between insulin requirement and serum IGF-1-SDS. Although these preliminary data were obtained in a significant sample size, longitudinal data are needed in order to confirm bone alterations in young patients with type 1 diabetes. This could be relevant for the clinician. In fact, given the critical role of bone mass accretion during pubertal years, monitoring of bone mineral content in young patients with type 1 diabetes, especially girls, is recommended.

Pre-type 1 diabetes dysmetabolism: maximal sensitivity achieved with both oral and intravenous glucose tolerance testing

Barker JM, McFann K, Harrison LC, Fourlanos S, Krischer J, Cuthbertson D, Chase HP, Eisenbarth GS
Barbara Davis Center for Childhood Diabetes, University of Colorado Health, Sciences Center, Denver, Colo., USA
jennifer.barker@uchsc.edu
J Pediatr 2007;150:31–36

Background: To determine the relationship of intravenous (IVGTT) and oral (OGTT) glucose tolerance test abnormalities to diabetes development in a high-risk prediabetic cohort and to identify an optimal testing strategy for detecting preclinical diabetes.

Methods: Diabetes Prevention Trial-Type 1 Diabetes (DPT-1) randomized subjects to oral ($n = 372$) and parenteral ($n = 339$) insulin prevention trials. Subjects were followed with IVGTTs and OGTTs. Factors associated with progression to diabetes were evaluated.

Results: Survival analysis revealed that higher quartiles of 2-hour glucose and lower quartiles of first-phase insulin response (FPIR) at baseline were associated with decreased diabetes-free survival. Cox proportional hazards modeling showed that baseline body mass index (BMI), FPIR, and 2-hour glucose levels were significantly associated with an increased hazard for diabetes. On testing performed within 6 months of diabetes diagnosis, 3% (1/32) had normal FPIR and normal 2-hour glucose on OGTT. The sensitivities for impaired glucose tolerance (IGT) and low FPIR performed within 6 months of diabetes diagnosis were equivalent (76 vs. 73%).

Conclusions: Most (97%) subjects had abnormal IVGTTs and/or OGTTs before the development of diabetes. The highest sensitivity is achieved using both tests.

Type 1 diabetes is a chronic autoimmune disease characterized by T-cell autoreactivity to pancreatic islets. β-Cell loss starts several months or years before the clinical onset of diabetes [1]. Thus, several early markers capable of reliably detecting patients at higher risk of diabetes are under investigation. In order to develop an optimal preclinical testing strategy to identify patients who eventually develop diabetes, the authors performed IVGTT and OGTT glucose tolerance tests in a high-risk pre-diabetic cohort participating in the Diabetes Prevention Trial-Type 1 Diabetes (DPT-1) [19]. In the present study, 258 subjects who developed diabetes and an additional 453 who were diabetes-free by the end of the study were followed with serial IVGTTs and OGTTs. Abnormalities of 2-hour glucose on OGTT and of first-phase insulin release during the IVGTT within 6 months before diabetes diagnosis were useful to identify individuals at high risk for clinical diabetes. Maximal sensitivity was achieved when both tests were used. First-phase insulin release <10th percentile for age was not specific for diabetes and a significant proportion of the subjects who did not develop diabetes during a 2-year follow-up had an abnormal IVGTT. Furthermore, despite abnormalities of 2-hour glucose on OGTT, the majority of subjects maintained a normal fasting plasma glucose. A significant proportion of subjects had a normal OGTT (24%) or IVGTT (22%) in the 6 months before the onset of diabetes. A very small subset (3%) of patients had normal results at both tests 6 months before diabetes onset. The large size and longitudinal follow-up provide important results for the interpretation of metabolic tests in antibody-positive relatives of patients with type 1 diabetes.

Clinical trials, new treatments

Insulin detemir compared with NPH insulin in children and adolescents with type 1 diabetes

Robertson KJ, Schoenle E, Gucev Z, Mordhorst L, Gall MA, Ludvigsson J
The Royal Hospital for Sick Children, Glasgow, UK
kjr@diabetes-scotland.org
Diabet Med 2007;24:27–34

Background: This study compared the effect of insulin detemir on glycemic control (HbA1c, fasting plasma glucose and variability thereof) with that of Neutral Protamine Hagedorn human isophane (NPH) insulin, both combined with insulin aspart, in children with type 1 diabetes mellitus, and compared the safety of these treatments.

Methods: In this 26-week, open-label, randomized (2:1), parallel-group study, 347 (140 prepubertal and 207 pubertal) children with type 1 diabetes, aged 6–17 years, received insulin detemir (n = 232) or NPH insulin (n = 115) once or twice daily, according to the prestudy regimen, plus premeal insulin aspart.

Results: The mean HbA1c decreased by approximately 0.8% with both treatments. After 26 weeks, the mean difference in HbA1c was 0.1% (95% confidence interval 0.1–0.3) (insulin detemir 8.0%, NPH insulin 7.9%). Within-subject variation in self-measured fasting plasma glucose was significantly lower with insulin detemir than with NPH insulin (SD 3.3 vs. 4.3, $p < 0.001$), as was mean fasting plasma glucose (8.4 vs. 9.6 mmol/l, p = 0.022). The risk of nocturnal hypoglycemia was 26% lower with insulin detemir (p = 0.041) and the risk of 24-hour hypoglycemia was similar with the two treatments (p = 0.351). The mean body mass index (BMI) z-score was lower with insulin detemir ($p < 0.001$).

Conclusions: Basal-bolus treatment with insulin detemir or NPH insulin and premeal insulin aspart in children and adolescents with type 1 diabetes mellitus improved HbA1c to a similar degree. The lower and more predictable fasting plasma glucose, lower risk of nocturnal hypoglycemia and lower BMI observed with insulin detemir are clinically significant advantages compared with NPH insulin.

To date, basal bolus multiple insulin injections are recommended in young patients with type 1 diabetes in order to improve metabolic control and reduce the risk for microvascular complications [20]. During the past decade the importance of the 24-hour glycemic profile has stimulated the development of new basal insulin analogs (insulin glargine, insulin detemir) in order to reproduce the physiological serum insulin changes and obtain stable and predictable blood glucose levels [21]. The basal insulin analog detemir is an acylated derivative of human insulin which has been shown to result in a lower risk of hypoglycemia and in a predictable glycemic control with less day-to-day variation compared with NPH insulin in adult diabetic patients [22]. This multicenter open-label, randomized (2:1), parallel-group study in children with type 1 diabetes (140 prepubertal and 207 pubertal) investigated the efficacy and safety of detemir compared with NPH insulin. It was observed that transfer from NPH to detemir can be performed on a 1:1 insulin unit basis. Basal-bolus treatment for 26 weeks with insulin detemir plus premeal insulin aspart was associated with lower risk of nocturnal hypoglycemia but did not improve metabolic control. Although only few nocturnal time points are used in this study, insulin detemir could be useful in young patients with recurrent hypoglycemia. Furthermore, treatment with insulin detemir resulted in lower and more predictable fasting glucose levels. This could make titration towards more ambitious plasma glucose levels easier and safer, especially in children with a highly variable lifestyle. In conclusion, insulin detemir represents an encouraging new alternative for basal bolus therapy in children with diabetes, especially in those who experienced recurrent hypoglycemia or with a highly variable lifestyle. However, further studies are needed in children and adolescents.

Feasibility of automating insulin delivery for the treatment of type 1 diabetes

Steil GM, Rebrin K, Darwin C, Hariri F, Saad MF
Medtronic MiniMed, Northridge, Calif., USA
garry.steil@medtronic.com
Diabetes 2006;55:3344–3350

Background and Methods: An automated closed-loop insulin delivery system based on subcutaneous glucose sensing and subcutaneous insulin delivery was evaluated in 10 subjects with type 1 diabetes (2 men, 8 women, mean ($\pm$SD) age 43.4 $\pm$ 11.4 years, duration of diabetes 18.2 $\pm$ 13.5 years). Closed-loop control was assessed over approximately 30 h and compared with open-loop control assessed over 3 days. Closed-loop insulin delivery was calculated using a model of the β-cell's multiphasic insulin response to glucose.
Results: Plasma glucose was 160 $\pm$ 66 mg/dl at the start of closed loop and was thereafter reduced to 71 $\pm$ 19 by 1:00 p.m. (preprandial lunch). Fasting glucose the subsequent morning on closed loop was not different from target (124 $\pm$ 25 vs. 120 mg/dl, respectively; p > 0.05). Mean glucose levels were not different between the open and closed loop (133 $\pm$ 63 vs. 133 $\pm$ 52 mg/dl, respectively; p > 0.65). However, glucose was within the range 70–180 mg/dl 75% of the time under closed loop vs. 63% for open loop. Incidence of biochemical hypoglycemia (blood glucose <60 mg/dl) was similar under the two treatments. There were no episodes of severe hypoglycemia.
Conclusions: The data provide proof of concept that glycemic control can be achieved by a completely automated external closed-loop insulin delivery system.

The clear association between metabolic control and risk of microvascular complications implies new methodological approaches to mimic physiological insulin variations and to obtain stable and predictable blood glucose levels around the clock [23]. Insulin pump delivery appears to be a suitable and practical method for the treatment of patients with type 1 diabetes. The recent availability of a real-time glucose sensor has raised the possibility of automated closed-loop systems capable of abolishing the operator-dependent link between glucose variations and insulin delivery. This study assessed a complex system comprising a real-time subcutaneous glucose sensor, an external insulin-delivery pump and a processor capable of reproducing the β-cell multiphasic glucose-induced insulin release. In 10 adult patients with diabetes, this closed-loop system was effective and able to achieve glucose levels similar to continuous subcutaneous insulin infusion with reduced variance. Furthermore, although no statistical differences were documented in terms of incidence of hypoglycemia, the system automatically suspended insulin delivery in all instances of hypoglycemia. However, postprandial levels were higher than in non-diabetic individuals. Although several improvements are needed, this is an important step ahead in the treatment of patients with type 1 diabetes. The availability of a closed-loop system which is able to integrate glucose levels automatically and translate them into insulin delivery should optimize glycemic control and reduce the risk of hypoglycemia, particularly during the night.

Longitudinal lipid screening and use of lipid-lowering medications in pediatric type 1 diabetes

Maahs DM, Wadwa RP, McFann K, Nadeau K, Williams MR, Eckel RH, Klingensmith GJ
Barbara Davis Center for Childhood Diabetes and Department of Medicine, University of Colorado Health Sciences Center, Aurora, Colo., USA
David.Maahs@uchsc.edu
J Pediatr 2007;150:146–150

Background: Because cardiovascular disease (CVD) is the leading cause of death in patients with type 1 diabetes, and dyslipidemia is an important CVD risk factor, the authors investigated dyslipidemia and its treatment in children with type 1 diabetes.
Methods: Subjects had type 1 diabetes (n = 360), repeated lipid measurements (n = 1,095, mean 3.04 ± 0.94, range 2–11), and were seen between 1994 and 2004. Total cholesterol (TC), high-density lipoprotein cholesterol (HDL), and non-HDL cholesterol (non-HDL) were categorized on the basis of published guidelines. Age, diabetes duration, sex, body mass index, HbA1c, and lipid-lowering medication use were recorded. Predictors of TC, HDL, and non-HDL were determined.
Results: Sustained abnormalities existed for TC ≥ 200 mg/dl (16.9%); HDL < 35 mg/dl (3.3%), and non-HDL ≥ 130 mg/dl (27.8%), ≥160 mg/dl (10.6%), and ≥190 mg/dl (3.3%). Lipid-lowering medications were started on 23 patients. In mixed model longitudinal data analyses, HbA1c was significantly related to TC and non-HDL. Body mass index z-score was inversely related to HDL.
Conclusions: In this retrospective, longitudinal study of pediatric patients with type 1 diabetes with repeated lipid measurements, sustained abnormal levels for TC, HDL, and non-HDL were present. Prospective longitudinal data for dyslipidemia in youth with type 1 diabetes are needed.

The improvement in diabetes care has resulted in a decrease of microangiopathy and in a paradoxical increase of diabetes-related long-term angiopathy later in life. Several studies, including some in children and adolescents, have demonstrated a direct role of dyslipidemia in diabetes-related arterial wall changes [24]. However, despite the role of abnormal lipid contents as a cardiovascular risk factor, several diet or lifestyle intervention studies have failed to normalize lipid profiles. These results have supported the use of lipid-lowering medication in children and adolescents [25]. This retrospective longitudinal study evaluated a total of 1,095 lipid measurements and tested the effect and safety of lipid-lowering medications. The prevalence of abnormal lipid levels was elevated: 18.9% of patients had total cholesterol ≥200 mg/dl, 4.2% had HDL cholesterol <35 mg/dl. Non-HDL cholesterol was ≥130 mg/dl in 34.2%, ≥160 mg/dl in 11.4%, and ≥19.0 mg/dl in 5.8%. Furthermore, higher total cholesterol levels were associated with a poor glycemic control and with older age. 23 of 360 patients who started lipid-lowering medication had a decrease of total and non-HDL cholesterol and an increase in HDL cholesterol; no significant side effects were reported. Although several limitations (inability to evaluate compliance with medications, differences in diet and lifestyle, differences in diabetes control, lipid profile evaluated in different laboratories), this study provides important information on lipid profiles in children and adolescents with diabetes. Further prospective longitudinal studies on the natural history of dyslipidemia and on the safety and efficacy of lipid-lowering medications are now needed.

TRPV1+ sensory neurons control β-cell stress and islet inflammation in autoimmune diabetes

Razavi R, Chan Y, Afifiyan FN, Liu XJ, Wan X, Yantha J, Tsui H, Tang L, Tsai S, Santamaria P, Driver JP, Serreze D, Salter MW, Dosch HM

Neurosciences and Mental Health Program, The Hospital for Sick Children, Research Institute, University of Toronto, Toronto, Ont., Canada
hmdosch@sickkids.ca
Cell 2006;127:1123–1135

Background: In type 1 diabetes, T-cell-mediated death of pancreatic β cells produces insulin deficiency. However, what attracts or restricts broadly autoreactive lymphocyte pools to the pancreas remains unclear.

Methods and Results: The authors report that transient receptor potential vanilloid-1+ pancreatic sensory neurons control islet inflammation and insulin resistance. Eliminating these neurons in diabetes-prone NOD mice prevents insulitis and diabetes, despite systemic persistence of pathogenic T-cell pools. Insulin resistance and β-cell stress of prediabetic NOD mice are prevented when transient receptor potential vanilloid-1+ neurons are eliminated. Transient receptor potential vanilloid-1 (NOD), localized to the Idd4.1 diabetes-risk locus, is a hypofunctional mutant, mediating depressed neurogenic inflammation. Delivering the neuropeptide substance P by intra-arterial injection into the NOD pancreas reverses abnormal insulin resistance, insulitis, and diabetes for weeks. Concordantly, insulin sensitivity is enhanced in trpv1$^{-/-}$ mice, whereas insulitis/diabetes-resistant NOD × B6Idd4-congenic mice, carrying wild-type transient receptor potential vanilloid-1, show restored transient receptor potential vanilloid-1 function and insulin sensitivity.

Conclusions: These data uncover a fundamental role for insulin-responsive transient receptor potential vanilloid-1+ sensory neurons in β-cell function and diabetes pathoetiology.

Type 1 diabetes in humans and NOD mice results from T-cell-mediated autoimmune destruction of insulin-producing β cells [1]. The disease is initiated by polyclonal activation of T cells to multiple specific antigens caused by a breakdown in normal tolerance to the β cell. Autoreactive T lymphocytes progressively infiltrate pancreatic islets of Langerhans reaching a complete and progressive destruction of β cells and overt diabetes. Several theories have been proposed in order to explain the mechanism involved in the recruitment and activation of autoreactive T lymphocytes in mediating islet cell destruction. Recent studies have supposed a role of nervous system failure defined by the function of the primary sensory afferent neuron and immune system failure in autoimmune diseases [26]. In particular, a non-specific cation channel, the transient receptor potential vanilloid-1 protein expressed in sensory neurons, has been shown to play an important role in proinflammatory reactions. This study evaluated whether sensory neurons may have a role in type 1 diabetes. It was clearly shown that transient receptor potential vanilloid-1 sensory neurons appear critical for the immune-cell accumulation in the pancreas playing a pivotal role in the initiation and progression of islet inflammation mediated in part by the primary afferent neurons. This study represents the first evidence for a direct role of sensory neurons in islet physiology, opening new perspectives for therapeutic strategies to prevent progression of β cell failure.

A genome-wide association study of non-synonymous SNPs identifies a type 1 diabetes locus in the interferon-induced helicase (IFIH1) region

Smyth DJ, Cooper JD, Bailey R, Field S, Burren O, Smink LJ, Guja C, Ionescu-Tirgoviste C, Widmer B, Dunger DB, Savage DA, Walker NM, Clayton DG, Todd JA

Juvenile Diabetes Research Foundation/Wellcome Trust Diabetes and Inflammation Laboratory, Cambridge Institute for Medical Research, Addenbrooke's Hospital, Cambridge, UK
john.todd@cimr.cam.ac.uk

Nat Genet 2006;38:617–619

Background and Methods: In this study the authors report convincing statistical support for a sixth type 1 diabetes (T1D) locus in the innate immunity viral RNA receptor gene region IFIH1 (also known as mda-5 or Helicard) on chromosome 2q24.3.

Results: The authors found the association in an interim analysis of a genome-wide non-synonymous SNP (nsSNP) scan, and validated it in a case-control collection and replicated it in an independent family collection. In 4,253 cases, 5,842 controls and 2,134 parent-child trio genotypes, the risk ratio for the minor allele of the nsSNP rs1990760 A $\rightarrow$ G (A946T) was 0.86 (95% confidence interval 0.82–0.90) at $P = 1.42 \times 10^{-10}$.

Several epidemiological studies have focused the important role of genetic susceptibility on the development of type 1 diabetes. During the past decades, genetic analyses sustained by convincing and reproducible statistical support have identified five main type 1 diabetes susceptibility loci: the HLA class II genes, the insulin gene, the CTLA4 locus, PTPN22 and the relatively recently reported locus in the IL2RA/CD25 region on chromosome 10p15 [27–31]. Adopting a genome-wide nsSNP scan approach using a highly multiplexed, high-throughput molecular inversion probe (MIP) technology (Affymetrix), this study reports a new type 1 diabetes susceptibility locus in the chromosome 2q24.3 (risk ratio for the minor allele G = 0.86; $P = 1.42 \times 10^{10}$) in a total of 12,229 subjects (case, controls and parent-child). This locus is involved in the innate immunity viral RNA receptor gene region IFIH1. This gene is an early type I interferon (IFN) β-responsive gene, which may contribute to the apoptosis of virally infected cells in antiviral immune responses, thus making it a sensor or pathogen recognition receptor for viral infection. The large sample size based on large case-control and family collections and the convincing statistical analysis justifies further genetic analysis of the region in other populations, association analyses of other infectious and chronic diseases, and functional studies to assess if IFIH1 is the causal gene in the locus and A946T is the substitution responsible for the disease association. Furthermore, the genetic association between type 1 diabetes and IFIH1 could provide a molecular link between the development of diabetes and its previously reported associations with viral infections.

An ATP-binding mutation (G334D) in KCNJ11 is associated with a sulfonylurea-insensitive form of developmental delay, epilepsy, and neonatal diabetes

Masia R, Koster JC, Tumini S, Chiarelli F, Colombo C, Nichols CG, Barbetti F

Department of Cell Biology and Physiology, Washington University School of Medicine, St. Louis, Mo., USA
cnichols@wustl.edu

Diabetes 2007;56:328–336

Background: Mutations in the pancreatic ATP-sensitive K$^+$ channel (K(ATP) channel) cause permanent neonatal diabetes mellitus (PNDM) in humans. All of the K(ATP) channel mutations examined result in decreased ATP inhibition, which in turn is predicted to suppress insulin secretion.

Methods and Results: Here the authors describe a patient with severe PNDM, which includes developmental delay and epilepsy, in addition to neonatal diabetes (developmental delay, epilepsy, and neonatal diabetes (DEND)), due to a G334D mutation in the Kir6.2 subunit of K(ATP) channel. The patient was wholly unresponsive to sulfonylurea therapy (up to $1.14\,\mathrm{mg} \cdot \mathrm{kg}^{-1} \cdot \mathrm{day}^{-1}$) and remained insulin-dependent. Consistent with the putative role of G334 as an ATP-binding residue, reconstituted homomeric and mixed WT+G334D channels exhibit absent or reduced ATP sensitivity but normal gating behavior in the absence of ATP. In disagreement with the sulfonylurea insensitivity of the affected patient, the G334D mutation has no effect on the sulfonylurea inhibition of reconstituted channels in excised patches. However, in macroscopic rubidium-efflux assays in intact cells, reconstituted mutant channels do exhibit a decreased, but still present, sulfonylurea response.

Results: The results demonstrate that ATP-binding site mutations can indeed cause DEND and suggest the possibility that sulfonylurea insensitivity of such patients may be a secondary reflection of the presence of DEND rather than a simple reflection of the underlying molecular basis.

The continuously increasing knowledge on the genetic mechanism underlying neonatal diabetes mellitus has recently improved the treatment opportunity of both the permanent and transient form of neonatal diabetes mellitus. In particular, evidence for a direct and primary role of the pancreatic ATP-sensitive K channel (K_{ATP}) mutation in the development of permanent neonatal diabetes mellitus has increased the interest of sulfonylurea compounds as an alternative treatment to insulin injections in many patients with K_{ATP}-induced diabetes [32]. However, treatment effectiveness and clinical features appear to be strongly related to the different mutations. In fact, convincing evidence exists for a genotype-phenotype relationship in which the severity of the mutation correlates with the severity of the disease. Ranging from mild to strong activating mutation of the K_{ATP}, clinical features vary from transient neonatal diabetes mellitus with no neurological symptoms to a severe multisystemic pathology defined by developmental delay, epilepsy, and neonatal diabetes (DEND). In the present study a novel human ATP-binding mutation (G334D) in KCNJ11 (Kir6.2) associated with DEND was identified. Structurally, K_{ATP} channels are hetero-octomers, consisting of four subunits each of the pore-forming Kir6.2 subunit (KCNJ11) and four regulatory sulfonylurea receptor subunits (SUR1, ABCC8). ATP inhibits the channel by directly interacting with Kir6.2 where binding of ATP at one of the four subunits is sufficient to close the channel. SUR1 mediates stimulation of channel activity by Mg-nucleotide as well as inhibition by sulfonylureas. The mutation described here determines absent or reduced ATP sensitivity, but normal gating behavior in the absence of ATP. This characteristic mutation appears to cause the unresponsiveness to sulfonylureas reported in this patient. This new mutation provides evidence of the tight relationship between genotype-phenotype-dependent clinical features and pharmacological susceptibility.

New hormones

Adiponutrin gene is regulated by insulin and glucose in human adipose tissue

Moldes M, Beauregard G, Faraj M, Peretti N, Ducluzeau PH, Laville M, Rabasa-Lhoret R, Vidal H, Clement K
Department of Endocrinology, Cancer and Metabolism, Institut Cochin, Paris, INSERM, U567, Paris, France
Eur J Endocrinol 2006;155:461–468

Background: Adiponutrin is a new transmembrane protein specifically expressed in adipose tissue. In obese subjects, short- or long-term calorie restriction diets were associated with a reduction in adiponutrin gene expression. Adiponutrin mRNA level was previously shown to be negatively correlated with fasting glucose plasma levels and associated with insulin sensitivity of non-diabetic obese and non-obese subjects. The purpose of the present work was to get more insight into the regulation of adiponutrin gene expression by insulin and/or glucose using clamp studies and to examine its potential dysregulation in subjects with a deterioration of glucose homeostasis.

Methods: Adiponutrin gene expression was quantified by reverse transcriptase-quantitative PCR in s.c. adipose tissue of healthy lean subjects after an euglycemic hyperinsulinemic clamp (EGHI), a hyperglycemic euinsulinemic clamp, and a hyperglycemic hyperinsulinemic (HGHI) clamp. Adiponutrin gene expression was also analyzed in patients with different levels of insulin resistance.

Results: During EGHI, insulin infusion induced adiponutrin gene expression 8.4-fold (p = 0.008). Its expression was also induced by glucose infusion, although to a lesser extent (2.2-fold, p = 0.03). Infusion of both insulin and glucose (HGHI) had an additive effect on the adiponutrin expression

(10-fold, p = 0.008). In a pathological context, adiponutrin gene was highly expressed in the adipose tissue of type 1 diabetic patients with chronic hyperglycemia compared with healthy subjects. Conversely, adiponutrin gene expression was significantly reduced in type 2 diabetics (p = 0.01), but remained moderately regulated in these patients after the EGHI clamp (2.5-fold increase).

Conclusions: These results suggest a strong relationship between adiponutrin expression, insulin sensitivity, and glucose metabolism in human adipose tissue.

Adipose tissue is now universally considered an endocrine tissue which is able to synthesize several endocrine and paracrine factors [33]. To date, several studies have documented their direct role in insulin sensitivity and metabolism. The metabolic influence of adipose-tissue-derived adipokines should play an important role on the metabolic state in patients with type 1 diabetes, especially during puberty. In fact, it is well known that puberty is characterized by insulin resistance and increased insulin requirement. This study evaluated the relationship between a novel adipocyte-expressed transmembrane protein (adiponutrin) and insulin sensitivity and glucose metabolism. A clamp study with different insulin and/or glucose infusion was performed in healthy males, in adults with type 1 diabetes and in patients with type 2 diabetes; adiponutrin gene expression and modulation was evaluated in subcutaneous adipose tissue. It was shown that adiponutrin gene expression is markedly stimulated by insulin and hyperglycemia, although less efficiency was shown in diabetic subjects. Insulin was shown to amplify the glucose-mediated gene expression. Furthermore, adiponutrin gene expression was increased in patients with type 1 diabetes, reduced in patients with type 2 diabetes and unmodified in obese subjects. Although the physiological role of adiponutrin in metabolism remains to be completely clarified, this study gives a relevant contribution in understanding adiponutrin effects. According to these data, a complete explanation of the metabolic effects of this new transmembrane protein is further needed in order to clarify its role in glucose homeostasis of patients with type 1 diabetes.

Reviews

Cardiovascular risk reduction in high-risk pediatric patients: a scientific statement from the American Heart Association Expert Panel on Population and Prevention Science; the Councils on Cardiovascular Disease in the Young, Epidemiology and Prevention, Nutrition, Physical Activity and Metabolism, High Blood Pressure Research, Cardiovascular Nursing, and the Kidney in Heart Disease, and the Interdisciplinary Working Group on Quality of Care and Outcomes Research: endorsed by the American Academy of Pediatrics

Kavey RE, Allada V, Daniels SR, Hayman LL, McCrindle BW, Newburger JW, Parekh RS, Steinberger J
National Heart, Lung, and Blood Institute, NIH, Bethesda, Md., USA
Circulation 2006;114:2710–2738

Background: Although for most children the process of atherosclerosis is subclinical, dramatically accelerated atherosclerosis occurs in some pediatric disease states, with clinical coronary events occurring in childhood and very early adult life. As with most scientific statements about children and the future risk for cardiovascular disease (CVD), there are no randomized trials documenting the effects of risk reduction on hard clinical outcomes. A growing body of literature, however, identifies the importance of premature CVD in the course of certain pediatric diagnoses and addresses the response to risk factor reduction.

Methods and Results: For this scientific statement, a panel of experts reviewed what is known about very premature CVD in 8 high-risk pediatric diagnoses and, from the science base, developed practical recommendations for management of cardiovascular risk.

Several studies have demonstrated a clear association between CVD risk markers and risk of developing micro- and macrovascular complications in young patients with type 1 diabetes. Although evident during adulthood, it is universally accepted that atherosclerosis begins early in life [34]. In fact, the exposure during childhood to diabetes-related metabolic alterations may induce changes in the arteries contributing to the development of atherosclerosis in adulthood. Several new markers have been associated with atherosclerotic vascular changes. Evaluating the published studies on premature CVD in 8 high-risk pediatric conditions, this scientific statement, endorsed by the American Academy of Pediatrics, provides relevant recommendations for the detection of cardiovascular risk in conditions like type 1 and type 2 diabetes or familial hypercholesterolemia.

Food for thought

Effects of high-dose vitamin E supplementation on oxidative stress and microalbuminuria in young adult patients with childhood-onset type 1 diabetes mellitus

Giannini C, Lombardo F, Curro F, Pomilio M, Bucciarelli T, Chiarelli F, Mohn A
Department of Pediatrics, University of Chieti, Italy
amohn@unich.it
Diabetes Metab Res Rev 2007 Feb [Epub ahead of print]

Background: The aim of this study was to evaluate the effects of high-dose vitamin E supplementation (1,200 mg/day) on reducing both microalbuminuria (MA) and oxidative stress in patients with type 1 diabetes mellitus (T1DM) and persistent MA.

Methods: The authors performed a 12-month, randomized, placebo-controlled, double-blind cross-over trial in 10 young Caucasian adults (7 m/3 f; mean age 18.87 ± 2.91 years) with T1DM and persistent MA. At baseline and at the end of the treatment period, determination of albumin excretion rate (AER) and HbA1c and evaluation of the oxidant/antioxidant status were performed.

Results: At the beginning of the study, AER and HbA1c were not significantly different between the vitamin E and placebo group. No differences in terms of oxidant and antioxidant status were found between the two groups. This was associated with no significantly different urinary VEGF and TGF-β levels. After 6 months, no significant differences in AER were observed between the two groups ($p = 0.59$). However, plasma and LDL-vitamin E content were significantly higher in the vitamin E group compared to the placebo group ($p = 0.0001$ and $p = 0.004$, respectively). This was associated with a significantly longer lag phase ($p = 0.002$) and lower MDA ($p = 0.049$). However, no statistically significant differences were detected in terms of VEGF and TGF-β urinary levels.

Conclusions: These data demonstrate that high-dose vitamin E supplementation reduces markers of oxidative stress and improves antioxidant defense in young patients with T1DM. However, although it positively affects the oxidant/antioxidant status, vitamin E supplementation does not reduce AER in patients with T1DM and persistent MA.

Previous studies have clarified the role of chronic hyperglycemia on microvascular complications showing a direct positive correlation between poor metabolic control and the development of diabetes complications [11]. However, microvascular complications may also occur in some patients with satisfactory glycemic control; these observations have paved the way for better studying the mechanisms involved in endothelial dysfunction in order to provide new approaches to prevent or reduce microvascular damage in patients with type 1 diabetes. The present study investigated whether microalbuminuria and oxidative stress could be affected by high-dose vitamin E supplementation (1,200 mg/day) given orally, in a group of young adult patients with childhood-onset type 1 diabetes and persistent microalbuminuria. This is the first randomized, placebo-controlled, double-blind cross-over trial with vitamin E in young adult Caucasian patients with type 1 diabetes. Although the small sample size population is a major flaw of this study, it is clinically relevant that orally supplemented high-dose vitamin E has no effects on glomerular functional changes in patients with type 1 diabetes and persistent microalbuminuria. During the 6-month period, no significant changes in albumin excretion rate occurred. In the past decades, the pathophysiological course and anatomic changes which occur in diabetic kidney have been characterized, ruling out the importance role of microalbuminuria on predicting later overt diabetic nephropathy. Furthermore, several studies have shown that antioxidant treatment might reduce heart disease morbidity and mortality in the general population. It is well known that chronic hyperglycemia causes alteration in the oxidant/antioxidant status in patients with type 1 diabetes, especially in those with overt vascular complications. However, the lack of effects on albumin excretion rate in patients enrolled in this study show that antioxidant treatment allows a significant improvement in the oxidant-antioxidant status without affecting the established functional glomerular abnormalities. All patients enrolled in this study had persistent microalbuminuria, therefore limiting the conclusions of this study to this specific group of patients. Further studies are therefore needed to evaluate the effect of antioxidant treatment in patients with type 1 diabetes.

References

1. Tisch R, McDevitt H: Insulin-dependent diabetes mellitus. Cell 1996;85:291–297.
2. Rus H, Pardo CA, Hu L, Darrah E, Cudrici C, Niculescu T, et al: The voltage-gated potassium channel Kv1.3 is highly expressed on inflammatory infiltrates in multiple sclerosis brain. Proc Natl Acad Sci USA 2005;102:11094–11099.
3. Ryan EA, Bigam D, Shapiro AM: Current indications for pancreas or islet transplant. Diabetes Obes Metab 2006;8:1–7.
4. Tam PP, Williams EA, Chan WY: Gastrulation in the mouse embryo: ultrastructural and molecular aspects of germ layer morphogenesis. Microsc Res Tech 1993;26:301–328.
5. Liew CG, Moore H, Ruban L, Shah N, Cosgrove K, Dunne M, et al: Human embryonic stem cells: possibilities for human cell transplantation. Ann Med 2005;37:521–532.
6. Rother KI, Harlan DM: Challenges facing islet transplantation for the treatment of type 1 diabetes mellitus. J Clin Invest 2004;114:877–883.
7. Calafiore R: Alginate microcapsules for pancreatic islet cell graft immunoprotection: struggle and progress towards the final cure for type 1 diabetes mellitus. Expert Opin Biol Ther 2003;3:201–205.
8. Reichard P, Britz A, Carlsson P, Cars I, Lindblad L, Nilsson BY, et al: Metabolic control and complications over 3 years in patients with insulin-dependent diabetes (IDDM): the Stockholm Diabetes Intervention Study (SDIS). J Intern Med 1990;228:511–517.
9. Bangstad HJ, Osterby R, Dahl-Jorgensen K, Berg KJ, Hartmann A, Hanssen KF: Improvement of blood glucose control in IDDM patients retards the progression of morphological changes in early diabetic nephropathy. Diabetologia 1994;37:483–490.
10. Home PD, Alberti KG, Rodger NW, Burrin JM: Conference on insulin pump therapy in diabetes. Multicenter study of effect on microvascular disease. The Central Biochemistry Laboratory in the Multicenter Kroc Study. Problems and proposals. Diabetes 1985;34(suppl 3):17–21.
11. Diabetes Control and Complications Trial Research Group: The effect of intensive treatment of diabetes on the development and progression of long-term complications in insulin-dependent diabetes mellitus. N Engl J Med 1993;329:977–986.
12. Hirsch IB, Brownlee M: Should minimal blood glucose variability become the gold standard of glycemic control? J Diabetes Complications 2005;19:178–181.
13. American Diabetes Association: Postprandial blood glucose. Diabetes Care 2001;24:775–778.
14. Mauer M, Zinman B, Gardiner R, Drummond KN, Suissa S, Donnelly SM, et al: ACE-I and ARBs in early diabetic nephropathy. J Renin Angiotensin Aldosterone Syst 2002;3:262–269.
15. Amin R, Turner C, van Aken S, Bahu TK, Watts A, Lindsell DR, et al: The relationship between microalbuminuria and glomerular filtration rate in young type 1 diabetic subjects: the Oxford Regional Prospective Study. Kidney Int 2005;68:1740–1749.
16. O'Bryan GT, Hostetter TH: The renal hemodynamic basis of diabetic nephropathy. Semin Nephrol 1997;17:93–100.
17. Bak M, Thomsen K, Christiansen T, Flyvbjerg A: Renal enlargement precedes renal hyperfiltration in early experimental diabetes in rats. J Am Soc Nephrol 2000;11:1287–1292.
18. Dunger DB, Acerini CL: IGF-1 and diabetes in adolescence. Diabetes Metab 1998;24:101–107.
19. Skyler JS, Krischer JP, Wolfsdorf J, Cowie C, Palmer JP, Greenbaum C, et al: Effects of oral insulin in relatives of patients with type 1 diabetes: The Diabetes Prevention Trial – Type 1. Diabetes Care 2005;28:1068–1076.
20. Standards of medical care in diabetes – 2006. Diabetes Care 2006;29(suppl 1):S4–S42.
21. Heise T, Nosek L, Ronn BB, Endahl L, Heinemann L, Kapitza C, et al: Lower within-subject variability of insulin detemir in comparison to NPH insulin and insulin glargine in people with type 1 diabetes. Diabetes 2004;53:1614–1620.
22. Vague P, Selam JL, Skeie S, De Leeuw I, Elte JW, Haahr H, et al: Insulin detemir is associated with more predictable glycemic control and reduced risk of hypoglycemia than NPH insulin in patients with type 1 diabetes on a basal-bolus regimen with premeal insulin aspart. Diabetes Care 2003;26:590–596.
23. Hovorka R: Continuous glucose monitoring and closed-loop systems. Diabet Med 2006;23:1–12.
24. Soedamah-Muthu SS, Chaturvedi N, Toeller M, Ferriss B, Reboldi P, Michel G, et al: Risk factors for coronary heart disease in type 1 diabetic patients in Europe: the EURODIAB Prospective Complications Study. Diabetes Care 2004;27:530–537.
25. Management of dyslipidemia in children and adolescents with diabetes. Diabetes Care 2003;26:2194–2197.
26. Carrillo J, Puertas MC, Alba A, Ampudia RM, Pastor X, Planas R, et al: Islet-infiltrating B-cells in nonobese diabetic mice predominantly target nervous system elements. Diabetes 2005;54:69–77.
27. Cucca F, Lampis R, Congia M, Angius E, Nutland S, Bain SC, et al: A correlation between the relative predisposition of MHC class II alleles to type 1 diabetes and the structure of their proteins. Hum Mol Genet 2001;10:2025–2037.
28. Barratt BJ, Payne F, Lowe CE, Hermann R, Healy BC, Harold D, et al: Remapping the insulin gene/IDDM2 locus in type 1 diabetes. Diabetes 2004;53:1884–1889.
29. Ueda H, Howson JM, Esposito L, Heward J, Snook H, Chamberlain G, et al: Association of the T-cell regulatory gene CTLA4 with susceptibility to autoimmune disease. Nature 2003;423:506–511.
30. Smyth D, Cooper JD, Collins JE, Heward JM, Franklyn JA, Howson JM, et al: Replication of an association between the lymphoid tyrosine phosphatase locus (LYP/PTPN22) with type 1 diabetes, and evidence for its role as a general autoimmunity locus. Diabetes 2004;53:3020–3023.

31. Vella A, Cooper JD, Lowe CE, Walker N, Nutland S, Widmer B, et al: Localization of a type 1 diabetes locus in the IL2RA/CD25 region by use of tag single-nucleotide polymorphisms. Am J Hum Genet 2005;76:773–779.
32. Pearson ER, Flechtner I, Njolstad PR, Malecki MT, Flanagan SE, Larkin B, et al: Switching from insulin to oral sulfonylureas in patients with diabetes due to Kir6.2 mutations. N Engl J Med 2006;355:467–477.
33. Trayhurn P, Wood IS: Adipokines: inflammation and the pleiotropic role of white adipose tissue. Br J Nutr 2004;92: 347–355.
34. Kavey RE, Daniels SR, Lauer RM, Atkins DL, Hayman LL, Taubert K: American Heart Association guidelines for primary prevention of atherosclerotic cardiovascular disease beginning in childhood. Circulation 2003;107:1562–1566.

Obesity and Weight Regulation

Martin Wabitsch, Malaika Fuchs, Sina Horenburg, Christian Denzer,
Julia von Puttkamer, Anja Moss, Georgia Lahr and Pamela Fischer-Posovszky

Pediatric Endocrinology, Diabetes and Obesity Unit, Department of Pediatrics and Adolescent Medicine,
University of Ulm, Ulm, Germany

The last 12 months have shown once more that obesity and weight regulation are among the most interesting biomedical fields of science. The number of high-quality papers reflects the multiple research activities which now can be documented at many places around the world. The last 12 months have also demonstrated that different governments in Europe have taken over some responsibility of the obesity epidemic as demonstrated by the European Charter on counteracting obesity (www.iotf.org). The aim of the Charter is to address the growing challenge posed by the epidemic of obesity on health, economies and development. The Charter has been established by the WHO European Ministerial Conference on Counteracting Obesity (Istanbul, Turkey, November 15–17, 2006). It acknowledges that the prevalence of obesity has risen up to threefold in the last two decades. Half of all adults and 1 in 5 children in the WHO European Region are overweight. Of these, one third is already obese, and numbers are increasing fast. Overweight and obesity contribute to a large proportion of non-communicable diseases, shortening life expectancy and adversely affecting the quality of life. More than 1 million deaths in the Region annually are due to diseases related to excess body weight. The trend is particularly alarming in children and adolescents, thus passing the epidemic into adulthood and creating a growing health burden for the next generation. The annual rate of increase in the prevalence of childhood obesity has been rising steadily and is currently up to ten times higher than it was in 1970. This Charter will also help scientists and physicians to stimulate experimental and clinical studies as well as preventive activities in their countries. This Charter should be known by every ESPE member.

For the yearbook selection this year, only articles published in journals with an impact factor of more than 4 were considered, assuming that relevant findings were published in these journals. The top findings of the last year lay within the areas of endocrinology of body weight regulation and endocrinology of the adipocyte. Two well-written reviews which are not included as an extensive summary are mentioned here:

Genetics of obesity in humans

Farooqi IS, O'Rahilly S
University Departments of Medicine and Clinical Biochemistry, Addenbrooke's Hospital, Cambridge, UK
So104@medschl.cam.ac.uk
Endocr Rev 2006;27:710–718

In this review, human monogenic obesity syndromes with single gene defects that disrupt the molecules in the leptin-melanocortin pathway are reviewed. It is then shown how far the characterization of these patients has improved our understanding of the physiological role of leptin and the melanocortins in the regulation of human body weight and neuroendocrine function. The discovery of these genetic disorders has helped destigmatize human obesity and allow it to be seen as a medical condition rather than simply a moral failing. The genetic defects found to date all affect the drive to eat, resulting in hyperphagia in affected subjects. Thus, human food intake should not be considered as an entirely voluntarily controllable phenomenon, but rather one driven by powerful biological signals. It is likely that further discovery of causative genetic defects in humans and experimental animals will continue to highlight other molecular elements of the pathways involved in the regulation of body weight.

Emerging therapeutic strategies for obesity

Foster-Schubert KE, Cummings DE
University of Washington, Veterans Administration Puget Sound Health Care System, Seattle, Wash., USA
davidec@u.washington.edu
Endocr Rev 2006;27:779–793

Medications approved so far to treat obesity promote no more than 5–7% loss of body weight, which is a drop in the ocean for the severely obese. New conceptual strategies are desperately needed. This review provides an expanding list of molecular targets for novel, rationally designed anti-obesity phar- maceuticals. Many of the target molecules which we have described in earlier yearbooks [1–3] are included and open new hope for the development of better anti-obesity medications. Dieting and exer- cise remain the cornerstones of obesity therapy. However, more effective medicines to augment the impact of these efforts would be welcome among obese individuals as they fight against their energy homeostasis systems.

BMI z-score in children and risk factors

Increasing body mass index z-score is continuously associated with complications of overweight in children, even in the healthy weight range

Bell LM, Byrne S, Thompson A, Ratnam N, Blair E, Bulsara M, Jones TW, Davis EA
Princess Margaret Hospital, Subiaco, W.A., Australia
Elizabeth.davis@health.wa.gov.au
J Clin Endocrinol Metab 2007;92:517–522

Background: Most analyses of the complications of childhood overweight and obesity have categorized both child's weight (e.g. 'obese' or 'overweight') and the complications (e.g. 'presence' or 'absence') using arbitrary, percentile-based criteria. This study has the aim to show that BMI z-score is a continu- ous variable associated with risk factors and complications.
Methods: A total of 177 children were recruited from the community- and hospital-based arms of a larger growth and development study at the University of Western Australia. Children were recruited from the community through randomly selected primary schools. Overweight children seeking treatment were recruited through tertiary senders.
Results: Adjusted regression analysis showed that there was a linear relationship with BMI z-scores of sys- tolic and diastolic blood pressure, fasting insulin, and ALT and a curvilinear relationship with insulin concentrations at 60 and 120 min of the oral glucose tolerance test, fasting C-peptide, HDL cholesterol and triglycerides, demonstrating a more unfavorable profile at the extremes of BMI z-score. In addi- tion, musculoskeletal pain, obstructive sleep apnea symptoms, headaches, depression, anxiety, bullying, and acanthosis nigricans increased with child BMI z-score.
Conclusion: The z-score of the children was related to complications of overweight and obesity in a linear or curvilinear fashion, most complications increase across the entire range of BMI values and are not defined by thresholds.

This is one of the few studies showing that the risk of comorbidity in children is seen to increase con- tinuously across the whole spectrum of childhood BMI z-scores, and is not limited to obese subjects. A child's BMI z-score is independently linearly or curvilinearly related to insulin resistance, liver enzymes and many medical complications. Interestingly, even in the so-called normal range of BMI this progression of risk factors is evident. These findings support recent recommendations of pedi- atric societies to screen children with an elevated BMI z-score for the occurrence of risk factors and complications. The threshold for such a screening might be lower than originally thought. In fact, this study tells us that all children, overweight or not, need to exercise and control their diet. Since the ethnical background is important for the occurrence of risk factors in association with increasing BMI z-scores in children, it is important that each country defines thresholds for such clinic programs on the basis of its own epidemiological data. The finding of this study will have implications for public health programs since it is obvious that decreasing the BMI of whole populations of children will decrease future disease burden.

Separation of human adipocytes by size: hypertrophic fat cells display distinct gene expression

Jernas M, Palming J, Sjöholm K, Jennische E, Svensson PA, Gabrielsson BG, Levin M, Sjögren A, Rudemo M, Lystig TC, Carlsson B, Carlsson LMS, Lönn M
Research Centre for Endocrinology and Metabolism, Division of Body Composition and Metabolism, Department of Internal Medicine, Göteborg, Sweden
Malin.lonn@medic.gu.se
FASEB J 2006;20:1540–1542

Background: Adipocytes are known to release a variety of factors including cytokines, chemokines, and other biologically active molecules, commonly called adipokines. Obese individuals are known to exhibit elevated circulating levels of inflammation markers closely related to adipokines secreted in adipose tissue. A few studies have suggested that cytokine release within adipose tissue correlates with adipocyte size.
Methods: Adipocytes were isolated from subcutaneous adipose tissue samples. Separation of two adipocyte fractions with different size was achieved by several steps using suspension, washing, and filtrations. Microarray analysis of gene expression in small and large adipocytes was performed.
Results: 14 genes have been identified with a more than 4-fold expression in large cells as compared to small cells. Two of these genes were serum amyloid A (SAA) and transmembrane 4 L six family member 1 (TM4SF1) which were 19- and 22-fold higher expressed in large cells.
Conclusion: This study has identified genes with markedly higher expression in large, compared with small human adipocytes. These genes may link hypertrophic obesity to insulin resistance and type 2 diabetes.

Relationship between adipocyte size and adipokine expression and secretion

Skurk T, Alberti-Huber C, Herder C, Hauner H
Else Kröner-Fresenius Centre for Nutritional Medicine, Technical University Munich, Freising-Weihenstephan, Germany
Nutritional.medicine@wzw.tum.de
J Clin Endocrin Metab 2007;92:1023–1033

Background: Adipocytes are known to release factors that may contribute to the proinflammatory state characteristic for obesity. The study was performed to get a better insight into possible underlying mechanisms investigating the effect of adipocyte size on adipokine production and secretion.
Methods: Adipose tissue was obtained from individuals undergoing elective plastic surgery. Isolated adipocytes were separated into four fractions (small, medium, large, and very large) by flotation. Adipokine release into medium was measured by highly sensitive sandwich ELISAs, and mRNA expression of adipokines was measured after RNA isolation from isolated cells.
Results: The secretion of the adipokines leptin, IL-6, IL-8, TNF-α, MCP-1, IP-10, MIP-1β, G-CSF, IL-1ra, and adiponectin was positively correlated with the size of the adipocytes. After correction for cell surface, there was still a significant difference for leptin, IL-6, IL-8, MCP-1, and G-CSF between very large and small cells.
Conclusion: The fractionation of adipocytes according to cell size revealed that the very large adipocytes show a markedly impaired adipokine secretion which may promote inflammation in human adipose tissue.

The above-mentioned papers showed two simple methods for separating human adipocytes from adipose tissue samples into several populations according to their size. The findings in these two studies provide novel insight into the molecular connection between hypertrophic obesity and insulin resistance as well as type 2 diabetes. Obesity is characterized by an increase in fat cell number and fat cell size. Human fat cells can change 20-fold in diameter and several thousand-fold in volume. The hypertrophy of adipocytes in obese patients has been suggested to be critical for the occurrence of a chronic inflammatory state. Originally, Weisberg et al. [4] showed that with increasing adipocyte size the proportion of cells expressing CD68, a macrophage marker, increases in human adipose tissue. It has recently also been shown that adipocyte size correlates strongly with circulating leptin levels [5–7]. In turn, weight loss results in a reduced adipocyte volume and a subsequent alteration in secretary activity, e.g. for leptin.

Adipocyte hypertrophy appears to cause a differentially impaired secretion between pro- and anti-inflammatory adipokines shifting the immunological balance towards the expression of proinflammatory proteins. It appears desirable to prevent adipocyte hypertrophy and/or to strive for a rapid removal of enlarged adipocytes.

The relationship between adipocyte size and macrophage accumulation suggests that hypertrophic adipocytes secrete factors that attract monocytes. The acute-phase protein serum amyloid A (SAA) is derived from hypertrophic adipocytes and may be involved in the process of attracting monocytes because SAA activates the chemotactic formyl peptide receptor like-1, which results in migration of blood monocytes and neutrophils [8, 9]. IL-8, also found to be expressed at high levels in hypertrophic adipocytes, may act as another potential monocyte recruiting factor in adipose tissue. Accumulation of macrophages in adipose tissue is likely to further increase the levels of inflammatory cytokines in adipose tissue and thereby increase insulin resistance [10].

Lipases: hormone-sensitive lipase is not the only one

Variation in the adiponutrin gene influences its expression and associates with obesity

Johansson LE, Hoffstedt J, Parikh H, Carlsson E, Wabitsch M, Bondeson AG, Hedenbro J, Tornqvist H, Groop L, Ridderstrale M
Department of Clinical Sciences Malmö, Clinical Obesity, Lund University, Wallenberg Laboratory, Malmö University Hospital, Malmö, Sweden
Lovisa.johansson@med.lu.se
Diabetes 2006;55:826–833

Background: Recent findings have identified three different proteins that seem to complement hormone-sensitive lipase (HSL), concerning triacylglycerol hydrolysis. One of these proteins is a membrane-associated protein called adiponutrin. The aim of the present study was to investigate the expression of adiponutrin in human obesity and its regulation in human adipocytes. Furthermore, it has been studied whether polymorphisms in the gene are associated with mRNA expression and function.

Results: Experiments in human adipocytes (SGBS cells) confirmed that the gene is upregulated in response to insulin in a glucose-dependent fashion. Adiponutrin mRNA expression levels are increased in obese subjects in subcutaneous and visceral adipose tissue. Two polymorphisms of adiponutrin have been identified showing an association with obesity. Carriers of these polymorphisms showed a lower adiponutrin mRNA expression and an increased basal lipolysis.

Conclusion: Genetic variation in adiponutrin is associated with obesity. The gene is upregulated in obese subjects. Its regulation is dependent on insulin and glucose. The results suggest that adiponutrin plays a so far unknown important role in the regulation of lipolysis and seems to be a candidate gene for obesity.

The release of energy from an adipocyte is controlled mostly by insulin, cortisol, growth hormone, and catecholamines, regulating the rate of lipolysis. So far, HSL has been believed to be the rate-limiting enzyme in the lipolytic process. Recently, three other proteins have been identified which participate in triacylglycerol hydrolysis at least under non-stimulated conditions. These proteins also exhibit transacylase activity in the catabolism of branched-chain amino acids [11–15].

The observation that HSL knockout mice retain a lean phenotype, residual lipase activity, and accumulation of diacylglycerol rather than triacylglycerol supports the hypothesis of the existence of complementary lipases.

Adiponutrin, which is identical to calcium-independent phospholipase $A_{2\varepsilon}$, along with two other recently discovered lipases, desnutrin (identical to adipose triglyceride lipase or $iPLA_{2\zeta}$) and GS-2 (identical to $iPLA_{2\eta}$), are prime candidates for this lipase activity.

The results of the present study show that adiponutrin is a candidate for an important player in the regulation of basal adipocyte lipolysis. The effect of carbohydrates on *adiponutrin gene* mRNA expression is dependent on insulin. The relative contribution of this lipase requires however further investigations. In particular, the associations of obesity with two polymorphisms in adiponutrin should be viewed with caution until replicated in other populations.

Adipose tissue: reviews on new functions of the bodies energy store

Adipocytes as regulators of energy balance and glucose homeostasis

Rosen ED, Spiegelman BM
Dana-Farber Cancer Institute, Boston, Mass., USA
Bruce_spiegelman@dfci.harvard.edu
Nature 2006;444:847–885

Role of adipose tissue as an inflammatory organ in human diseases

Schäffler A, Müller-Ladner U, Schölmerich J, Büchler C
Department of Internal Medicine 1, University of Regensburg, Regensburg, Germany
Andreas.schaeffler@klinik.uni-regensburg.de
Endocrine Reviews 2006;27:449–467

Adipose tissue: from lipid storage compartment to endocrine organ

Scherer PE
Diabetes Research and Training Center, Albert Einstein College of Medicine, Bronx, N.Y., USA
scherer@aecom.yu.edu
Diabetes 2006;55:1537–1545

These three reviews are high-quality papers summarizing and interpreting recent findings on adipose tissue biology.

The review by Philip E. Scherer represents the Lilly lecture 2005. It summarizes findings on recently discovered adipokines and the secretory pathway of adipocytes. Furthermore, it shows the physiological impact of an acute loss of adipose tissue in relation to the consecutive lack of adipokines.

The review by Rosen and Spiegelman shows that adipose tissue serves as a crucial integrator of glucose homeostasis. It briefly examines the transcriptional basis of adipocyte development, and discusses energy homeostasis in mammals and how adipocytes regulate components of that system. The authors provide evidence that adipocytes have a crucial role in regulating glucose homeostasis through a series of endocrine and non-endocrine mechanisms. These involve adipose-derived secreted molecules, known as adipokines, neural connections and changes in whole-body physiology. Adipocytes have been a popular model for studying cell differentiation since the development of the murine adipose 3T3 cell culture system by Green and colleagues. Recently a human pre-adipocyte cell strain has been characterized with high capacity for adipocyte differentiation [16]. These cells now represent a unique model for studying human adipocyte differentiation and adipocyte biology, especially the regulation of adipokines. In the past decade, adipose tissue has moved from being a minor participant to having a central role in diverse homeostatic processes. These findings led to the idea that manipulation of adipocyte biology may be a useful therapeutic strategy in metabolic diseases, such as obesity and type 2 diabetes. Enhancement of leptin and adiponectin synthesis, and secretion and promotion of intra-adipocyte lipid oxidation are examples of approaches that might be expected to benefit patients.

Finally, the review by Schäffler et al. addresses the inflammatory role of adipose tissue outside the field of metabolism. In contrast to numerous and excellent publications describing the role of adipose tissue and adipokines in metabolism, reviews on the inflammatory role of adipose tissue outside this field are rare. The review summarizes and discusses the inflammatory role of adipocytokines and special types of regional adipocytes, such as retroorbital, synovial, visceral, subdermal, peritoneal, and bone marrow adipocytes in different diseases, demonstrating another new and important role of the fat cell.

It remains to be seen how well we will translate these discoveries to our patients, but hopes for breakthrough therapies for obesity and diabetes are as high as they have ever been.

Central regulation of energy homeostasis – some new findings

Identification of nesfatin-1 as a satiety molecule in the hypothalamus

Oh-I S, Shimizu H, Satoh T, Okada S, Adachi S, Inoue K, Eguchi H, Yamamoto M, Imaki T, Hashimoto K, Tsuchiya T, Monden T, Horiguchi K, Yamada M, Mori M

Department of Medicine and Molecular Science, Gunma University Graduate School of Medicine, Maebashi, Japan
mmori@med.gunma-u.ac.jp
Nature 2006;443:709–712

Background: The brain hypothalamus contains certain secreted molecules that are important in regulating feeding behavior. Most of these molecules are also expressed in peripheral adipose tissue.

Methods: It was attempted to identify any new appetite-regulating molecule by using a subtraction-cloning assay of peroxisome proliferator-activated receptor-γ activator-stimulated genes in SQ-5 cells. The aim of the present study was to identify such new genes expressed in both brain medulloblastoma and 3T3-L1 adipocyte cells.

Results: Nine genes meeting these criteria were identified. Sequencing of the gene with the most profound stimulation by troglitazone demonstrated that it corresponds to a gene encoding DNA-binding/ EF-hand/acidic protein (NEFA) or NUCB2. NUCB2 is composed of a signal peptide of 24 amino acids and a protein structure containing 396 amino acids. The homology of the amino-acid sequence of NUCB2 is highly conserved in humans, mice and rats. NUCB2 belongs to a homologous gene family together with nucleobindin1 (NUCB1). These two genes might have arisen from a single EF-hand ancestor and are so far of unknown function. NUCB2 is expressed in the appetite-control hypothalamic nuclei in rats. Nesfatin-1, an amino-terminal fragment derived from NUCB2, is present in cerebrospinal fluid and its expression is decreased under starvation. Injection of nesfatin-1 intracerebroventricularly decreases food intake in a dose-dependent manner. Conversion of NUCB2 to nesfatin-1 is necessary to induce feeding suppression. Nesfatin-1-induced anorexia in Zucker rats carrying a leptin-receptor mutation, and an anti-nesfatin-1 antibody, does not block leptin-induced anorexia. Furthermore, α-MSH elevates NUCB2 gene expression, and satiety by nesfatin-1 is abolished by an antagonist of the melanocortin-3/4 receptor.

Conclusion: This paper shows that nesfatin-1 is a newly discovered satiety molecule that is associated with melanocortin signalling in the hypothalamus.

This work has identified a novel anorexigenic molecule, nesfatin, derived from NUCB2 in the hypothalamus. NUCB2 is as a prohormone that can be processed to generate bioactive fragments, such as nesfatin-1, located in the N-terminus of NUCB2. This molecule induces satiety. Nesfatin-1 might be a potential target for the development of drug therapies to treat obese persons.

There are complex but integrated interconnections among the hypothalamic nuclei in regulating feeding. Leptin and proopiomelanocortin (POMC)-derived α-MSH are key anorectic molecules in the hypothalamus. Studies in Zucker rats indicate a possible lack of involvement of hypothalamic leptin signalling in the induction of anorexia by nesfatin-1. In contrast, central injection of α-MSH stimulated the expression of NUCB2. Furthermore, an antagonist specific for the melanocortin-3/4 receptor abolished nesfatin-1-induced satiety. These findings show that hypothalamic nesfatin-1 signalling might involve a leptin-independent melanocortin signalling system.

Since nesfatin-1 might also be secreted by adipocytes it will be important to study its regulation and its possible involvement in the cross-talk between the energy stores of the body and the central regulatory system for energy balance.

Critical role for peptide YY in protein-mediated satiation and body-weight regulation

Batterham RL, Heffron H, Kapoor S, Chivers JE, Chandarana K, Herzog H, Le Roux CW, Thomas EL, Bell JD, Withers DJ

Centre for Diabetes and Endocrinology, Department of Medicine, University College London, UK
r.batterham@ucl.ac.uk

Cell Metabolism 2006;4:223–233

Background: The satiating effect of dietary protein requires the gut-endocrine axis, since suppression of food intake is observed only when protein is administered enterally. It is not yet clear which hormones are involved in the transmission of this specific signal. Therefore, studies in normal and obese humans as well as in rodents were performed to investigate the effect of meal macronutrient composition on hunger scores and plasma concentrations of candidate hormones as there are PYY, ghrelin and GLP-1.
Results: In normal-weight and obese humans high-protein intake induced the greatest release of the anorectic hormone peptide YY (PYY) and the most pronounced satiety. When mice were fed with increased amounts of dietary protein, increased plasma PYY levels, decreased food intake, and reduced adiposity were found. In PYY null mice, protein had no satiating or weight-reducing effect, however treatment with exogenous PYY resulted in comparable effects as the high-protein diet in normal mice.
Conclusions: These results suggest that PYY is responsible for the satiating effect of dietary protein. Furthermore, it can be hypothesized that modulating the release of endogenous PYY through alteration of the diet could help to treat obesity more efficiently.

High-protein content meals have been shown to increase satiety and decrease food intake [17–19], resulting in both improved weight loss and weight loss maintenance [20–22]. Recently a number of gut-derived hormonal signals have been characterized [2]. PYY is produced by intestinal L-cells and is released into circulation after food intake. Circulating PYY3-36 inhibits appetite by acting directly on the arcuate nucleus via the Y2-receptor to which the hormone has a high affinity.

The present investigations aimed at understanding the effects of macronutrients on satiation and body weight in humans. They demonstrated that high-protein meals caused the greatest reduction in hunger coupled with the greatest increase in PYY. In the performed rodent studies, further support was generated for the hypothesis that PYY is a specific signal for the protein content of the diet. PYY null mice were resistant to the satiating effects of high-protein diets. In contrast, altering the fat and carbohydrate content of the diets while keeping the protein content constant resulted in a similar change in feeding, suggesting that deletion of PYY specifically affects the satiating effects of proteins. Further studies in humans are required to show that this specific effect of PYY can be critical for long-term body weight development.

Clinical and molecular genetic spectrum of congenital deficiency of the leptin receptor

Farooqi SI, Wangensteen T, Collins S, Kimber W, Matarese G, Keogh JM, Lank E, Bottomley B, Lopez-Fernandez J, Ferraz-Amaro I, Dattani MT, Ercan O, Myhre AG, Retterstol L, Stanhope R, Edge JA, McKenzie S, Lessan N, Ghodsi M, De Rosa V, Perna F, Fontana S, Barroso I, Undlien DE, O'Rahilly S

University Department of Clinical Biochemistry, Addenbrooke's Hospital, Cambridge, UK
lsf20@cam.ac.uk

N Engl J Med 2007;356:237–247

Background: So far only one mutation in the leptin-receptor gene (LEPR) has been reported. The 3 patients are characterized by severe early-onset obesity and very elevated serum leptin levels. The present study determined the prevalence of pathogenic mutations in the leptin receptor in a large cohort of patients with severe, early-onset obesity.
Methods: The leptin receptor was sequenced in 300 patients, characterized by severe obesity of early-onset (90 subjects out of a cohort from consanguineous families). Evaluation of metabolic, endocrine, and immune function in affected probands, relatives and controls was performed.
Results: Five nonsense and four missense mutations in 8 of the 300 patients were identified. The missense mutations resulted all in impaired receptor signalling. The phenotype of the affected subjects was characterized by hyperphagia, severe and early-onset obesity, delayed puberty, as well as alterations in the

immune function. Interestingly in these cases, serum leptin levels were within the range given for the elevated fat mass.

The mean BMI standard deviation score for the affected subjects was 5.1 ± 1.6, as compared with 6.8 ± 2.1 for subjects with congenital leptin deficiency and 5.0 ± 1.5 for MC4R-deficient subjects.

Conclusions: In this cohort of patients with severe obesity the prevalence of pathogenic leptin-receptor mutations was about 3%. Therefore, congenital leptin-receptor deficiency should be considered in the differential diagnosis in any child with hyperphagia and severe obesity.

Although the prevalence of leptin-receptor mutations in this highly selected cohort is unlikely to reflect that in unrelated populations of obese subjects or in populations in which the age and the onset of obesity is more heterogeneous, the diagnosis of a pathogenic leptin-receptor mutation should be considered in children of early-onset extreme obesity, hyperphagia and eventually also in adolescents with extreme obesity and delayed puberty.

All frameshift mutations occurred in the N-terminal domain of the leptin receptor and were predicted to result in the loss of all leptin-receptor isoforms. The authors examined the functional properties of receptors with missense mutations and could show that in three of the missense mutations a complete loss of signalling (leptin-stimulated phosphorylation of STAT3) was found, whereas one missense mutation encodes a receptor with some residual ability to phosphorylate STAT3 in response to leptin.

The clinical phenotype of the affected patients was impressing: during an ad libitum test meal the probands with leptin-receptor mutations consumed almost three times the amount of energy that control subjects consumed. Interestingly, all 4 adults (all of them were female) had clinical evidence of hypogonadism, with a lack of pubertal growth spurt and reduced expression of secondary sexual characteristics; 3 had no menses until after 20 years of age. Furthermore, the children among them had more frequent childhood infections than did their siblings with wild-type leptin receptor. The premature deaths of 2 obese children in these families were associated with acute respiratory tract infections. It may be worth mentioning that leptin-deficient ob/ob mice exhibit several metabolic and immune abnormalities, including thymus atrophy and markedly reduced inflammatory responses, and that leptin normalized the metabolic, immune and inflammatory parameters in ob/ob mice.

Classically, patients with genetic obesity syndromes have been identified in childhood as a result of associated mental retardation and developmental abnormalities. In the present monogenetic disorders with leptin-receptor deficiency, obesity itself is the predominant presenting feature. This is comparable to cases with monogenetic disorders as leptin deficiency or melanocortin-4-receptor deficiency. These disorders result from disruption of the hypothalamic leptin-melanocortin signalling pathway. The described phenotypes of the subjects with leptin-receptor deficiency are comparable to the characteristic features of leptin deficiency including hyperphagia, obesity, hypogonadism, and impaired T-cell-mediated immunity.

The enemy is inside us – gut bacteria and weight gain

An obesity-associated gut microbiome with increased capacity for energy harvest

Turnbaugh PJ, Ley RE, Mahowald MA, Magrini V, Mardis ER, Gordon JI
Center for Genome Sciences, Washington University, St. Louis, Mo., USA
Jgordon@wustl.edu
Nature 2006;444:1027–1031

Background: The understanding of energy balance is the basis for the understanding of the development of obesity. The present article presents studies which determined if microbial community gene content correlates with and is a potential contributing factor to obesity in mice.

Methods: Distal gut microbiomes of ob/ob, ob/+ and +/+ littermates by random shot sequencing of their cecal microbial DNA were characterized. The predicted increased capacity for dietary energy harvest by the ob/ob microbiome was subsequently validated using biochemical assays and by transplantation of lean and obese cecal microbiotas into germ-free wild-type mouse recipients.

Results: Changes in relative abundance of two dominant bacterial divisions, the Bacteroidetes and the Firmicutes have been found in association with genetically obese mice (decreased ratio Bacteroidetes/Firmicutes) and their lean littermates (increased ratio Bacteroidetes/Firmicutes). Through metagenomic and biochemical analysis it has been shown that these changes affect the metabolic potential of the mouse gut microbiota. The microbiomes of obese mice have an increased capacity to harvest energy from the diet. Interestingly, this trait is transmissible and germ-free mice colonized with the microbiota show increases in their total body fat.

Conclusion: The results identified gut microbiota as an additional contributing factor to the pathophysiology of body weight regulation.

Human gut microbes associated with obesity

Ley RE, Turnbaugh PJ, Klein S, Gordon JI
Washington University School of Medicine, St. Louis, Mo., USA
Jgordon@wustl.edu
Nature 2006;444:1022–1023

Background: Two groups of beneficial bacteria are dominant in the human gut, the Bacteroidetes and the Firmicutes. Earlier findings have proposed that the microbiota of obese individuals may be more efficient at extracting energy from a given diet than microbiota of lean individuals.

Methods: To investigate the relation between gut microbial ecology and body fat in humans, 12 obese people were studied on either a fat-restricted or a carbohydrate-restricted low-calorie diet. The composition of the gut microbiota was monitored over the course of 1 year by sequencing 16S ribosomal RNA genes from the stool samples.

Results: The relative proportion of Bacteroidetes is decreased in obese people when compared to lean people. The proportion of Bacteroidetes increases with weight loss on two types of low-calorie diet.

Conclusion: The findings indicate that obesity has a microbial component which might have potential therapeutic implications.

Much has been written about the sequencing of the human genome. However, our own genome is not the only one with which we need to be concerned. The human 'metagenome' is a composite of *Homo sapiens* genes and genes present in the genomes of the trillions of microbes that colonize our adult bodies. The latter genes are thought to outnumber the former by several orders of magnitude [23]. Our microbial genomes (the microbiome) encode metabolic capacities that have not evolved wholly on their own and remain largely unexplored. These include degradation of otherwise indigestible components of our diet, and therefore may have an impact on our energy balance.

The Firmicutes and the Bacteroidetes are divisions within the domain bacteria. The microbiota of the human gut is dominated by their members, most of which are benign. The Firmicutes is the largest bacterial phylum and contains more than 250 genera, including *Lactobacillus*, *Mycoplasma*, *Bacillus* and *Clostridium*. The Bacteroidetes include about 20 genera.

Colonization of adult germ-free mice with a distal gut microbial community harvested from conventionally raised mice produces a dramatic increase in body fat within 10–14 days, despite an associated decrease in food consumption. The change involves several linked mechanisms: microbial fermentation of dietary polysaccharides that cannot be digested by the host, subsequent intestinal absorption of monosaccharides and short-chain fatty acids, their conversion to more complex lipids in the liver and microbial regulation of host genes that promote deposition of the lipids in adipocytes.

The work described in the two articles raises the possibility that our gut bacteria is another factor that contributes to differences in body weight among individuals. The reports suggest that the differences in the efficiency of caloric extraction from food may be determined by the composition of the microbiota which in turn may contribute to differential body weights.

This is a potentially revolutionary idea that could change our views of what causes obesity and how we depend on the bacteria that inhabit our gut. However, many questions remain unanswered. Most notably, it is not clear whether such small changes in caloric extraction can actually contribute to the meaningful differences in body weight in humans. Furthermore, the questions about how and why the composition of gut microbiota is regulated will have to be answered. After these answers we are tempted to consider how we might manipulate the microbiotic environment to treat or prevent obesity.

The two papers open up an intriguing line of scientific inquiry that will allay microbiologists with nutritionists, physiologists and neuroscientists in the fight against obesity.

Obesity in Children and Adolescents: recent treatment trials

Randomised, controlled trial of metformin for obesity and insulin resistance in children and adolescents: improvement in body composition and fasting insulin

Srinivasan S, Ambler GR, Baur LA, Garnett SP, Tepsa M, Yap F, Ward GM, Cowell CT
Institute of Endocrinology and Diabetes, The Children's Hospital at Westmead, Westmead, N.S.W., Australia
Shubhas@chw.edu.au
J Clin Endocrinol Metab 2006;9:2074–2080

Background: Insulin resistance associated with obesity in children and adolescents has become an increasing challenge in pediatric endocrinology. Metformin is a well-established, oral hypoglycemic agent in the treatment of adults with type 2 diabetes and other conditions with insulin resistance. The aim of the present study was to clarify the role of metformin therapy in pediatric patients with obesity.
Methods: 28 patients (13 males) aged 9–18 years were included in a crossover, randomized, controlled trial. The advantage of this kind of study design is that each patient acts as his own control, thereby minimizing inaccuracies in case-control matching and variability in adherence between patients on metformin vs. placebo.
Results: Metformin showed a significant treatment effect over placebo for weight (difference −4.35 kg), for body mass index (−1.26 kg/m^2), for waist circumference (difference −2.8 cm). Subcutaneous abdominal adipose tissue (MRI) was also significantly reduced, whereas visceral abdominal adipose tissue was not differentially influenced by the treatment. Fasting insulin decreased more than in the placebo group (difference −2.2 mU/l).
Conclusion: The study demonstrates that metformin therapy for insulin resistance in obese children and adolescents is safe and well tolerated and has a beneficial effect on weight, BMI, waist circumference, subcutaneous abdominal fat, and fasting insulin.

The beneficial role of metformin in young patients with type 2 diabetes has been demonstrated in a randomized, controlled trial [24]. Metformin is also beneficial in pediatric patients with type 1 diabetes mellitus and insulin resistance [25–27]. There is also a positive treatment effect of metformin on girls with polycystic ovarian syndrome [28–31] and on children with non-alcoholic fatty liver disease [32]. The primary mechanism of action of metformin is by suppression of hepatic glucose production through activation of the insulin receptor, preferentially through insulin receptor substrate-2.

The effect on weight loss and insulin concentrations in obese children was first shown in a study by Lutjens and Smit [33]. Subsequent studies in children have shown that metformin is able to improve body mass index, fasting serum glucose, insulin, lipid profile.

In the present study a number of patients had also improved insulin sensitivity as measured by the minimal model, this however did not reach statistical significance. This might be due to the small number of patients and due to the fact that several patients underwent a change in their pubertal stage which is associated with a change in the physiological insulin resistance.

This double-blind, placebo-controlled, crossover trial increases our knowledge about effectiveness and safety of metformin (2 × 1 g/day) in children and adolescents with insulin resistance associated with obesity. The study results help to guide the clinician in the management of insulin resistance. The impact of metformin and any other drug tested so far was around 5% weight loss. There seems to be an inhibiting mechanism to surpass that magic number.

This study has to be taken in the right context: a very small cohort of obese children with questionable compliance to therapy. Several other studies, albeit less strict in their design, failed to show a positive metformin effect on either weight or insulin resistance.

The effect of sibutramine on energy expenditure and body composition in obese adolescents

Van Mil E, Westerterp KR, Kester ADM, Delemarre-van de Waal HA, Gerver WJM, Saris WHM
Department of Pediatrics, Subdivision of Pediatric Endocrinology, VU University Medical Center, Amsterdam, The Netherlands
e.vanmil@vumc.nl

J Clin Endocrinol Metab 2007;92:1409–1414

Background: Recently, two randomized controlled trials in obese adolescents were published, demonstrating the additional effect of sibutramine in a 6-month treating program comprising changing the daily diet and increasing daily physical activity. The present study was designed to evaluate the effect of sibutramine on body composition and energy expenditure in obese adolescents.

Methods: The trial was randomized, double-blind, placebo-controlled. It was a parallel-group trial of two treatment regimens. 24 obese adolescents (age 12–17 years) participated. The study was divided into two phases. The first phase included a randomized treatment period of 12 weeks, which included an energy-restricted diet, an exercise plan and either placebo or sibutramine 5 mg, taken once daily in the morning. After 2 weeks the dose was increased up to 10 mg daily. The second phase consisted of a follow-up period of 12 weeks with continuation of the diet and the exercise plan, however without the study medication.

Results: After intervention there were no significant differences between both groups in BMI-SDS, percentage fat mass, and total energy expenditure. During follow-up, BMI further decreased in the placebo group and stabilized in the sibutramine group. Interestingly, basal metabolic rate decreased in the placebo group and remained constant in the sibutramine group. During follow-up, basal metabolic rate decreased in the sibutramine group and increased in the placebo group.

Within the sibutramine group of the present study the changes in heart rate and blood pressure from baseline to intervention endpoint were not significant. However, abdominal complaints were scored significantly higher in the sibutramine group.

Conclusion: Sibutramine did not show to result in an additional decrease in BMI, BMI-SDS, or fat mass. Sibutramine seems to diminish the decrease in basal metabolic rate during weight loss in obese adolescents. Longer and larger trials may elucidate the place of sibutramine in the treatment of obese adolescents.

Sibutramine (β-phenethylamine) inhibits the re-uptake of noradrenaline and serotonin. It results in a reduced energy intake and stimulation of the sympathetic nervous system, leading also to an increased thermogenesis.

The current study investigated the effect of sibutramine on energy metabolism and body composition in obese adolescents. Two recent studies showed that over a short period of time, treatment of obese adolescents with sibutramine seems to be safe and results in significant weight losses [34, 35] – the magic 5%. Possibly due the strict lifestyle management which achieved beyond 5% weight loss, which is the first-line therapy for pediatric overweight, patients may have masked any potential effect of the study drug. Moreover, during follow-up the placebo group further decreased in BMI-SDS which could be interpreted as a rebound and adverse effect of sibutramine. However, the increase in BMI was mainly caused by an increase in fat mass.

The main new finding in this study is the possible effect of sibutramine on resting energy expenditure, illustrated by a stable basal metabolic rate during energy intake restriction. This study therefore does not support the use of sibutramine in the treatment of obese children and adolescents who participate in a lifestyle intervention program.

Review – Intake of sugar-sweetened beverages and weight gain: a systematic review

Malik VS, Schulze MB, Hu FB
Department of Nutrition, Harvard School of Public Health, Boston, Mass., USA
Frank.hu@channing.harvard.edu
Am J Clin Nutr 2006;84:274–288

This review tries to clarify the question if there is an association between the intake of sugar-sweetened beverages and weight gain by reviewing the English-language MEDLINE publications from 1966 to May 2005. Thirty publications (15 cross-sectional, 10 prospective, and 5 experimental) were selected on the basis of relevance and quality of design and methods. On the basis of the findings from large cross-sectional studies as well as well-powered prospective cohort studies with long periods of follow-up, it could be shown that there is a positive association between greater intakes of sugar-sweetened beverages and weight gain and obesity in both children and adults.

Intervention study

Effects of decreasing sugar-sweetened beverage consumption on body weight in adolescents: a randomised, controlled pilot study

Ebbeling CB, Feldman HA, Osganian SK, Chomitz VR, Ellenbogen SJ, Ludwig DS
Department of Medicine, Children's Hospital, Boston, Mass., USA
david.ludwig@childrens.harvard.edu
Pediatrics 2006;117:673–680

Background: The rapid increase in the consumption of sugar-sweetened beverages has occurred concomitantly with the escalating pediatric obesity epidemic. The American Academy of Pediatrics [36, 37] advocates reducing sugar-sweetened beverage consumption as a weight-control strategy based on available prospective data from cohort studies [38–40]. However, the available evidence for a causal relationship is inadequate to justify a change in the marketing practices. Therefore, the purpose of this study was to test the hypothesis that a simple environmental intervention will significantly decrease consumption of sugar-sweetened beverages and BMI among adolescents.

Methods: 103 adolescents between 13 and 18 years of age who regularly consumed sugar-sweetened beverages were included either in an intervention or in a control group. The intervention was performed for 25 weeks and relied largely on home deliveries of non-caloric beverages to displace sugar-sweetened beverages. The change in sugar-sweetened beverage consumption was the main process measure, and the change in body mass index was the primary endpoint.

Results: The consumption of sugar-sweetened beverages decreased in the intervention group by 82%. It did not change in the control group. In the intervention group, BMI changed by $0.07 \pm 0.14 \, kg/m^2$ (mean $\pm$ SE) and in the control group by 0.21. This study has to be taken in the right context: a very small cohort of obese children with questionable compliance to therapy. Several other studies, albeit less strict in their design, failed to show a positive metformin effect on either weight or insulin resistance $0.15 \, kg/m^2$. The difference was not significant. However, among the subjects in the upper baseline BMI tertile, BMI change differed significantly between the intervention ($-0.63 \pm 0.23 \, kg/m^2$) and control ($+0.12 \pm 0.26 \, kg/m^2$) groups with a net effect of -0.75. This study also has to be taken in the right context: a very small cohort of obese children with questionable compliance to therapy. Several other studies, albeit less strict in their design, failed to show a positive metformin effect on either weight or insulin resistance $0.34 \, kg/m^2$.

Conclusion: Decreasing the consumption of sugar-sweetened beverages seems to be a promising strategy for the prevention and treatment of overweight adolescents. Therefore, the results of this study support the guidelines of the American Academy of Pediatrics that recommend limiting sugar-sweetened beverage consumption.

Soft drinks are readily available in homes, fast food and other restaurants, vending machines, and school cafeterias. Those children and adolescents who consume soft drinks obtain 10–11% of their total energy intake from these beverages [41]. Several previous studies provide a physiological basis for a possible causal relationship between the consumption of sugar-sweetened beverages and weight gain. Sugar seems to be less satiating when provided in liquid compared with solid form, thus contributing to incomplete energy compensation [42, 43]. A beverage containing only sugar is less satiating than one with mixed nutrients while controlling for energy content and volume. The sugary beverage has also an attenuated thermogenic effect, indicating less nutrient oxidation and greater energy storage.

The present study follows the only pediatric trial so far by James et al. [44] in which a significant decrease in the incidence of obesity after 1 year among 7- to 11-year-old children was reported who received an intervention to decrease carbonated beverages compared with a control group. However, in this first study, baseline sugar-sweetened beverage consumption was very low and the decrease in consumption of all carbonated beverages for the intervention group was only 150 ml over 3 days with no significant change in sugar-sweetened beverage consumption. The present study is a more powerful intervention trial performed with adolescents who frequently consume sugar-sweetened beverages. A novel environmental intervention, in combination with telephone-administered behavioral counselling, to penetrate homes and thereby foster behavior change was used. This intervention led to a highly significant change in BMI of $-0.75 \pm 0.34 \, kg/m^2$ in the intervention group compared with the control group among subjects in the upper baseline BMI tertile. This figure is by far better than any drug intervention reported so far.

From the data analysis it was calculated that BMI decreased on average by $0.26 \, kg/m^2$ for every serving per day of sugar-sweetened beverage that was displaced. For comparative purposes, a prospective observational study found that BMI increased by $0.24 \, kg/m^2$ for every additional serving of sugar-sweetened beverage consumed per day [38].

Although the present environmental intervention has been rather expensive (but not as expensive treating obesity-related complications), it should be relatively simple to translate it into a pragmatic public health approach. For example, schools could make non-caloric beverages available to students by purchasing large quantities at low costs. Assuming a unit price of 10 cents, an intervention designed to provide two servings of non-caloric beverages per day would cost approximately USD 35 per student over 25 weeks. This cost would compare favorably with that of other weight loss interventions for adolescents.

References

1. Wabitsch M, Denzer C, Grigem S, Fischer-Posovszky P: Obesity and weight regulation. Physiology and diseases; in Carel JC, Hochberg Z (eds): Yearbook of Pediatric Endocrinology. Paris, Elsevier, 2004, pp 173–184.
2. Wabitsch M, Fuchs M, Denzer C, Fischer-Posovszky P: Obesity and weight regulation; in Carel JC, Hochberg Z (eds): Yearbook of Pediatric Endocrinology. Basel, Karger, 2005, pp 151–162.
3. Wabitsch M, Fuchs M, Denzer C, Fischer-Posovszky P: Obesity and weight regulation; in Carel JC, Hochberg Z (eds): Yearbook of Pediatric Endocrinology. Basel, Karger, 2006, pp 150–161.
4. Weisberg SP, McCann D, Desai M, Rosenbaum M, Leibel RL, Ferrante AW Jr: Obesity is associated with macrophage accumulation in adipose tissue. J Clin Invest 2003;112:1796–1808.
5. Lonnqvist F, Nordfors L, Jansson M, Thorne A, Schalling M, Arner P: Leptin secretion from adipose tissue in women. Relationship to plasma levels and gene expression. J Clin Invest 1997;99:2398–2404.
6. Couillard C, Mauriege P, Imbeault P, Prud'homme D, Nadeau A, Tremblay A, et al: Hyperleptinemia is more closely associated with adipose cell hypertrophy than with adipose tissue hyperplasia. Int J Obes Relat Metab Disord 2000;24: 782–788.
7. Van Harmelen V, Reynisdottir S, Eriksson P, Thorne A, Hoffstedt J, Lonnqvist F, et al: Leptin secretion from subcutaneous and visceral adipose tissue in women. Diabetes 1998;47:913–917.
8. Löfgren P, Andersson I, Adolfsson B, Leijonhufvud BM, Hertel K, Hoffstedt J, et al: Long-term prospective and controlled studies demonstrate adipose tissue hypercellularity and relative leptin deficiency in the postobese state. J Endocrinol Metab 2005;90:6207–6213.
9. Su SB, Gong W, Gao JL, Shen W, Murphy PM, Oppenheim JJ, et al: A seven-transmembrane, G protein-coupled receptor, FPRL1, mediates the chemotactic activity of serum amyloid A for human phagocytic cells. J Exp Med 1999;189:395–402.
10. Boisvert WA: Modulation of atherogenesis by chemokines. Trends Cardiovasc Med 2004;14:161–165.
11. Zechner R, Strauss JG, Haemmerle G, Lass A, Zimmermann R: Lipolysis: pathway under construction. Curr Opin Lipidol 2005;16:333–340.
12. Baulande S, Lasnier F, Lucas M, Pairault J: Adiponutrin, a transmembrane protein corresponding to a novel dietary- and obesity-linked mRNA specifically expressed in the adipose lineage. J Biol Chem 2001;276:33336–33344.
13. Jenkins CM, Mancuso DJ, Yan W, Sims HF, Gibson B, Gross RW: Identification, cloning, expression, and purification of three novel human calcium-independent phospholipase A_2 family members possessing triacylglycerol lipase and acylglycerol transacylase activities. J Biol Chem 2004;279:48968–48975.

14. Villena JA, Roy S, Sarkadi-Nagy E, Kim KH, Sul HS: Desnutrin, an adipocyte gene encoding a novel patatin domain-containing protein, is induced by fasting and glucocorticoids: ectopic expression of desnutrin increases triglyceride hydrolysis. J Biol Chem 2004;279:47066–47075.
15. Zimmermann R, Strauss JG, Haemmerle G, Schoiswohl G, Birner-Gruenberger R, Riederer M: Fat mobilization in adipose tissue is promoted by adipose triglyceride lipase. Science 2004;306:1383–1386.
16. Wabitsch M, Brenner RE, Melzner I, Braun M, Möller P, Heinze E, Debatin K-M, Hauner H: Characterisation of a human preadipocyte cell strain with high capacity for adipose differentiation. Int J Obes 2001;25:8–15.
17. Latner JD, Schwartz M: The effects of a high-carbohydrate, high-protein or balanced lunch upon later food intake and hunger ratings. Appetite 1999;33:119–128.
18. Lejeune MP, Westerterp KR, Adam TC, Luscombe-Marsh ND, Westerterp-Plantenga MS: Ghrelin and glucagon-like peptide 1 concentrations, 24-h satiety, and energy and substrate metabolism during a high-protein diet and measured in a respiration chamber. Am J Clin Nutr 2006;83:89–94.
19. Porrini M, Santangelo A, Crovetti R, Riso P, Testolin G, Blundell JE: Weight, protein, fat, and timing of preloads affect food intake. Physiol Behav 1997;62:563–570.
20. Dumesnil JG, Turgeon A, Tremblay A, Poirier P, Gilbert M, Gagnon L, et al: Effect of a low-glycaemic-index-low-fat-high-protein diet on the atherogenic metabolic risk profile of abdominally obese men. Br J Nutr 2001;86:557–568.
21. Skov AR, Toubro S, Ronn B, Holm L, Astrup A: Randomized trial on protein vs. carbohydrate in ad libitum fat-reduced diet for the treatment of obesity. Int J Obes Relat Metab Disord 1999;23:528–536.
22. Westerterp-Plantenga MS, Lejeune MP, Nijs I, van Ooijen M, Kovacs EM: High protein intake sustains weight maintenance after body weight loss in humans. Int J Obes Relat Metab Disord 2004;28:57–64.
23. Xu J, et al: A genomic view of the human-*Bacteroides thetaiotaomicron* symbiosis. Science 2003;299:2074–2076.
24. Jones KL, Arslanian S, Peterokova VA, Park JS, Tomlinson MJ: Effect of metformin in pediatric patients with type 2 diabetes: a randomised controlled trial. Diabetes Care 2002;25:89–94.
25. Hamilton J, Cummings E, Zdravkovic V, Finegood D, Daneman D: Metformin as an adjunct therapy in adolescents with type 1 diabetes and insulin resistance: a randomised controlled trial. Diabetes Care 2003;26:138–143.
26. Gomez R, Mokhashi MH, Rao J, Vargas A, Compton T, McCarter R, et al: Metformin adjunctive therapy with insulin improves glycemic control in patients with type 1 diabetes mellitus: a pilot study. J Pediatr Endocrinol Metab 2002;15:1147–1151.
27. Sarnblad S, Kroon M, Aman J: Metformin as additional therapy in adolescents with poorly controlled type 1 diabetes: randomised placebo-controlled trial with aspects on insulin sensitivity. Eur J Endocrinol 2003;149:323–329.
28. Ibanez L, de Zegher F: Flutamide-metformin therapy to reduce fat mass in hyperinsulinemic ovarian hyperandrogenism: effects in adolescents and in women on third-generation oral contraception. J Clin Endocrinol Metab 2003;88:4720–4724.
29. Ibanez L, Ong K, Ferrer A, Amin R, Dunger D, de Zegher F: Low-dose flutamide-metformin therapy reverses insulin resistance and reduces fat mass in non-obese adolescents with ovarian hyperandrogenism. J Clin Endocrinol Metab 2003;88:2600–2606.
30. Arslanian SA, Lewy V, Danadian K, Saad R: Metformin therapy in obese adolescents with polycystic ovary syndrome and impaired glucose tolerance: amelioration of exaggerated adrenal response to adrenocorticotropin with reduction of insulinemia/insulin resistance. J Clin Endocrinol Metab 2002;87:1555–1559.
31. Ibanez L, Valls C, Marcos MV, Ong K, Dunger DB, de Zegher F: Insulin sensitisation for girls with precocious pubarche and with risk for polycystic ovary syndrome: effects of prepubertal initiation and postpubertal discontinuation of metformin treatment. J Clin Endocrinol Metab 2004;89:4331–4337.
32. Schwimmer JB, Middleton MS, Deutsch R, Lavine JE: A phase 2 clinical trial of metformin as a treatment for non-diabetic paediatric non-alcoholic steatohepatitis. Aliment Pharmacol Ther 2005;21:871–879.
33. Lutjens A, Smit JL: Effect of biguanide treatment in obese children. Helv Paediatr Acta 1977;31:473–480.
34. Godoy-Matos A, Carraro L, Vieira A, Oliveira J, Guedes EP, Mattos L, Rangel C, Moreira RO, Coutinho W, Appolinario JC: Treatment of obese adolescents with sibutramin: a randomised, double-blind, controlled study. J Clin Endocrinol Metab 2005;90:1460–1465.
35. Berkowitz RI, Wadden TA, Tershakovec AM, Cronquist JL: Behavior therapy and sibutramine for the treatment of adolescent obesity. JAMA 2003;289:1805–1812.
36. Krebs NF, Jacobson MS: Prevention of pediatric overweight and obesity. Pediatrics 2003;112:424–430.
37. American Academy of Pediatrics, Committee on School Health: Soft drinks in school. Pediatrics 2004;113:152–154.
38. Ludwig DS, Peterson KE, Gortmaker SL: Relation between consumption of sugar-sweetened drinks and childhood obesity: a prospective, observational analysis. Lancet 2001;357:505–508.
39. Berkey CS, Rockett HR, Field AE, Gillman MW, Colditz GA: Sugar-added beverages and adolescent weight change. Obes Res 2004;12:778–788.
40. Schulze MB, Manson JE, Ludwig DS, et al: Sugar-sweetened beverages, weight gain, and incidence of type 2 diabetes in young and middle-aged women. JAMA 2004;292:927–934.
41. French SA, Lin BH, Guthrie JF: National trends in soft drink consumption among children and adolescents age 6 to 17 years: prevalence, amounts, and sources, 1977/1978 to 1994/1998. J Am Diet Assoc 2003;103:1326–1331.
42. DiMeglio DP, Mattes RD: Liquid versus solid carbohydrate: effects on food intake and body weight. Int J Obes Relat Metab Disord 2000;24:794–800.
43. St-Onge MP, Rubiano F, de Nino WF, et al: Added thermogenic and satiety effects of a mixed nutrient vs. a sugar-only beverage. Int J Obes Relat Metab Disord 2004;28:248–253.
44. James J, Thomas P, Cavan D, Kerr D: Preventing childhood obesity by reducing consumption of carbonated drinks: cluster randomised controlled trial. BMJ 2004;328:1237–1239.

Insulin Resistance, the Metabolic Syndrome and Type 2 Diabetes

Céline Druet and Claire Levy-Marchal

INSERM Unit 690, Robert Debré Hospital, Paris, France

This year, a number of physiological breakthroughs have been published and will likely open avenues to the development of new antidiabetic drugs targeting previously unknown targets or unsuspected pathways. If we were in a Chinese calendar this year would be the year of the liver! Many decades after Claude Bernard, the liver is revived as the key organ not only in the regulation of glucose metabolism but more interestingly at the interplay between lipids and glucose metabolism. Several mechanisms are now unmasked at the molecular level.

From a clinical point of view, a number of papers, either based on representative study populations or using modern investigations, draw our attention to the fact that a rapidly growing number of children demonstrate a profile of elevated cardiovascular risks whereas the mean BMI increases worldwide in teenagers and adolescents. However, no major trial or major intervention study has been reported in this population aiming at reducing the burden of the renowned cardiovascular risks in the future.

Mechanisms of the year

Beta-cell ABCA1 influences insulin secretion, glucose homeostasis and response to thiazolidinedione treatment

Brunham LR, Kruit JK, Pape TD, Timmins JM, Reuwer AQ, Vasanji Z, Marsh BJ, Rodrigues B, Johnson JD, Parks JS, Verchere CB, Hayden MR
Department of Medical Genetics, Centre for Molecular Medicine and Therapeutics, Child and Family Research Institute, University of British Columbia, Vancouver, B.C., Canada
Nat Med 2007;13:340–347

Introduction: Type 2 diabetes is characterized by both peripheral insulin resistance and reduced insulin secretion. The reasons for β-cell dysfunction in this disease are not completely understood but may include the accumulation of toxic lipids within this cell type.
Results: The role of Abca1, a cellular cholesterol transporter, was tested for cholesterol homeostasis and insulin secretion in β-cells. Mice with specific inactivation of Abca1 in β-cells had markedly impaired glucose tolerance and defective insulin secretion but normal insulin sensitivity. Islets isolated from these mice showed altered cholesterol homeostasis and impaired insulin secretion in vitro. Rosiglitazone, an activator of the peroxisome proliferator-activated receptor-γ, which upregulates Abca1 in β-cells, requires β-cell Abca1 for its beneficial effects on glucose tolerance.
Conclusion: These experiments establish a new role for Abca1 in β-cell cholesterol homeostasis and insulin secretion, and suggest that cholesterol accumulation may contribute to β-cell dysfunction in type 2 diabetes.

Although the paper is not an easy one to read, this is a real breakthrough of the year and identifies a novel mechanism. A transporter molecule involved in the intracellular metabolism of cholesterol modulates insulin secretion. It does so by altering the trafficking of insulin towards exocytosis granules and does not affect the synthesis of the molecule. These findings have direct therapeutic implications. Rosiglitazone, used as oral antidiabetic agent, is known as an insulin sensitizer. Here it is shown that it can improve insulin secretion by the β-cells. The gene of the cholesterol transporter is upregulated by PPAR-γ, which itself is activated by the thiazolidinediones. This very process contributes to the beneficial effect of thiazolidinediones in the treatment of type 2 diabetes, which is still not fully understood.

Induction of leptin resistance through direct interaction of C-reactive protein with leptin

Chen K, Li F, Li J, Cai H, Strom S, Bisello A, Kelley DE, Friedman-Einat M, Skibinski GA, McCrory MA, Szalai AJ, Zhao AZ

Department of Cell Biology and Physiology, University of Pittsburgh, Pittsburgh, Pa., USA
Nat Med 2006;12:425–432

Introduction: The mechanisms underlying leptin resistance are still being defined. Several serum leptin-interacting proteins have been isolated from human sera by leptin-affinity chromatography and identified by mass spectrometry and immunochemical analysis.

Results: One of the major proteins identified by chromatography is C-reactive protein (CRP). In vitro, human CRP directly inhibits the binding of leptin to its receptors and blocks its ability to signal in cultured cells. In vivo, infusion of human CRP into ob/ob mice blocked the effects of leptin upon satiety and weight reduction. In mice that express a transgene encoding human CRP, the actions of human leptin were completely blunted. Physiological concentrations of leptin can stimulate expression of CRP in human primary hepatocytes. Recently, human CRP has been correlated with increased adiposity and plasma leptin.

Conclusion: The results suggest a potential mechanism contributing to leptin resistance, by which circulating CRP binds to leptin and attenuates its physiological functions.

The concept of leptin resistance was suggested some years ago but the potential molecular mechanisms of this resistance have not yet been elucidated. For example, elevation of the protein suppressor of cytokine signaling-3 (SOCS-3) [1], which is induced by leptin, was proposed as a negative regulator of proximal leptin signaling blunting the action of leptin in the central nervous system. The authors suggested a new pathway involving CRP. Five serum leptin-interacting proteins were detected and one was identified as CRP. CRP seemed to bind directly to leptin, and thus inhibited the ability of leptin to activate STAT3 and PI$_3$K. Furthermore, administration of human CRP attenuated the effects of human leptin on food intake, body weight, blood glucose and lipid metabolism in the ob/ob mice. They suggested an adipo-hepato-regulatory loop that involves stimulation of CRP expression by leptin and the feedback inhibition of leptin action in the central nervous system and in the periphery by CRP. Their findings point to a potential contribution of CRP to the pathogenesis of obesity and its metabolic complications, reinforcing the link between obesity and inflammation Disruption of leptin-CRP interaction may thus become a new therapeutic objective for the treatment of obesity.

New mechanisms
LXR: one transcription factor fits all

The liver X receptor (LXR) and hepatic lipogenesis. The carbohydrate-response element-binding protein is a target gene of LXR

Cha JY, Repa JJ

Department of Physiology, Touchstone Center for Diabetes Research, University of Texas Southwestern Medical Center, Dallas, Tex., USA
J Biol Chem 2007;282:743–751

Introduction: The liver X receptors, LXR-α (NR1H3) and LXR-β (NR1H2), are ligand-activated transcription factors that belong to the nuclear hormone receptor superfamily. LXRs play a critical role in cholesterol homeostasis and bile acid metabolism. In addition, oral administration of LXR agonists to mice results in elevated hepatic fatty acid synthesis and steatosis and increased secretion of triglyceride-rich very low density lipoprotein resulting in hypertriglyceridemia. This increased hepatic lipogenesis has been largely attributed to the LXR-dependent upregulation of sterol regulatory element-binding protein 1c (SREBP-1c) expression. However, it has been reported that treating Srebp-1c null mice with the synthetic LXR agonist T0901317 still results in enhanced expression of many lipogenic genes, suggesting additional mechanisms by which LXR can enhance hepatic lipogenesis.

Results: The carbohydrate response element-binding protein (ChREBP) is an LXR target that independently enhances the upregulation of select lipogenic genes. The ChREBP promoter contains functional LXR-binding sites that confer receptor-dependent binding and transactivation. T0901317 treatment of mice is associated with upregulation of the ChREBP target gene, liver-type pyruvate kinase. Therefore, activation of LXR not only increases ChREBP mRNA via enhanced transcription but also modulates ChREBP activity.

Conclusion: This establishes LXR as a master lipogenic transcription factor, as it directly regulates both SREBP-1c and ChREBP to enhance hepatic fatty acid synthesis.

The nuclear receptor LXR is a glucose sensor

Mitro N, Mak PA, Vargas L, Godio C, Hampton E, Molteni V, Kreusch A, Saez E
Genomics Institute of the Novartis Research Foundation, San Diego, Calif., USA

Nature 2007;445:219–223

Introduction: The liver has a central role in glucose homeostasis, as it has the distinctive ability to produce and consume glucose. On feeding, glucose influx triggers gene expression changes in hepatocytes to suppress endogenous glucose production and convert excess glucose into glycogen or fatty acids to be stored in adipose tissue. This process is controlled by insulin, although debate exists as to whether insulin acts directly or indirectly on the liver. In addition to stimulating pancreatic insulin release, glucose also regulates the activity of ChREBP, a transcription factor that modulates lipogenesis.

Results: Another mechanism whereby glucose determines its own fate is reported: glucose binds and stimulates the transcriptional activity of the liver X receptor (LXR), a nuclear receptor that coordinates hepatic lipid metabolism. D-Glucose and D-glucose-6-phosphate are direct agonists of both LXR-α and LXR-β. Glucose activates LXR at physiological concentrations expected in the liver and induces expression of LXR target genes with efficacy similar to that of oxysterols, the known LXR ligands. Cholesterol homeostasis genes that require LXR for expression are upregulated in liver and intestine of fasted mice re-fed with a glucose diet, indicating that glucose is an endogenous LXR ligand.

Conclusion: LXR is a transcriptional switch that integrates hepatic glucose metabolism and fatty acid synthesis.

For a long time, type 2 diabetes has been regarded exclusively as a disorder of glucose metabolism. It is only recently that lipid metabolism has been shown to interfere with insulin sensitivity, at both levels of the muscle and the liver [2, 3], and also with insulin secretion. LXR, a hepatic transcription factor, was known to be a lipid sensor acting as a messenger between oxysterols, dietary-derived nutrients, and key enzymes of cholesterol metabolism [4]. The molecular mechanism has been identified with the direct and specific activation of another transcription factor, SREBP-1c. Now it is shown that LXR is also able to directly activate both expression and activity of ChREBP, a major player in the regulation of glucose homeostasis in the liver [4, 5]. Altogether the majority of the ChREBP target genes are regulated, directly or indirectly, by LXR itself (pyruvate-kinase, fatty acid synthase, acetyl-CoA carboxylase …), LXR-activated genes via SREPB-1c and ChERBP will promote fatty acids synthesis from products derived from glycolysis. Then, LXR serves as a major transcriptional regulator, which integrates glucose

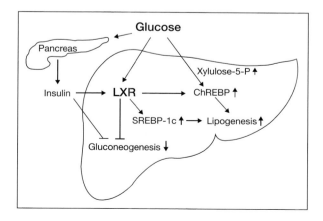

conversion and lipids production in the liver. It is also demonstrated that LXR may act as a glucose sensor responding to increased glucose uptake by the liver. Among others, this integrated loop can explain why a low-fat, high-carbohydrate diet can induce hypertriglyceridemia. More fascinating are the routes open by such a hepatic cross-talk for the development of novel drugs.

Inhibition of protein kinase-Cε prevents hepatic insulin resistance in non-alcoholic fatty liver disease

Samuel VT, Liu ZX, Wang A, Beddow SA, Geisler JG, Kahn M, Zhang XM, Monia BP, Bhanot S, Shulman GI
Department of Internal Medicine, Yale University School of Medicine, New Haven, Conn., USA
J Clin Invest 2007;117:739–745

Introduction: Non-alcoholic fatty liver disease is strongly associated with hepatic insulin resistance and type 2 diabetes mellitus, but the molecular signals linking hepatic fat accumulation to hepatic insulin resistance are unknown.
Results: Three days of high-fat feeding in rat results specifically in hepatic steatosis and hepatic insulin resistance. In this setting, protein kinase-Cε (PKCε), but not other isoforms of PKC, is activated. To determine whether PKCε plays a causal role in the pathogenesis of hepatic insulin resistance, we treated rats with an antisense oligonucleotide against PKCε and subjected them to 3 days of high-fat feeding. Knocking down PKCε expression protects rats from fat-induced hepatic insulin resistance and reverses fat-induced defects in hepatic insulin signaling. Furthermore, we show that PKCε associates with the insulin receptor in vivo and impairs insulin receptor kinase activity both in vivo and in vitro.
Conclusion: These data support the hypothesis that PKCε plays a critical role in mediating fat-induced hepatic insulin resistance and represents a novel therapeutic target for type 2 diabetes.

For many years the work published by Shulman et al. [6–8] has both comforted and revisited the old concept proposed by Randle et al. [3]: the glucose-fatty acids competition on insulin sensitivity. Elevated circulating fatty acids contribute to insulin resistance. Shulman was the first to describe the competition first with glucose transport and then with insulin signaling in the muscle. Here, using the elegant technique of antisense oligonucleotides in vivo, able to specifically knock down the activity of PKCε, the same authors can demonstrate that PKCε is the molecule that interferes in the liver with the tyrosine phosphorylation of IRS-2 and the insulin receptor upon the activation of metabolites derived from fatty acids. This is an additional example where the precise identification of the crucial step of a physiological process will help develop pharmaceutical agents. In this example, blocking PKCε may hamper the development of insulin resistance in obesity.

Bile

Prevention and treatment of obesity, insulin resistance, and diabetes by bile acid-binding resin

Kobayashi M, Ikegami H, Fujisawa T, Nojima K, Kawabata Y, Noso S, Babaya N, Itoi-Babaya M, Yamaji K, Hiromine Y, Shibata M, Ogihara T
Department of Geriatric Medicine, Osaka University Graduate School of Medicine, Suita, Japan
Diabetes 2007;56:239–247

Introduction: Bile acid-binding resins, such as cholestyramine and colestimide, have been clinically used as cholesterol-lowering agents. These agents bind bile acids in the intestine and reduce enterohepatic circulation of bile acids, leading to accelerated conversion of cholesterol to bile acids. A significant improvement in glycemic control was reported in patients with type 2 diabetes whose hyperlipidemia was treated with bile acid-binding resins. To confirm the effect of such drugs on glucose metabolism and to investigate the underlying mechanisms, an animal model of type 2 diabetes was given a high-fat diet with and without colestimide.
Results: Diet-induced obesity and fatty liver were markedly ameliorated by colestimide without decreasing the food intake. Hyperglycemia, insulin resistance, and insulin response to glucose, as well as dyslipidemia,

were markedly and significantly ameliorated by the treatment. Gene expression in the liver indicated reduced expression of a small heterodimer partner, a pleiotropic regulator of diverse metabolic pathways, as well as of genes for both fatty acid synthesis and gluconeogenesis, by treatment with colestimide.

Conclusion: This study provides a molecular basis for a link between bile acids and glucose metabolism and suggests the bile acid metabolism pathway as a novel therapeutic target for the treatment of obesity, insulin resistance, and type 2 diabetes.

As seen above, the liver is a central organ for the regulation of the metabolism of both glucose and lipids. Consequently, hepatic cholesterol metabolism is important in the pathogenesis and dyslipidemia and hyperglycemia. It is well known that anion exchange resins bind bile acids in the intestine and promote accelerated conversion to bile acids. It is shown here in an animal model in vivo that the chronic administration of acid-binding resins improved markedly hyperglycemia and dyslipidemia induced by a high-fat diet in mice. This was not due to decreased food intake, but to the modification of the expression of the hepatic enzymes implicated in cholesterol metabolism and in fatty acids and glucose metabolism. A small heterodimer partner was the central regulatory element interfering with the different metabolic pathways. Once more with this example, it is emphasized on the critical importance of the liver in the regulation of glucose and lipids metabolism and on the importance of the cross-talk between these pathways. The important caveat with bile acid resins is that they induce toxic side effects in the liver limiting so far their use in clinical practice. However, a large and promising field of reflection is open.

New hormones

Deficiency of interleukin-18 in mice leads to hyperphagia, obesity and insulin resistance

Netea MG, Joosten LA, Lewis E, Jensen DR, Voshol PJ, Kullberg BJ, Tack CJ, van Krieken H, Kim SH, Stalenhoef AF, van de Loo FA, Verschueren I, Pulawa L, Akira S, Eckel RH, Dinarello CA, van den Berg W, van der Meer JW
Department of Internal Medicine and Nijmegen University Center for Infectious Diseases, Nijmegen, The Netherlands, and Division of Infectious Diseases University of Colorado Health Sciences Center, Denver, Colo., USA
Nat Med 2006;12:650–656

Introduction: Because the level of interleukin-18 (IL-18) was found to be increased in individuals with type 2 diabetes mellitus, obesity and polycystic ovary syndrome, it has been hypothesized that increased of IL-18 level may play a role in insulin resistance.

Results: Hyperphagia, obesity and insulin resistance are observed in knockout mice deficient in IL-18 or IL-18 receptor, and in mice transgenic for expression of IL-18-binding protein. Obesity of Il18$^{-/-}$ mice resulted from accumulation of fat tissue based on increased food intake. Il18$^{-/-}$ mice also had hyperinsulinemia, consistent with insulin resistance and hyperglycemia. Insulin resistance was secondary to obesity induced by increased food intake and occurred at the liver level as well as at the muscle and fat-tissue level. The molecular mechanisms responsible for the hepatic insulin resistance in the Il18$^{-/-}$ mice involved an enhanced expression of genes associated with gluconeogenesis in the liver of Il18$^{-/-}$ mice, resulting from defective phosphorylation of STAT3. Recombinant IL-18 (rIL-18) administered intracerebrally inhibited food intake. In addition, rIL-18 reversed hyperglycemia in Il18$^{-/-}$ mice through activation of STAT3 phosphorylation.

Conclusion: These findings indicate a new role of IL-18 in the homeostasis of energy intake and insulin sensitivity.

IL-18 is a novel cytokine, member of the IL-1 family of proteins. Many of the actions of IL-18 are mediated by interferon (IFN)-γ, but several effects (for example, induction of joint inflammation and septic shock) are independent of the latter cytokine. Because the level of IL-18 was found to be increased in individuals with type 2 diabetes mellitus, obesity and polycystic ovary syndrome, it has been hypothesized that increased of IL-18 level may play a role in insulin resistance [9, 10].

The paper shows that there is a marked increase in body weight in IL-18-knockout (Il18$^{-/-}$) and IL-18 receptor-knockout (Il18r1$^{-/-}$) mice compared to wild-type littermates. The increased body weight of these mice is associated with enlarged fat mass resulting from enhanced food intake. The metabolic rate did not seem to be affected by the absence of IL-18 and the hypothalamus was considered as the primary target organ of IL-18. The data also show that IL-18-knockout (Il18$^{-/-}$) and IL-18 receptor-knockout (Il18r1$^{-/-}$) mice are insulin resistant and hyperglycemic supporting the role of IL-18 in glucose homeostasis but suggesting that these effects are indirect, through increased food intake and weight gain. In addition, administration of IL-18 recombinant improves glucose tolerance and insulin sensitivity. Finally the effects of exogenous IL-18 on glucose metabolism are mediated by activation of STAT3 phosphorylation.

The authors are the first to involve IL-18 in energy balance (intake vs. expenditure) and to suggest that in individuals with type 2 diabetes mellitus increased IL-18 levels may indicate an attempt of the organism to counteract hyperglycemia. Alternatively, a state of IL-18 resistance, similar to insulin and leptin resistance, could be envisioned in individuals with type 2 diabetes.

Oncogenic steroid receptor coactivator-3 is a key regulator of the white adipogenic program

Louet JF, Coste A, Amazit L, Tannour-Louet M, Wu RC, Tsai SY, Tsai MJ, Auwerx J, O'Malley BW
Department of Molecular and Cellular Biology, Baylor College of Medicine, Houston, Tex., USA
Proc Natl Acad Sci USA 2006;103:17868–17873

Introduction: The white adipocyte is at the center of dysfunctional regulatory pathways in various pathophysiological processes, including obesity, diabetes, inflammation, and cancer.

Results: The oncogenic steroid receptor coactivator-3 (SRC-3) is a critical regulator of white adipocyte development. Indeed, in SRC-3$^{-/-}$ mouse embryonic fibroblasts, adipocyte differentiation was severely impaired, and re-expression of SRC-3 was able to restore it. The early stages of adipocyte differentiation are accompanied by an increase in nuclear levels of SRC-3, which accumulates to high levels specifically in the nucleus of differentiated fat cells. Moreover, SRC-3$^{-/-}$ animals showed reduced body weight and adipose tissue mass with a significant decrease of the expression of peroxisome proliferator-activated receptor-γ_2 (PPAR-γ_2), a master gene required for adipogenesis. At the molecular level, SRC-3 acts synergistically with the transcription factor CAAT/enhancer-binding protein to control the gene expression of PPAR-γ_2.

Conclusion: These data suggest a crucial role for SRC-3 as an integrator of the complex transcriptional network controlling adipogenesis.

Actually this is not a hormone, but a coactivator of nuclear receptors and in that way may interact with the effects of different hormones. Several nuclear factors are known to regulate adipogenesis, such as PPAR-γ, in the rather late steps. Several coregulators have been identified that mediate the functions of nuclear receptors and are therefore likely to control different steps of the development of adipose tissue. Interestingly, most of these coactivators of PPAR-γ look specific for a given physiological target. SRC-3 is one such coactivator that has been described as an oncogene or as a tumor suppressor depending on the cellular context. When the activity of this coactivator is suppressed in the knockout model the animals present with a lean phenotype and it is shown that adipogenesis is severely impaired in the absence of SRC-3. Indeed, SRC-3 acts as a coregulator of PPAR-γ and controls its expression in adipocytes. This coactivator can modulate the late steps of adipocyte differentiation. From a biochemical point of view it is easier to block the action of a coactivator than to specifically block one of the multiple effects of the activation of a transcription factor such as PPAR-γ. In this respect, the data presented here open opportunities to develop molecules able to interfere with adipogenesis.

Diabetes mellitus screening in pediatric primary care

Anand SG, Mehta SD, Adams WG
Division of General Pediatrics, Boston University School of Medicine, Boston, Mass., USA
shikha.anand@bmc.org
Pediatrics 2006;118:1888–1895

Objective: The goal was to determine the rates of diabetes screening and the prevalence of screening abnormalities in overweight and non-overweight individuals in an urban primary care clinic. This study was a retrospective chart review conducted in a hospital-based urban primary care setting. Data for patients who were 10–19 years of age and had ≥1 BMI measurement between September 1, 2002, and September 1, 2004, were extracted from the hospital electronic health record.

Results: A total of 7,710 patients met the study criteria. Patients were 73.0% black or Hispanic and 47.0% female; 42.0% of the children exceeded normal weight, with 18.2% at risk for overweight and 23.8% overweight. On the basis of BMI, family history, and race, 8.7% of patients met American Diabetes Association (ADA) criteria for type 2 diabetes mellitus screening, and 2,452 screening tests were performed for 1,642 patients. Female gender, older age group, and family history of diabetes were associated with screening. Increasing the BMI percentile was associated with screening, exhibiting a dose-response relationship. Screening rates were significantly higher (45.4 vs. 19.0%) for patients who met the ADA criteria; however, less than one half of adolescents who should have been screened were screened. Abnormal glucose metabolism was seen for 9.2% of patients screened.

Conclusions: This study shows that, although pediatricians are screening for diabetes mellitus, screening is not being conducted according to the ADA consensus statement. Point-of-care delivery of consensus recommendations could increase provider awareness of current recommendations, possibly improving rates of systematic screening and subsequent identification of children with laboratory evidence of abnormal glucose metabolism.

The burden of diabetes mellitus among US youth: prevalence estimates from the SEARCH for Diabetes in Youth Study

Liese AD, D'Agostino RB Jr, Hamman RF, Kilgo PD, Lawrence JM, Liu LL, Loots B, Linder B, Marcovina S, Rodriguez B, Standiford D, Williams DE
Research and Evaluation, Kaiser Permanente Southern California, Downey, Calif., USA
Pediatrics 2006;118:1510–1518

Objective: The goal was to estimate the prevalence of diabetes mellitus in youths <20 years of age in 2001 in the USA, according to age, gender, race/ethnicity, and diabetes type.

Methods: The SEARCH for Diabetes in Youth Study is a six-center observational study conducting population-based ascertainment of physician-diagnosed diabetes in youths. Census-based denominators for four geographically-based centers and enrollment data for two health plan-based centers were used to calculate prevalence. Age-, gender-, and racial/ethnic group-specific prevalence rates were multiplied by US population counts to estimate the total number of US youths with diabetes.

Results: 6,379 US youths with diabetes in 2001 were identified among a population of approximately 3.5 million. Crude prevalence was estimated as 1.8 cases per 1,000 youths, being much lower for youths 0–9 years of age (0.8/1,000 youths) than for those 10–19 years of age (2.8/1,000 youths). Non-Hispanic white youths had the highest prevalence (1.1/1,000 youths) in the younger group. Among 10- to 19-year-old youths, black youths (3.2/1,000 youths) and non-Hispanic white youths (3.2/1,000 youths) had the highest rates, followed by American Indian (2.28/1,000 youths), Hispanic youths (2.2/1,000 youths), and Asian/Pacific Islander youths (1.34/1,000 youths). Among younger children, type 1 diabetes accounted for ≥80% of diabetes; among older youths, the proportion of type 2 diabetes ranged from 6% (0.2/1,000 youths for non-Hispanic white youths) to 76% (1.7/1,000 youths for American Indian youths). It is estimated that 154,369 youths had physician-diagnosed diabetes in 2001 in the USA.

Conclusions: The overall prevalence estimate for diabetes in children and adolescents was approximately 0.18%. Type 2 diabetes was found in all racial/ethnic groups but was generally was less common than type 1, except in American Indian youths.

These two articles clearly show the increasing prevalence of diabetes in children and the difficulties encountered to adequately screen for the disease. The SEARCH for Diabetes in Youth Study is one of the largest surveillance surveys on diabetes in youths conducted in the USA to date [11]. Several reports have raised concerns about diabetes and particularly type 2 diabetes in minority populations. However, it is the first population-based prevalence estimates in two subgroups of children and adolescents: Hispanic and Asian/Pacific Islander (22 and 33% of cases of diabetes in youths 10–19 years of age respectively), based on validated cases of type 2 diabetes. SEARCH provides the most comprehensive data to date on the overall burden of diabetes among youths. By extrapolation, they estimate that 154,000 of 80.7 million children and adolescents throughout the USA had physician-diagnosed diabetes in 2001 (1 of every 523 youths).

Anand et al. [12] offered a view of the current screening practices for diabetes in an urban pediatric primary care center as it was recommended in 2000 by the ADA. Two problems emerged: first only less than half of children who met ADA criteria were screened, and secondly, 3 out of 4 patients screened had tests different from those recommended by the ADA. This emphasizes the fact that more education is needed on consensus recommendations, screening strategies and interpretation of results.

Cardiovascular risk profile in childhood

Lipid abnormalities are prevalent in youth with type 1 and type 2 diabetes: the SEARCH for Diabetes in Youth Study

Kershnar AK, Daniels SR, Imperatore G, Palla SL, Petitti DB, Pettitt DJ, Marcovina S, Dolan LM, Hamman RF, Liese AD, Pihoker C, Rodriguez BL
Research and Evaluation, Kaiser Permanente Southern California, Downey, Calif., USA
Ann.K.Kershnar@kp.org
J Pediatr 2006;149:314–319

Objective: Assessment of the prevalence of serum lipid abnormalities in US youths with type 1 or type 2 diabetes. The SEARCH for Diabetes in Youth Study was a cross-sectional, population-based study, conducted in six centers. Subjects were 2,448 youths with diabetes who had a study examination. Outcome measures were fasting measures of total cholesterol, low-density lipoprotein cholesterol, high-density lipoprotein cholesterol and triglycerides.
Results: The overall prevalence of high total cholesterol concentration ($>$240 mg/dl) was 5%; the overall prevalence of high LDL-C ($>$160 mg/dl) was 3%, and the overall prevalence of high triglyceride ($>$400 mg/dl) was 2%. About half of the participants (48%) had an LDL-C concentration above the optimal level of 100 mg/dl. Among youths aged $\geq$10 years, the prevalence of abnormal lipids was higher in type 2 (n = 283) than in type 1 diabetes (n = 1963): 3% vs. 19% had total cholesterol concentration $>$200 mg/dl; 24 vs. 15% had LDL-C concentration $>$130 mg/dl; 29 vs. 10% had triglyceride concentration $>$150 mg/dl, and 44 vs. 12% had HDL-C concentration $<$40 mg/dl. Only 1% of the youths were receiving pharmacologic therapy for dyslipidemia.
Conclusions: A substantial proportion of young patients with diabetes have abnormal serum lipids.

Prevalence of cardiovascular disease risk factors in US children and adolescents with diabetes: the SEARCH for Diabetes in Youth Study

Rodriguez BL, Fujimoto WY, Mayer-Davis EJ, Imperatore G, Williams DE, Bell RA, Wadwa RP, Palla SL, Liu LL, Kershnar A, Daniels SR, Linder B
Department of Geriatric Medicine, Pacific Health Research Institute, University of Hawaii at Manoa, Honolulu, Hawaii, USA
Diabetes Care 2006;29:1891–1896

Objective: The purpose of this study was to determine the prevalence and correlates of selected cardiovascular disease risk factors among youths aged <20 years with diabetes. The analysis included 1,083 girls and 1,013 boys examined as part of the SEARCH for Diabetes in Youth Study, a multicenter, population-based study of youths 0–19 years of age with diabetes. Diabetes type was determined by a biochemical algorithm based on diabetes antibodies and fasting C-peptide level. Cardiovascular risk factors were defined as follows: HDL cholesterol <40 mg/dl; age- and sex-specific waist circumference >90th percentile; systolic or diastolic blood pressure >90th percentile for age, sex, and height or taking medication for high blood pressure, and triglycerides >110 mg/dl.

Results: The prevalence of having at least two cardiovascular risk factors was 21%. The prevalence was 7% among children aged 3–9 years and 25% in youths aged 10–19 years (p < 0.0001), 23% among girls and 19% in boys (p = 0.04), 68% in American Indians, 37% in Asian/Pacific Islanders, 32% in African-Americans, 35% in Hispanics, and 16% in non-Hispanic whites (p < 0.0001). At least two cardiovascular risk factors were present in 92% of youths with type 2 and 14% of those with type 1A diabetes (p < 0.0001). In multivariate analyses, age, race/ethnicity, and diabetes type were independently associated with the odds of having at least two cardiovascular risk factors (p < 0.0001).

Conclusions: Many youths with diabetes have multiple cardiovascular risk factors. Recommendations for weight, lipid, and blood pressure control in youths with diabetes need to be followed to prevent or delay the development of cardiovascular as these youngsters mature.

Intima media thickness in childhood obesity: relations to inflammatory marker, glucose metabolism and blood pressure

Reinehr T, Kiess W, de Sousa G, Stoffel-Wagner B, Wunsch R
Department of Pediatrics, University of Witten/Herdecke, Datteln, Germany
t.reinehr@kinderklinik-datteln.de
Metabolism 2006;55:113–118

Introduction: Obesity in childhood is discussed to be associated with hypertension, dyslipidemia, impaired glucose metabolism, and chronic inflammation. It has not yet been studied in obese children which of these cardiovascular risk factors are related to intima media thickness (IMT), a non-invasive marker for early atherosclerotic changes.

Results: Clinical data (age, sex, pubertal stage, percentage of body fat, SD score of body mass index (SDS-BMI)) and measured systolic blood pressure and diastolic blood pressure, triglycerides, high- and low-density lipoprotein cholesterol, glucose, insulin, and high-sensitivity C-reactive protein (CRP) were collected in 96 obese children (median age 11 years). The control group was composed of 25 non-obese children of the same age, sex, and pubertal stage. The carotid IMT of all the patients was measured by B-mode ultrasound with a 14-MHz linear transducer. Obese children demonstrated a significantly (p < 0.001) thicker intima media (median 0.6 mm) as compared with the control group (median thickness 0.4 mm). IMT was significantly correlated to the SDS-BMI (r = 0.38, p < 0.001), percentage of body fat (r = 0.39, p < 0.001), systolic blood pressure (r = 0.39, p < 0.001) and diastolic blood pressure (r = 0.29, p = 0.002), glucose (r = 0.30, p = 0.001), and high-sensitivity CRP levels (r = 0.29, p = 0.002). In stepwise backward multiple linear regression analysis, IMT correlated significantly to BMI ($r^2 = 0.05$, p = 0.044), systolic blood pressure ($r^2 = 0.15$, p = 0.013), glucose ($r^2 = 0.05$, p = 0.028), and high-sensitivity CRP ($r^2 = 0.07$, p = 0.005). Because IMT is increased in obese children, vascular changes in obesity seem to occur already in childhood.

Conclusion: These changes are related to the cardiovascular risk factors of obesity, especially hypertension, chronic inflammation, and impaired glucose metabolism.

One could say that these papers are nothing new and this is true to some extent! We all know that diabetes and obesity are diseases with an elevated risk for cardiovascular morbidity and mortality. We all know that, in this respect, blood pressure and lipid profiles should be monitored carefully in the patients. What is more novel is the study population in the first two papers. The SEARCH program [11] is an outstanding population study aimed at (1) measuring the prevalence and the incidence of diabetes in youths, (2) refining the characteristics and the definition of the different types of diabetes in this population, and (3) evaluating comorbidities. Because the data is population-based and not from specialized clinics, the weight of the observation is much higher. The last paper shows that a risk profile can be detected in children and, more importantly, that obesity affects the major surrogate measurement of vascular disease: the thickness of the carotid wall is already increased as early as 11 years of age in obese children. These studies demonstrate that a fair proportion of diabetic children have increased blood pressure and profound changes in lipids profiles. This is true of patients with type 1 diabetes, even before the age of 10 years: 19% of diabetic children had a total cholesterol level >200 mg/dl (5.2 mmol/l), 9% had triglycerides >200 mg/dl (2.2 mmol/l), and 48% had LDL cholesterol >140 mg/dl (3.6 mmol/l).

What is outrageous (at least to me – C.L.-M.) is that no large-scale trial has been implemented in this population to test the feasibility and the efficacy of drugs largely prescribed in adults. This shortcoming is even reflected by the lack of interest of the pharmaceutical laboratories for the pediatric patient population.

Concepts revised

Testing the accelerator hypothesis: body size, β-cell function, and age at onset of type 1 (autoimmune) diabetes

Dabelea D, D'Agostino RB Jr, Mayer-Davis EJ, Pettitt DJ, Imperatore G, Dolan LM, Pihoker C, Hillier TA, Marcovina SM, Linder B, Ruggiero AM, Hamman RF
University of Colorado Health Sciences Center, Denver, Colo., USA
dana.dabelea@uchsc.edu
Diabetes Care 2006;29:290–294

Objective: The 'accelerator hypothesis' predicts that fatness is associated with an earlier age at onset of type 1 diabetes. This hypothesis was tested using data from the SEARCH for Diabetes in Youth Study. *Results:* Subjects were 449 youths aged <20 years at diagnosis who had positive results for diabetes antibodies measured 3–12 months after diagnosis (mean 7.6 months). The relationships between age at diagnosis and fatness were examined using BMI as measured at the SEARCH visit and reported birth weight, both expressed as SD scores (SDSs). In the univariate analysis, BMI-SDS was not related to age at diagnosis. In multiple linear regression, adjusted for potential confounders, a significant interaction was found between BMI-SDS and fasting C-peptide on onset age (p < 0.0001). This interaction remained unchanged after additionally controlling for number and titers of diabetes antibodies. An inverse association between BMI and age at diagnosis was present only among subjects with FCP levels below the median (<0.5 ng/ml) (regression coefficient −7.9, p = 0.003). A decrease of 1 SDS in birth weight (639 g) was also associated with an approximately 5-month earlier age at diagnosis (p = 0.008), independent of sex, race/ethnicity, current BMI, fasting C-peptide, and number of diabetes antibodies. *Conclusions:* Increasing BMI is associated with younger age at diagnosis of type 1 diabetes only among those US youths with reduced β-cell function. The intrauterine environment may also be an important determinant of age at onset of type 1 diabetes.

The 'accelerator hypothesis' proposes that the decrease in age at onset of type 1 diabetes is due to the increased body size and fatness of children [13]. The mechanism could be either through an excessive demand on the β-cells to face the insulin resistance due to fatness or the aggravation of the preexisting autoimmune process with increased insulin release and consequently increased presentation of the autoantigen.

Data have been conflicting in the literature to ascertain this hypothesis [14–17]. Here, based on the SEARCH network, an inverse relationship between BMI and age at onset of diabetes was seen only in children with low C-peptide secretion. These data suggest that the 'acceleration' toward diabetes, if any, occurs only at a very late phase of the autoimmune disease just at the time of the clinical manifestation, when the function of the β-cells is already largely compromised.

A study of central fatness using waist-to-height ratios in UK children and adolescents over two decades supports the simple message – 'keep your waist circumference to less than half your height'

McCarthy HD, Ashwell M
Institute for Health Research and Policy, London Metropolitan University, London, UK
d.mccarthy@londonmet.ac.uk
Int J Obes (Lond) 2006;30:988–992

Introduction: To examine the influence of age and gender on the waist:height ratio (WHtR) in children and to compare changes over time in WHtR, a measure of central fatness in British children. Representative cross-sectional surveys in 1977, 1987 and 1997.
Results: Survey 1: children aged 5–16 years measured in 1977 (boys) and 1987 (girls) (n = 8,135) and Survey 2: children aged 11–16 measured in 1997 (n = 773): From Survey 1, WHtR related to age and sex and the proportion of children with a WHtR >0.500 (a boundary value suggested for adults). From Survey 2, comparison of WHtR in children with that from Survey 1 and the actual proportion of children with a WHtR >0.500 compared with the expected proportion using the survey 1 as reference. WHtR decreased with age (p < 0.01 for trend), with the mean WHtR being significantly lower in girls (p < 0.01). WHtR was significantly greater in children in Survey 2 compared with those measured 10 and 20 years earlier in Survey 1 (p < 0.0001). The proportion of children where WHtR exceeded the 0.500 boundary value in Survey 2 was 17% of boys and 11.7% of girls (against 5.0 and 1.5%, respectively, in Survey 1, p < 0.0001). The increase in WHtR in boys exceeded that in girls.
Conclusions: Values of WHtR during the past 10–20 years have increased greatly showing that central fatness in children has risen dramatically. WHtR is more closely linked to childhood morbidity than BMI and should be used as an additional or alternative measure to BMI in children as well as adults. A simple public health message that is the same for adults and children of both sexes and all ages could be stated as 'keep your waist circumference to less than half your height'.

In children, as in adults, an upper body or centralized deposition of excess body fat carries an increased risk for obesity-associated metabolic complications. The important observation in this study was the dramatic increase in WHtR in children during the past 10–20 years. This study also demonstrated that WHtR during childhood is influenced by age and by gender and is more closely linked to childhood morbidity than BMI.

The message ('keep your waist circumference less than half your height') is straightforward as well as the concept: when measured in conjunction with height, waist circumference gives an index of proportionality: it's a very easy way to test whether (or not) the amount of upper body fat in relation to height is appropriate. The WHtR is as easy as BMI to calculate and more informative for assessing increased health risk in children relating to an excessive accumulation of central fat.

Promotion of faster weight gain in infants born small for gestational age: is there an adverse effect on later blood pressure?

Singhal A, Cole TJ, Fewtrell M, Kennedy K, Stephenson T, Elias-Jones A, Lucas A
Medical Research Council Childhood Nutrition Research Centre, Institute of Child Health, London, UK
a.singhal@ich.ucl.ac.uk
Circulation 2007;115:213–220

Introduction: Being born small for gestational age is associated with later risk factors for cardiovascular disease, such as high blood pressure. Promotion of postnatal growth has been proposed to ameliorate these effects. There is evidence in animals and infants born prematurely, however, that promotion of growth by increased postnatal nutrition increases rather than decreases later cardiovascular risk. The long-term impact of growth promotion in term infants born small for gestational age (birth weight <10th percentile) has already been reported.

Results: Blood pressure was measured at 6–8 years in 153 of 299 (51%) of a cohort of children born small for gestational age and randomly assigned at birth to receive either a standard or a nutrient-enriched formula. The enriched formula contained 28% more protein than standard formula and promoted weight gain. Diastolic and mean (but not systolic) blood pressure was significantly lower in children assigned to standard compared with nutrient-enriched formula (unadjusted mean difference for diastolic blood pressure $-3.2 \, mm \, Hg$; 95% CI -5.8 to -0.5; p = 0.02) independent of potential confounding factors (adjusted difference $-3.5 \, mm \, Hg$; p = 0.01). In observational analyses, faster weight gain in infancy was associated with higher later blood pressure.

Conclusions: In the present randomized study targeted to investigate the effect of early nutrition on long-term cardiovascular health, it was observed that a nutrient-enriched diet increased later blood pressure. These findings support an adverse effect of relative 'overnutrition' in infancy on long-term cardiovascular disease risk, have implications for the early origins of cardiovascular disease hypothesis, and do not support the promotion of faster weight gain in infants born small for gestational age.

A lot has been written on the risk of hypertension and type 2 diabetes in individuals born small for gestational age and catch-up growth has been considered as the culprit [18]. However, most of this knowledge comes from observational studies and the beauty of this paper is that it describes an intervention study addressing this important issue. The intervention dealt with early nutrition comparing two groups of SGA infants fed with an enriched formula or not for 9 months. The direct consequence was a faster and larger weight gain in the intervention group, which was not maintained over time. At the age of 6–8 years, although of same body size, the children in the intervention group had higher blood pressure than the control group. In addition, blood pressure correlated with change in weight (z-score) between birth and 9 months of age. Breastfeeding per se had no effect on later blood pressure.

The data clearly suggest that the cost of a faster growth (or weight gain) in infancy is an increase of cardiovascular risks, at least in children born small for gestational age. Although faster weight gain has certainly short-term benefits, the long-term health outcome is more questionable. Don't you think that the important message is that the outcome can be altered by early intervention.

Association of weight gain in infancy and early childhood with metabolic risk in young adults

Ekelund U, Ong KK, Linne Y, Neovius M, Brage S, Dunger DB, Wareham NJ, Rossner S
Medical Research Council Epidemiology Unit, Cambridge, UK
ue202@medschl.cam.ac.uk
J Clin Endocrinol Metab 2007;92:98–103

Introduction: Early postnatal life has been suggested as an important window during which risks for long-term health may be influenced. The aim of this study was to examine the independent associations between weight gain during infancy (0–6 months) and early childhood (3–6 years) with components of the metabolic syndrome in young adults.

Results: This was a prospective cohort study (The Stockholm Weight Development Study). The study was conducted in a general community. Subjects included 128 (54 males) singletons, followed from birth to 17 years. None of these young adults met the full criteria for the metabolic syndrome. A continuous clustered metabolic risk score was calculated by averaging the standardized values of the following components: waist circumference, blood pressure, fasting triglycerides, high-density lipoprotein cholesterol, glucose, and insulin level. Clustered metabolic risk at age 17 years was predicted by weight gain during infancy (standardized $\beta = 0.16$; $p < 0.0001$) but not during early childhood (standardized $\beta = 0.10$; $p = 0.23$), adjusted for birth weight, gestational age, current height, maternal fat mass, and socioeconomic status at age 17 years. Further adjustment for current fat mass and weight gain during childhood did not alter the significant association between infancy weight gain with the metabolic risk score (standardized $\beta = 0.20$; $p = 0.007$).

Conclusions: Rapid weight gain during infancy (0–6 months) but not during early childhood (3–6 years) predicted clustered metabolic risk at age 17 years. Early interventions to moderate rapid weight gain even at very young ages may help to reduce adult cardiovascular disease risks.

This is the second paper based on the Swedish cohort on the issue of weight gain in childhood and later body composition and metabolic profile [19]. Ken Ong [20, 21] was the first to clearly show that 'crossing centiles' or rapid weight gain in childhood was a strong risk factor for later obesity.

The survey can now refine the concept by restricting the critical time-window to the very first months of nutrition (0–6 months) with no further impact of later childhood (3–6 years). Not only overnutrition in this very period may induce permanent and deleterious changes in body composition, but they also induce parallel changes in the metabolic profile. The association of the metabolic 'score' at age 17 and early weight gain was independent of birth weight, gestational age, maternal fat mass and socioeconomic condition. The sweet, chubby baby is nice for his mother but not for its heart!

Consequences of being born small for gestational age

Relationships of maternal and paternal birth weights to features of the metabolic syndrome in adult offspring: an inter-generational study in South India

Veena SR, Geetha S, Leary SD, Saperia J, Fisher DJ, Kumaran K, Coakley P, Stein CE, Fall CH
Holdsworth Memorial Hospital, Mysore, Karnataka, India
Diabetologia 2007;50:43–54

Introduction: The association between lower birth weight and metabolic syndrome may result from fetal undernutrition (fetal programming hypothesis) and/or genes causing both low birth weight and insulin resistance (fetal insulin hypothesis). Associations between the birth weight of parents and metabolic syndrome in the offspring were looked for in an Indian cohort.

Results: Men and women (aged 35–68 years), who had been born in Holdsworth Memorial Hospital, Mysore, India, were identified together with the offspring (20–46 years) of these men and women. In total, 283 offspring of 193 mothers and 223 offspring of 144 fathers were studied. Investigations included anthropometry, oral glucose tolerance, plasma insulin and lipid concentrations and blood pressure. The metabolic syndrome was defined using WHO criteria. Among the offspring, lower birth weight was associated with an increased risk of glucose intolerance (impaired glucose tolerance, impaired fasting glucose or type 2 diabetes) and higher cholesterol and triacylglycerol concentrations ($p < 0.05$ for all adjusted for sex and age). Most outcomes in the offspring, including most individual components of the metabolic syndrome, were unrelated to parental birth weight. However, both maternal and paternal birth weight were inversely related to offspring metabolic syndrome (odds ratio 0.36 per kg, $p = 0.053$ for mother-offspring pairs; odds ratio 0.26, $p = 0.04$ for father-offspring pairs, adjusted for offspring age, sex, BMI and socioeconomic status). Maternal birth weight was inversely related to offspring systolic blood pressure ($\beta = -2.5$ mm Hg per kg maternal birth weight; $p = 0.052$).

Conclusions: Factors in both parents may influence the risk of metabolic syndrome in their offspring. There are several possible explanations, but the findings are consistent with the fetal insulin (genetic) hypothesis.

A summary of the findings would be nice. Several models have been proposed to explain the association of restricted fetal growth with later diseases development. The 'thrifty genotype' concept, first proposed by Neel [21], stated that populations have been selected for alleles favoring insulin resistance, which would be advantageous in terms of survival by reducing glucose uptake and limiting body growth at the time of famine but would become detrimental when food supply is abundant. This concept is further developed as 'fetal insulin hypothesis', which proposes that genetically determined insulin resistance results in impaired fetal growth as well as insulin resistance in adult life [22]. As a purely genetic model cannot explain reported effects of human famine during gestation and in experimental animal models, Barker and colleagues [23] proposed the alternative 'thrifty phenotype' model. According to a 'programming' process, they proposed that alteration in fetal nutrition and endocrine status resulted in developmental adaptations that permanently change structure, physiology and metabolism, thereby predisposing individuals to cardiovascular, metabolic and endocrine diseases in adult life [24].

References

1. Bjorbæk C, El-Haschimi K, Frantz JD, Flier JS: The role of SOCS-3 in leptin signaling and leptin resistance. J Biol Chem 1999;274:30059–30065.
2. McGarry JD: What if Minkowski had been ageusic? An alternative angle on diabetes. Science 1992;258:766–770.
3. Randle PJ, Newsholme EA, Garland PB: Regulation of glucose uptake by muscle. 8. Effects of fatty acids, ketone bodies and pyruvate, and of alloxan-diabetes and starvation, on the uptake and metabolic fate of glucose in rat heart and diaphragm muscles. Biochem J 1964;93:652–665.
4. Yamashita H, Takenoshita M, Sakurai M, Bruick RK, Henzel WJ, Shillinglaw W, Arnot D, Uyeda K: A glucose-responsive transcription factor that regulates carbohydrate metabolism in the liver. Proc Natl Acad Sci USA 2001;98: 9116–9121.
5. Dentin R, Benhamed F, Hainault I, Fauveau V, Foufelle F, Dyck JR, Girard J, Postic C: Liver-specific inhibition of ChREBP improves hepatic steatosis and insulin resistance in ob/ob mice. Diabetes 2006;55:2159–2170.
6. Cline GW, Petersen KF, Krssak M, Shen J, Hundal RS, Trajanoski Z, Inzucchi S, Dresner A, Rothman DL, Shulman GI: Impaired glucose transport as a cause of decreased insulin-stimulated muscle glycogen synthesis in type 2 diabetes. N Engl J Med 1999;341:240–246.
7. Petersen KF, Laurent D, Rothman DL, Cline GW, Shulman GI: Mechanism by which glucose and insulin inhibit net hepatic glycogenolysis in humans. J Clin Invest 1998;101:1203–1209.
8. Roden M, Price TB, Perseghin G, Petersen KF, Rothman DL, Cline GW, Shulman GI: Mechanism of free fatty acid-induced insulin resistance in humans. J Clin Invest 1996;97:2859–2865.
9. Escobar-Morreale HF, Botella-Carretero JI, Villuendas G, Sancho J, San Millan JL: Serum interleukin-18 concentrations are increased in the polycystic ovary syndrome: relationship to insulin resistance and to obesity. J Clin Endocrinol Metab 2004;89:806–811.
10. Moriwaki Y, Yamamoto T, Shibutani Y, Aoki E, Tsutsumi Z, Takahashi S, Okamura H, Koga M, Fukuchi M, Hada T: Elevated levels of interleukin-18 and tumor necrosis factor-α in serum of patients with type 2 diabetes mellitus: relationship with diabetic nephropathy. Metabolism 2003;52:605–608.
11. 2004 SEARCH for Diabetes in Youth: A multicenter study of the prevalence, incidence and classification of diabetes mellitus in youth. Control Clin Trials 2004;25:458–471.
12. Fagot-Campagna A, Saaddine JB, Engelgau MM: Is testing children for type 2 diabetes a lost battle? Diabetes Care 2000;23:1442–1443.
13. Wilkin TJ: The accelerator hypothesis: weight gain as the missing link between type 1 and type 2 diabetes. Diabetologia 2001;44:914–922.
14. Betts P, Mulligan J, Ward P, Smith B, Wilkin T: Increasing body weight predicts the earlier onset of insulin-dependant diabetes in childhood: testing the 'accelerator hypothesis' (2). Diabet Med 2005;22:144–151.
15. Fourlanos S: Insulin resistance in children and adolescents with type 1 diabetes mellitus: relation to obesity. Pediatr Diabetes 2005;6:3–4.
16. Littorin B, Nystrom L, Gullberg B, Rastam L, Ostman J, Arnqvist HJ, Bjork E, Blohme G, Bolinder J, Eriksson JW, Schersten B, Sundkvist G: Increasing body mass index at diagnosis of diabetes in young adult people during 1983–1999 in the Diabetes Incidence Study in Sweden (DISS). J Intern Med 2003;254:251–256.
17. Porter JR, Barrett TG: Braking the accelerator hypothesis? Diabetologia 2004;47:352–353.
18. Levy-Marchal C, Czernichow P: Small for gestational age and the metabolic syndrome: which mechanism is suggested by epidemiological and clinical studies? Horm Res 2006;65(suppl 3):123–130.
19. Ekelund U, Ong K, Linne Y, Neovius M, Brage S, Dunger DB, Wareham NJ, Rossner S: Upward weight percentile crossing in infancy and early childhood independently predicts fat mass in young adults: the Stockholm Weight Development Study (SWEDES). Am J Clin Nutr 2006;83:324–330.
20. Ong KK, Ahmed ML, Emmett PM, Preece MA, Dunger DB: Association between postnatal catch-up growth and obesity in childhood: prospective cohort study. BMJ 2000;320:967–971.
21. Neel JV: Diabetes mellitus: a 'thrifty' genotype rendered detrimental by 'progress'? Am J Hum Genet 1962;14:353–362.
22. Hattersley AT, Tooke JE: The fetal insulin hypothesis: an alternative explanation of the association of low birth weight with diabetes and vascular disease. Lancet 1999;353:1789–1792.
23. Phipps K, Barker DJP, Hales CN, Fall CHD, Osmond C, Clark PMS: Fetal growth and impaired glucose tolerance in men and women. Diabetologia 1993;36:225–228.
24. Lucas A: Programming by early nutrition in man. Ciba Found Symp 1991;156:38–55.

Population Genetics and Pharmacogenetics

Ken Ong

Medical Research Council Epidemiology Unit and Department of Paediatrics, University of Cambridge, Cambridge, UK

With 10 million single nucleotide polymorphisms (SNPs) to choose from it is little wonder that the vast majority of candidate-SNP- or candidate-gene-driven genetic association studies turned up negative or misleading false-positive results. The leading investigators and funding bodies in this field have therefore now committed their resources to very large studies in the range of 5,000–10,000 individuals and also employing Genomewide association SNP chips that genotype hundreds of thousands of SNPs, which in turn 'tag', or are markers for, the majority of all the common variants in the HapMap [1]. These 'high-stakes' approaches are now paying dividends. In the last year alone:

- a common SNP in a T-cell transcription factor gene TCF7L2 has been repeatedly confirmed in numerous large studies as a consistent genetic marker of type 2 diabetes (T2DM) risk (see Helgason et al. below)
- the first Genomewide association study for T2DM claims to have explained 70% of the disease risk (see Sladek et al. below)
- the first Genomewide association study for type 1 diabetes has led to convincing statistical evidence for a sixth susceptibility locus at the interferon inducer IFIH1 (see Smyth et al. in Chapter 7 [2])
- most recently a Genomewide association study for T2DM unearthed a major common variant associated with obesity at the TFO gene (see Frayling et al. below).

It may be debatable whether such findings will truly generate new drug targets. However, as the number of such validated genetic markers increases, we will hopefully be able to understand much more about the genetic epidemiology of various diseases, including much better refinement of individual disease risk prediction, how genetic susceptibility interacts with environmental factors, and eventually individual-level selection of optimal drug therapies or lifestyle interventions.

New hope – genomewide association studies

A genome-wide association study identifies novel risk loci for type 2 diabetes

Sladek R, Rocheleau G, Rung J, Dina C, Shen L, Serre D, Boutin P, Vincent D, Belisle A, Hadjadj S, Balkau B, Heude B, Charpentier G, Hudson TJ, Montpetit A, Pshezhetsky AV, Prentki M, Posner BI, Balding DJ, Meyre D, Polychronakos C, Froguel P
Department of Human Genetics, McGill University and Genome Quebec Innovation Centre, Montreal, Que., Canada
Polychronakos@McGill.ca
Nature 2007;44:881–885

Background: Type 2 diabetes (T2DM) results from the interaction between various environmental factors with a number of genetic variants, most of which are yet unknown. The recent development of high-density arrays allows the genotyping of hundreds of thousands of polymorphisms, and thereby allows a systematic search for T2DM susceptibility variants.
Methods: 392,935 single-nucleotide polymorphisms were tested in a French case-control cohort of 1,363 individuals. 59 markers with the most significant difference in genotype frequencies between cases of T2DM and controls were fast-tracked for testing in a second case-control study of 5,511 individuals.
Results: In addition to confirming the known association with the TCF7L2 gene, the second stage study identified four further loci containing variants that confer T2DM risk. These loci include a non-synonymous polymorphism in the zinc transporter SLC30A8, which is expressed exclusively in insulin-producing β-cells, and two linkage disequilibrium blocks that contain genes potentially involved in β-cell development or function (IDE-KIF11-HHEX and EXT2-ALX4).

Conclusions: These four novel genetic loci together with TCF7L2 explained a substantial 70% of the risk of T2DM. These findings constitute proof of principle for the genome-wide approach to the elucidation of complex genetic traits.

This is the first reported Genomewide association study in T2DM and it demonstrates the advantages of a hypothesis-free approach to SNP selection. The authors initially tested 392,935 SNPs in the smaller case-control study, where cases were enriched for genetic susceptibility by having a first-degree family history of diabetes, early age at onset and non-obese range BMI. They then took forward to the second stage larger study in more representative cases only those SNPs that reached Genomewide association after stringent correction for multiple testing. In addition to extremely convincing evidence for the T-cell transcription factor gene TCF7L2 (p value = 1.5×10^{-34}), the study found four new genes or loci related to T2DM risk. These include SLC30A8 on chromosome 8, which encodes a zinc transporter expressed only in the secretory granules of β-cells, and HHEX, a homeodomain protein which is essential for hepatic and pancreatic development. Further studies need to confirm these novel findings and results from other Genomewide association studies for T2DM are expected shortly. Interestingly, zinc deficiency that often accompanies fetal growth retardation, which in turn has been linked to later development of T2DM in adulthood, was associated with hypomethylation and hyperacetylation of genomic DNA in brain and liver of IUGR fetal and juvenile rats [3].

The authors speculate that the results may lead to the development of new dietary and pharmacological approaches to treating and preventing diabetes, for example with zinc supplementation. Other notable findings of this groundbreaking study were that these genetic markers explained 70% of the population-attributable risk of diabetes, which far exceeds previous estimates of the heritability of T2DM. Lastly, in 7 of the 8 SNPs associated with diabetes, the susceptibility allele was the ancestral, or older, allele. This supports the hypothesis that ancestral alleles were adapted to promote survival in the environments of ancient human history, but predispose to disease risk in today's affluent and obesogenic environments.

A common variant in the FTO gene is associated with body mass index and predisposes to childhood and adult obesity

Frayling TM, Timpson NJ, Weedon MN, Zeggini E, Freathy RM, Lindgren CM, Perry JR, Elliott KS, Lango H, Rayner NW, Shields B, Harries LW, Barrett JC, Ellard S, Groves CJ, Knight B, Patch AM, Ness AR, Ebrahim S, Lawlor DA, Ring SM, Ben-Shlomo Y, Jarvelin MR, Sovio U, Bennett AJ, Melzer D, Ferrucci L, Loos RJ, Barroso I, Wareham NJ, Karpe F, Owen KR, Cardon LR, Walker M, Hitman GA, Palmer CN, Doney AS, Morris AD, Davey-Smith G; The Wellcome Trust Case Control Consortium; Hattersley AT, McCarthy MI
Institute of Biomedical and Clinical Science, Peninsula Medical School, Exeter, UK
Andrew.Hattersley@pms.ac.uk
Science 2007 Apr 12 [Epub ahead of print]

Background: Obesity is a serious international health problem that increases the risk of several common diseases. The genetic factors predisposing to obesity are poorly understood.

Methods and Results: A genome-wide association study for type 2 diabetes-susceptibility genes identified a common variant SNP rs9939609 in the FTO gene that predisposes to diabetes through an effect on increasing body mass index (BMI). An additive association of the variant with BMI was replicated in 13 cohorts with 38,759 participants (p = 3×10^{-35}). The 16% of adults who are homozygous for the risk allele weighed ~3 kg more and had a 1.67-fold higher risk of obesity compared to those not inheriting a risk allele. This association was observed from age 7 years upwards and reflects a specific increase in fat mass.

Conclusions: Understanding how variation in the FTO gene region is associated with BMI and adiposity may provide insights into novel pathways involved in the control of adiposity.

This study surely represents the first true genetic signal for common obesity in adults and children. Family-based studies have long indicated a large genetic contribution to obesity, yet attempts to confirm initial promising reports of association with common variants (e.g. in GAD, ENPP1 and INSIG2 genes) have been disappointing. In this study, a Genomewide association study for T2DM firstly found that SNPs in the FTO gene region on chromosome 16 were strongly associated with T2DM. The diabetes-risk alleles were also strongly associated with increased BMI, and this completely explained the susceptibility to T2DM. They then studied the FTO gene variant in an additional 19,424 white

European adults and 10,172 white European children and confirmed the association with BMI in all 13 cohorts to an unprecedented level of significance ($p = 3 \times 10^{-35}$).

FTO is a gene of yet unknown function in an unknown pathway. It was originally cloned in a fused toe (Ft) mutant mouse arising from a large chromosomal deletion. Heterozygous animals are characterized by fused toes on the forelimbs and thymic hyperplasia, but no alteration in body weight or adiposity. However, the Ft mutant is a poor model for altered Fto activity as multiple genes are deleted. In humans, FTO is widely expressed in fetal and adult tissues with expression highest in the brain and pancreatic islet. Future studies will hopefully be quick to confirm its association with obesity in other populations and to explore this potentially novel causal pathway to obesity.

New paradigms – TCF7L2 in T2DM

Refining the impact of TCF7L2 gene variants on type 2 diabetes and adaptive evolution

Helgason A, Palsson S, Thorleifsson G, Grant SF, Emilsson V, Gunnarsdottir S, Adeyemo A, Chen Y, Chen G, Reynisdottir I, Benediktsson R, Hinney A, Hansen T, Andersen G, Borch-Johnsen K, Jorgensen T, Schafer H, Faruque M, Doumatey A, Zhou J, Wilensky RL, Reilly MP, Rader DJ, Bagger Y, Christiansen C, Sigurdsson G, Hebebrand J, Pedersen O, Thorsteinsdottir U, Gulcher JR, Kong A, Rotimi C, Stefansson K
deCODE genetics, Reykjavik, Iceland
agnar@decode.is
Nat Genet 2007;39:218–225

Background: This group recently reported association between risk of type 2 diabetes (T2DM) and common single nucleotide polymorphisms (SNPs) in the transcription factor 7-like 2 gene (TCF7L2), which explained a population-attributable risk (PAR) of 17%–28% in three populations of European ancestry. *Methods:* In order to refine the definition of the TCF7L2 diabetes susceptibility haplotype 'HapB(T2D)', replication studies were performed in West African and Danish T2DM case-control studies and in an expanded Icelandic study. *Results:* The T2DM susceptibility haplotype was narrowed to a single SNP, the ancestral T allele of rs7903146. These new data also identified another TCF7L2 variant 'HapA' that shows evidence of positive selection in East Asian, European and West African populations. Notably, HapA shows a suggestive association with body mass index and altered concentrations of the hunger-satiety hormones ghrelin and leptin in males. *Conclusions:* Selective advantage of HapA may have been mediated through effects on energy metabolism.

Since the original publication in January 2006 [4], TCF7L2, encoding the transcription factor 7-like 2, has proved to be the first consistent genetic marker of T2DM susceptibility. This association has been confirmed but only in very large studies, but also in various populations from around the world including Japanese, Indians and Mexican-Americans. The original study by this group identified strong association with an intron 3 microsatellite 'DG10S478'. While this has proved to be a good marker of disease risk, this was unlikely to be the actual causal or functional variation. The authors therefore went on in this study to try to refine the association with T2DM and identify the causal variation by genotyping a more genetically diverse West African population. Overall, these results rule out DG10S478 X and rs12255372 T as causal variants but identify rs7903146 T as either the risk variant itself or its closest known correlate.

The authors then went on to look at evolutionary selection of the various TCF7L2 haplotypes, however these results raise more questions than answers. Using HapMap data, they found two major lineages, HapA and HapB (which predisposes to diabetes). The frequency of HapA increased dramatically from African to European through to the East Asian populations, suggesting a strong selection pressure. There was weaker evidence that HapA predisposes to higher BMI, yet the strongest relationship was observed for HapA with ghrelin and the ghrelin-to-leptin ratio. These findings do not explain why East Asians should have lower BMI, and develop diabetes at lower levels of obesity compared to other populations, nor indeed what the survival advantage is of having HapA.

TCF7L2-gene polymorphisms confer an increased risk for early impairment of glucose metabolism and increased height in obese children

Korner A, Berndt J, Stumvoll M, Kiess W, Kovacs P
University Hospital for Children and Adolescents, Department of Internal Medicine III, University of Leipzig, Leipzig, Germany
J Clin Endocrinol Metab 2007 Feb 20 [Epub ahead of print]

Background: Variants in the transcription factor 7-like 2 (TCF7L2) gene have been associated with increased risk for type 2 diabetes (T2DM) in adults. This study evaluated whether TCF7L2 variants confer a higher risk for obesity and early impairment of glucose metabolism in children.

Methods: The five reported TCF7L2 risk variants were genotyped in a representative cohort of 1,029 Caucasian children and an independent cohort of 283 obese children.

Results: There was a significantly lower prevalence of the rs11196205 and rs7895340 T2DM risk alleles in the obese (n = 283) compared to lean (n = 672) children (0.40 vs. 0.45, p = 0.02). However, there were no significant associations between these genotypes and quantitative traits of obesity in either the normal or the obesity cohort. Obese children were significantly taller than lean children. This increase in height was independently associated with T2DM risk variants of the TCF7L2-gene, while in the normal representative cohort height appeared to be decreased in carriers of the minor alleles. In the obese cohort, three risk alleles (rs7901695, rs7903146, rs1225572) were significantly associated with higher fasting and 120-minute blood glucose levels independent of sex, age, pubertal stage, and BMI. Fasting and peak insulin levels and HOMA-IR appeared with a similar tendency but were not statistically significant.

Conclusions: These data indicate for the first time that TCF7L2 variants are associated with increased risk for early impairment of glucose metabolism in obese children. These findings are consistent with adult studies identifying TCF7L2 as a major diabetes susceptibility gene.

These authors found that the main genetic markers at TCF7L2 that confer T2DM susceptibility in adults are also associated with higher glucose levels in obese children. Such findings may help to discriminate which obese children are at most risk for diabetes and therefore need oral glucose tolerance testing. Furthermore, such studies in young non-diabetic subjects may also help to understand the functional consequences of variants in this gene that lead to T2DM risk. Unfortunately, despite looking at this in a large and representative childhood cohort no clear answers to this question were apparent. In adults, TCF7L2 variants show increasing associations with reduced insulin secretion and defective insulin processing rather than increased insulin resistance or greater obesity risk [5]. In contrast, in the current study, non-significant trends towards both higher fasting and peak insulin levels were seen. Two SNPs were weakly associated with reduced obesity risk, but these variants showed least association with glucose levels and the findings were not confirmed in the more powerful quantitative trait analyses. Finally, some associations were seen with childhood heights, but intriguingly these findings were in the opposite directions in their obese and representative cohorts. Further studies in other childhood cohorts with more detailed birth weight and growth data might help the identification of early pathways to T2DM.

New paradigms – childhood models of adult T2DM

Common variants in maturity-onset diabetes of the young genes contribute to risk of type 2 diabetes in Finns

Bonnycastle LL, Willer CJ, Conneely KN, Jackson AU, Burrill CP, Watanabe RM, Chines PS, Narisu N, Scott LJ, Enloe ST, Swift AJ, Duren WL, Stringham HM, Erdos MR, Riebow NL, Buchanan TA, Valle TT, Tuomilehto J, Bergman RN, Mohlke KL, Boehnke M, Collins FS
Genome Technology Branch, National Human Genome Research Institute, National Institutes of Health, Bethesda, Md., USA
francisc@mail.nih.gov
Diabetes 2006;55:2534–2540

Background: Previous studies have suggested that variants in the genes for maturity-onset diabetes of the young (MODY) may confer susceptibility to type 2 diabetes (T2DM). However, the results have been conflicting and coverage of the MODY genes has been incomplete. To complement previous studies of HNF4A, the other five known MODY genes were examined for association with T2DM in Finnish individuals.

Methods: The following single nucleotide polymorphism (SNP) selection criteria were used for each of the five genes: (1) tagging in linkage ($r^2 < 0.8$) with other SNPs from the HapMap database or another linkage disequilibrium map, (2) SNPs previously associated with T2DM, and (3) non-synonymous coding SNPs. In total, 128 SNPs were tested for association with T2DM in 786 index cases from T2DM families and 619 normal glucose-tolerant controls. 35 of the most significant SNPs were genotyped in a second study of 384 cases and 366 controls from Finland. Previously reported HNF4A results were extended by genotyping 12 SNPs on additional Finnish samples.

Results: After correcting for multiple testing, there was evidence of T2DM association with SNPs in five of the six known MODY genes: GCK, HNF1A, HNF1B, NEUROD1, and HNF4A.

Conclusions: These studies suggest that common variants in five of the six known MODY genes play a modest role in T2DM susceptibility.

Assessment of the role of common genetic variation in the transient neonatal diabetes mellitus region in type 2 diabetes: a comparative genomic and tagging single nucleotide polymorphism approach

Gloyn AL, Mackay DJ, Weedon MN, McCarthy MI, Walker M, Hitman G, Knight BA, Owen KR, Hattersley AT, Frayling TM
Diabetes Research Laboratories, Oxford Centre for Diabetes, Endocrinology and Metabolism, Oxford, UK
frayling@pms.ac.uk
Diabetes 2006;55:2272–2276

Background: Recent evidence supports the strong overlap between genes implicated in monogenic diabetes and susceptibility to type 2 diabetes (T2DM). Several T2DM linkage studies have reported linkage to chromosome 6q22-25. Transient neonatal diabetes mellitus (TNDM) is a rare disorder associated with overexpression of genes at a paternally expressed imprinted locus on chromosome 6q24. There are two overlapping genes in this region: the transcription factor zinc finger protein associated with cell cycle control and apoptosis (ZAC also known as PLAGL1) and HYMA1, which encodes an untranslated mRNA. This study tested the hypothesis that common genetic variants at this TNDM region may be associated with T2DM susceptibility.

Methods: In 47 individuals, new single nucleotide polymorphisms (SNP) in the TNDM gene region were identified by resequencing the ZAC coding regions and also regions of high conservation between human and mouse ZAC and 20-kb flanking sequences. The resulting tag SNPs were genotyped in a large UK Caucasian case-control (n = 3,594) and family-based (n = 1,654) study.

Results: 26 SNPs were identified. 15 tag SNPs were successfully genotyped, which captured 92% of the 26 SNPs with $r^2 > 0.5$. There was no evidence of association or overtransmission of any SNP to affected offspring or of a parent-of-origin effect.

Conclusions: In a study sufficiently powered to detect odds ratios of <1.2, common variation in the TNDM region does not appear to play an important role in the genetic susceptibility to T2DM in UK Caucasians.

These two papers explore the principle that the detailed study of rare childhood disorders may help the understanding of the etiology of common adult disease. The candidate gene approach to genetic association studies of common disease seems to have had greatest success by choosing genes in which rare, usually deleterious, mutations have already been shown to cause monogenic forms of those conditions. The above two studies have studied common variations in genes involved in MODY and TNDM for association with T2DM in adults. Interestingly, five of the six known MODY genes showed evidence of association with T2DM. One further variant in HNF4A associated with earlier age at diagnosis.

However, the effect sizes were modest, and the authors cited personal communications in the discussion that the findings with the MODY genes were not confirmed in a large cohort of Swedish, Finnish, Canadian and Polish individuals. Further large studies and meta-analyses may also conclude that the current findings are false positives. However it is not long ago that these different forms of MODY were clinically classified together with T2DM. Similarly, a subtype of early onset type 1 diabetes has recently been recognized to have a distinct monogenic cause and dramatic response to oral sulfonylurea therapy [6]. In addition to the large-study and large-scale genotyping approach, careful recognition of further clinical subtypes of disease are necessary to unravel the genetics of common diseases.

New genetic associations: with childhood obesity

A common genetic variant is associated with adult and childhood obesity

Herbert A, Gerry NP, McQueen MB, Heid IM, Pfeufer A, Illig T, Wichmann HE, Meitinger T, Hunter D, Hu FB, Colditz G, Hinney A, Hebebrand J, Koberwitz K, Zhu X, Cooper R, Ardlie K, Lyon H, Hirschhorn JN, Laird NM, Lenburg ME, Lange C, Christman MF
Department of Genetics and Genomics, Boston University Medical School, Boston, Mass., USA
aherbert@bu.edu
Science 2006;312:279–283

Background: Obesity is a heritable trait and is an important risk factor for several common diseases such as type 2 diabetes, heart disease, and hypertension.
Methods: In a dense whole-genome scan, 116,204 SNPs were genotyped in 694 participants from the Framingham Heart Study offspring cohort. After exclusions, 86,604 SNPs were tested for association with BMI.
Results: One SNP (rs7566605) near the INSIG2 gene reached overall significance for association with obesity at a genome-wide level. This association was subsequently replicated in four separate populations composed of individuals of Western European ancestry, African-Americans, and children. The obesity-predisposing genotype is present in 10% of individuals.
Conclusions: This study suggests that common genetic polymorphisms are important determinants of obesity.

This Genomewide association study using the Affymetrix 100K SNP chip found strong evidence for a new obesity-associated common genetic variant. A meta-analysis of all their case-control samples showed that the rs7566605 CC genotype conferred a mild increase in obesity risk in a recessive model with odds ratio of 1.22 (95% CI 1.05–1.42, p = 0.008). This variant lies 10 kb upstream of the insulin induced gene 2 (INSIG2), which includes a protein that inhibits synthesis of fatty acid and cholesterol, and is therefore an attractive biological candidate for further functional studies.

However, while the authors went to great lengths to show the consistency of their finding a wide range of other populations, the subsequent correspondence relating to this paper only a few months later in *Science* reveals that other investigators have failed to support the main finding of the original study. Loos et al. [7] if anything found the opposite tendency with BMI in two large UK Caucasian cohorts totalling 6,599 individuals; Dina et al. [8] also found no evidence for this association in 10,265 Caucasian individuals, and Rosskopf et al. [9] found no association with BMI in 4,089 German individuals. A major contribution of INSIG2 rs7566605 to the genetic risk of obesity in the West European population is therefore unlikely, however it remains possible that INSIG2 contributes to BMI variation in children and other ethnic groups.

The enormous analytical and computational capacity of modern technology requires special attention to old rules of statistics. Tossing a cube 100 thousand times, one would expect just by chance one gene with a p value of 10^{-5}.

ENPP1 variants and haplotypes predispose to early onset obesity and impaired glucose and insulin metabolism in German obese children

Bottcher Y, Korner A, Reinehr T, Enigk B, Kiess W, Stumvoll M, Kovacs P
Medical Department III, University of Leipzig, Leipzig, Germany
peter.kovacs@medizin.uni-leipzig.de
J Clin Endocrinol Metab 2006;91:4948–4952

Background: ENPP1 (nucleotide pyrophosphatase/phosphodiesterase-1) encodes a membrane-bound glycoprotein that inhibits the insulin-receptor tyrosine kinase activity, resulting in reduced insulin sensitivity. Common variants in this gene have previously been associated with obesity and insulin resistance. This study explored the role of ENPP1 genetic variants in obesity and related traits in a representative population of Caucasian children and in cohorts of obese children with detailed metabolic assessments.

Methods: The K121Q, IVS20delT-11, and A/G+1044TGA variants in ENPP1 were genotyped in 712 schoolchildren (346 boys and 366 girls; mean age 12 ± 3 years; BMI SD score 0.09 ± 0.04) and in independent cohorts of 205 obese children from Leipzig and 195 obese children from Datteln, Germany.

Results: Compared to a lean control group, there was an increased risk of obesity in Leipzig children carrying the 121Q variant (adjusted odds ratio 1.82; 95% CI 1.30–2.56, p = 0.0005) or the [Q-delT-G] haplotype [1.75 (1.17–2.62), p = 0.006]. These findings were replicated in another independent obesity/overweight cohort from Leipzig as well as obese children from Datteln. In addition, among obese children from Leipzig, the [Q-delT-G] haplotype was associated with higher 2-hour glucose levels, whereas the [K-delT-G] and [K-insT-A] haplotypes were associated with improved insulin sensitivity and glucose metabolism (all p < 0.05 after adjusting for age, gender, and BMI).

Conclusions: This study suggests a potential role of the K121Q polymorphism and ENPP1 haplotypes in conferring increased susceptibility to obesity and early impairment of glucose tolerance in children.

Recent studies summarized in *Yearbook 2006* [1] had raised the hope that ENPP1 might represent the first common genetic determinant of both obesity and T2DM, and might help to identify which obese individuals are at high risk of metabolic complications. However, as is often the case, subsequent large studies in adult populations have since found no evidence of the original associations [10, 11], and even findings in the opposite direction [12], indicating that the results may be false positive or are not easily generalizable.

In contrast to adults, the above study in German children does provide some support for a consistent association in children. The ENPP1 Q121 variant, proposed to impair insulin signaling (or a haplotype of Q121 plus two other variants), was associated with increased risk of obesity and glucose intolerance, while haplotypes with the K121 variant conferred improved insulin sensitivity and glucose homeostasis. These findings strongly resemble those published in French children [13] and obviously need to be confirmed in further large and well-characterized childhood cohorts. Early-onset obesity and childhood or adolescent T2DM may be determined by different or more specific risk factors compared to their adult counterparts, and the confirmation of their genetic risk factors should not be reliant on large-scale studies performed only in adults.

New genetic associations: with birth weight

Polymorphism in maternal LRP8 gene is associated with fetal growth

Wang L, Wang X, Laird N, Zuckerman B, Stubblefield P, Xu X
Program for Population Genetics, Harvard School of Public Health, Boston, Mass., USA
xin_xu@harvard.edu
Am J Hum Genet 2006;78:770–777

Background: Fetal growth restriction (FGR) affects >200,000 pregnancies in the USA annually and is associated with increased perinatal mortality and morbidity, as well as poorer long-term health for the infants. FGR appears to be a complex trait, and the role of genetic factors is largely unknown.

Methods: A candidate-gene association study of birth weight and FGR was performed in two independent study samples obtained at the Boston Medical Center. Firstly, association between maternal genotypes of 68 SNPs from 41 candidate genes and fetal growth was investigated in a sample of 204 black women selected for a previous study of preeclampsia, 92 of whom had preeclampsia (characterized by high blood pressure and the presence of protein in the urine).

Results: SNP rs2297660 in the LRP8 gene was significantly associated with birth weight. In a subsequent replication study, there was a similar association between LRP8 and FGR in a larger independent sample of 1,094 black women: the 'A' allele at rs2297660 was associated with a higher standardized birth weight and a lower risk of FGR. In an additive model, each additional copy of the 'A' allele reduced the risk of FGR by 33% (p < 0.05).

Conclusions: Results from two independent samples of black women provide consistent evidence that SNP rs2297660 in LRP8 is associated with fetal growth.

Many childhood cohorts are being studied in relation to the etiology of long-term health outcomes associated with low birth weight and related postnatal growth patterns. This study reminds us that the predisposition to producing low birth weight offspring is a heritable maternal trait and that candidate underlying factors may therefore reside in mother's genotype.

In this study all the candidate genes were selected based on biological plausibility, as they were potentially important in preeclampsia and chronic hypertension, which is a major pathogenic pathway of FGR. The author's definition of FGR was synonymous with small gestational age (SGA), being defined as birth weight below the 10th centile for sex and gestation. In their pooled analysis, each A allele at rs2297660 was associated with a 0.18 SD increase in birth weight and 0.67 relative risk of FGR.

LRP8 encodes the apolipoprotein E (ApoE) receptor 2, which mediates the cellular recognition and internalization of ApoE-containing lipoproteins and is highly expressed in the placenta. The authors did not directly report whether this variant was associated with maternal hypertension or preeclampsia, however further putative effects of the transmitted variant in the fetus could also contribute to links between low birth weight and long-term risk for adult disease.

A common haplotype of the glucokinase gene alters fasting glucose and birth weight: association in six studies and population-genetics analyses

Weedon MN, Clark VJ, Qian Y, Ben-Shlomo Y, Timpson N, Ebrahim S, Lawlor DA, Pembrey ME, Ring S, Wilkin TJ, Voss LD, Jeffery AN, Metcalf B, Ferrucci L, Corsi AM, Murray A, Melzer D, Knight B, Shields B, Smith GD, Hattersley AT, Di Rienzo A, Frayling TM
Institute of Biomedical and Clinical Science, Peninsula Medical School, Exeter, UK
Am J Hum Genet 2006;79:991–1001

Background: Fasting glucose is associated with future type 2 diabetes and ischemic heart disease risks and is tightly regulated despite considerable variations in food intake. During pregnancy, maternal fasting glucose concentration is an important determinant of offspring birth weight. The key determinant of fasting glucose is the enzyme glucokinase (GCK). Rare mutations of GCK cause fasting hyperglycemia and alter birth weight. The extent to which common variation of GCK explains normal variation of fasting glucose and birth weight is not known.

Methods: In order to comprehensively define the role of common genetic variation in GCK in the regulation of fasting glucose and birth weight, a tagSNP approach was studied in a total of 19,806 individuals from six population-based studies.

Results: Out of 22 tagSNPs, only the promoter variant rs1799884 was independently associated with fasting glucose levels. This association was seen at all ages in the normal population and exceeded genomewide levels of significance ($p = 10^{-9}$). rs3757840 was also highly significantly associated with fasting glucose ($p = 8 \times 10^{-7}$), but this was explained by linkage disequilibrium ($r^2 = 0.2$) with rs1799884. A maternal A allele at rs1799884 was associated with a 32-g (95% CI 11–53 g) increase in offspring birth weight ($p = 0.002$). Genetic variation influencing birth weight may have conferred a selective advantage in human populations. However, extensive population-genetics analyses revealed no evidence of recent positive natural selection on patterns of GCK variation.

Conclusions: This comprehensive analysis of common variation of the glucokinase gene shows that this is the first gene to be reproducibly associated with fasting glucose and fetal growth.

During pregnancy, maternal glucose concentration is an important determinant of offspring birth weight. Rare mutations in GCK cause the mild hyperglycemia phenotype of maturity-onset diabetes of the young type 2 (MODY2). The original study of the effects of these rare mutations on birth weight provided the original model for the fetal insulin hypothesis [14]; maternal mutations leading to gestational hypoglycemia increased birth weight, while fetal mutations leading to fetal insulin undersecretion lowered birth weight.

The authors have now comprehensively tested the hypothesis that common variants in GCK might contribute to the normal variation in glucose levels and birth weight. They performed new sequencing of the exons and surrounding gene region to identify the common tagSNPs, which were then genotyped in a huge combined population of 19,806 individuals. Overall minor allele carriers of rs1799884 had an average 0.06 mmol/l increase in fasting glucose (p = 10^{-9}), and mothers with this variant had babies with 32 g higher birth weights. However, no independent effect of fetal genotype was seen. The frequency of the variant was lower in a Sub-Saharan African population than in non-African populations cut, however further analyses did not show a significant deficit in haplotype variation.

The relevance of these findings remains to be fully established, however the study adds support the fruitfulness of studying common variants in genes where rare mutations are known to be deleterious.

A quantitative trait locus on chromosome 6q influences birth weight in two independent family studies

Arya R, Demerath E, Jenkinson CP, Goring HH, Puppala S, Farook V, Fowler S, Schneider J, Granato R, Resendez RG, Dyer TD, Cole SA, Almasy L, Comuzzie AG, Siervogel RM, Bradshaw B, DeFronzo RA, MacCluer J, Stern MP, Towne B, Blangero J, Duggirala R
Division of Clinical Epidemiology, University of Texas Health Science Center, San Antonio, Tex., USA
arya@uthscsa.edu
Hum Mol Genet 2006;15:1569–1579

Background: Low birth weight is an important cause of infant mortality and morbidity. Birth weight has also been shown to correlate inversely with adult obesity, type 2 diabetes and cardiovascular disease. However, little is known about the genetic factors influencing variation in birth weight and its association with diseases in later life.

Methods: A genome-wide linkage study was performed to identify genes that influence birth weight in Mexican-Americans using the data from the San Antonio Family Birth Weight Study participants (n = 840).

Results: Heritability of birth weight was estimated as 72.0 ± 8.4% (p < 0.0001) after adjusting for sex and gestation. Multipoint linkage analysis yielded the strongest evidence for linkage of birth weight (LOD = 3.7) between the markers D6S1053 and D6S1031 on chromosome 6q. This finding was replicated (LOD = 2.3) in an independent European-American population. Together, these findings provide substantial evidence (LOD_{adj} = 4.3) for a major locus influencing variation in birth weight. Positional candidate genes in this region include: chorionic gonadotropin, α-chain, collagen, type XIX, α_1-, and protein-tyrosine phosphatase, type 4A-1. In addition, potential evidence for linkage (LOD > or = 1.2) was found on chromosomes 1q, 2q, 3q, 4q, 9p, 19p and 19q with LODs ranging from 1.3 to 2.7.

Conclusions: This study found strong evidence for a major gene on chromosome 6q that influences variation in birth weight in both Mexican- and European-Americans.

This study complements the above two studies by searching for 'positional candidate genes' for birth weight in the mother's genotype. Not to be confused with the more recent Genomewide Association studies, this is an example of a Genomewide Linkage study where highly polymorphic markers are genotyped at a much greater interval of 10 cM density. These studies also differ by being based in family pedigrees, rather than unrelated individuals. The study found strong evidence for a common genetic variant on chromosome 6q and suggests that further studies of the candidate genes in this region may be fruitful. Interestingly, the candidate region on chromosome 6q contains the *hCG* gene, which stimulates progesterone secretion and acts as a growth factor that facilitates endometrial receptivity.

With the advent of Genomewide association studies, the further utility of Genomewide Linkage analyses is debated. The T2DM susceptibility gene TCF7L2 was discovered as a positional candidate gene through the latter approach, however the current Genomewide association studies also quickly detected its very strong signal (p value = 1.5×10^{-34} in Sladek et al. above). One clear further benefit of the family-based approach is the ability to estimate heritability. Indeed in the above study the heritability of birth weight as a continuous trait was very high at 72%, suggesting that further studies to identify the genetics of birth weight using either approach will be worthwhile.

Global variation in copy number in the human genome

Redon R, Ishikawa S, Fitch KR, Feuk L, Perry GH, Andrews TD, Fiegler H, Shapero MH, Carson AR, Chen W, Cho EK, Dallaire S, Freeman JL, Gonzalez JR, Gratacos M, Huang J, Kalaitzopoulos D, Komura D, MacDonald JR, Marshall CR, Mei R, Montgomery L, Nishimura K, Okamura K, Shen F, Somerville MJ, Tchinda J, Valsesia A, Woodwark C, Yang F, Zhang J, Zerjal T, Zhang J, Armengol L, Conrad DF, Estivill X, Tyler-Smith C, Carter NP, Aburatani H, Lee C, Jones KW, Scherer SW, Hurles ME

The Wellcome Trust Sanger Institute, Wellcome Trust Genome Campus, Hinxton, Cambridge, UK
steve@genet.sickkids.on.ca
Nature 2006;444:444–454

Background: Copy number variation (CNV) of DNA sequences is functionally significant but has yet to be fully ascertained. This report describes the construction of a first-generation CNV map of the human genome based on the HapMap population of 270 individuals from four populations with ancestry in Europe, Africa or Asia.

Methods: DNA from these individuals was screened for CNV using two complementary technologies: SNP genotyping arrays and clone-based comparative genomic hybridization.

Results: A total of 1,447 copy number variable regions (CNVRs) covering 360 megabases (12% of the genome) were identified in these populations. These CNVRs encompassed overlapping or adjacent gains or losses, and contained hundreds of genes, disease loci, functional elements and segmental duplications. Notably, the CNVRs encompassed more nucleotide content per genome than SNPs, underscoring the importance of CNV in genetic diversity and evolution.

Conclusions: These findings delineate linkage disequilibrium patterns for many CNVs, and reveal marked variation in copy number among populations. They also demonstrate the utility of this resource for genetic disease studies.

A comprehensive analysis of common copy-number variations in the human genome

Wong KK, deLeeuw RJ, Dosanjh NS, Kimm LR, Cheng Z, Horsman DE, MacAulay C, Ng RT, Brown CJ, Eichler EE, Lam WL

Department of Cancer Genetics and Developmental Biology, University of British Columbia, Vancouver, B.C., Canada
kwong@bccrc.ca
Am J Hum Genet 2007;80:91–104

Background: Segmental copy-number variations (CNVs) in the human genome are associated with developmental disorders and susceptibility to diseases. More importantly, CNVs may represent a major genetic component of human phenotypic diversity.

Methods: A whole-genome array comparative genomic hybridization assay was performed in 95 individuals.

Results: 3,654 autosomal segmental CNVs were identified, 800 of which appeared at a frequency of at least 3%. Of these frequent CNVs, 77% are novel. In the 95 individuals analyzed, the two most diverse genomes differed by at least 9 Mb in size or varied by at least 266 loci in content. Approximately 68% of the 800 polymorphic regions overlap with genes, which may reflect human diversity in senses (smell, hearing, taste, and sight), rhesus phenotype, metabolism, and disease susceptibility. Intriguingly, 14 polymorphic regions harbor 21 of the known human microRNAs, raising the possibility of the contribution of microRNAs to phenotypic diversity in humans.

Conclusions: This in-depth survey of CNVs across the human genome provides a valuable baseline for studies involving human genetics.

The first map of CNV in the human genome has been published. Copy CNVs are defined as DNA segments >1 kb that are present in variable copy number. Such variation can arise through various ways including: deletions, insertions, duplications and complex multisite variants such as gains or losses of homologous sequences at multiple sites in the genome. Several of these CNV-associated genes are related to the senses, including a group of olfactory receptor genes, multiple taste-receptor genes, and several genes related to sight or hearing.

It is known that rare genomic rearrangements are a cause of human disease, for example MODY5 [15], while other large structural variations have been described to occur commonly and may even confer some survival advantage or positive selection [16]. The current studies now help describe the full extent of CNVs in the human genome. The estimated average total length of CNV regions per genome was more than 20 million base pairs, which is far greater than the total variation due to SNPs alone. Furthermore, 285 out of the 1,961 (14.5%) genes in the OMIM database of genetic diseases overlapped with CNVs, indicating numerous possible disease associations.

Concepts revised: the insulin gene VNTR

Insulin gene variable number of tandem repeats (INS VNTR) genotype and metabolic syndrome in childhood obesity

Santoro N, Cirillo G, Amato A, Luongo C, Raimondo P, D'Aniello A, Perrone L, Miraglia del Giudice E
Department of Pediatrics, F. Fede Seconda Università di Napoli, Napoli, Italy
emanuele.miraglia@unina2.it
J Clin Endocrinol Metab 2006;91:4641–4644

Background: The insulin gene variable number of tandem repeats (INS VNTR) polymorphism has been associated with insulin levels in obese children. Hyperinsulinemia is a pivotal factor in the development of metabolic syndrome, an emerging complication in childhood obesity. This study tested the associations between INS VNTR genotype and the metabolic syndrome in juvenile-onset obesity.
Methods: A marker for INS VNTR allele class was genotyped in 320 obese children (152 girls, mean age 11.2 ± 2.3 years, mean z-score BMI 3.6 ± 1.1). All of them underwent a standard oral glucose tolerance test (OGTT); baseline measurements included blood pressure, plasma lipid profile and fasting insulin levels. Whole-body insulin sensitivity and the insulinogenic index were calculated from the OGTT data.
Results: The prevalence of metabolic syndrome was 39%. There was no difference in INS VNTR genotype distribution between obese and 200 lean, age- and sex-matched children (p = 0.7). However, among obese children, those who were homozygous for the class I allele showed higher insulin levels and insulinogenic index but lower whole-body insulin sensitivity than other obese children. Accordingly, among obese children the odds ratio for developing the metabolic syndrome was 2.5-fold higher (95% CI 1.5–3.9, p = 0.006) in obese children carrying the I/I genotype, compared to other obese children.
Conclusions: Class I/I homozygotes for the INS VNTR insulin promoter predisposes obese children to develop the metabolic syndrome.

The INS VNTR locus does not associate with smallness for gestational age (SGA) but interacts with SGA to increase insulin resistance in young adults

Vu-Hong TA, Durand E, Deghmoun S, Boutin P, Meyre D, Chevenne D, Czernichow P, Froguel P, Levy-Marchal C
Institut National de la Santé et de la Recherche Médicale, Unit 690, Robert Debré Hôpital, Paris, France
J Clin Endocrinol Metab 2006;91:2437–2440

Background: Both adverse intrauterine events and genetic background have been suggested to confer insulin resistance in individuals born small for gestational age (SGA). Insulin is a candidate gene that could potentially influence both fetal growth and glucose metabolism. However, the potential effect of the insulin gene VNTR (INS) on birth weight is yet controversial.
Methods: This study tested the contribution of the INS VNTR locus on birth weight and on the metabolic profile of young adults born SGA (mean age 22 years). Two groups were selected based their birth weights: SGA (birth weight <10th percentile, n = 735), and appropriate for gestational age (AGA; birth weight between 25th and 75th percentiles, n = 886). All individuals were genotyped for the rs689 A/T SNP, which is in complete linkage disequilibrium with the INS VNTR classes I and III, respectively.
Results: Class I allele frequencies were similar in the two groups (70% in AGA; 72% in SGA, p = 0.42), and the INS VNTR was not associated with mean birth weight in either SGA (p = 0.99) or AGA groups (p = 0.18). Although the INS VNTR genotype did not associate with indices of insulin resistance

in the AGA group, in the SGA group, INS VNTR class III allele was associated with higher insulin resistance (quantitative insulin sensitivity check index = 0.38 vs. 0.39, p = 0.05). Furthermore, there was a significant interaction between the SGA/AGA status and INS VNTR genotype on insulin resistance indices (p = 0.01) in a multivariate analysis.

Conclusions: The INS VNTR locus was not directly associated with SGA or birth weight in this French population. However, these data support an interaction between fetal growth restriction and INS VNTR genotype, which influences insulin resistance in young adults born SGA.

The INS VNTR polymorphism has occupied the literature for many years. It is a functional polymorphism that regulates insulin and insulin-like growth factor-2 transcription and class I alleles have been consistently shown to predispose to type 1 diabetes risk. In contrast, studies for T2DM and obesity risks in large adult populations have been inconsistent and are overall unconvincing. However, in addition to the above two recent studies, several childhood cohorts have also repeatedly shown that the genotype effects on insulin levels and adiposity in children are highly modified by birth weight, postnatal weight gain and childhood obesity [17–19].

These findings in children either represent multiple false-positive reports in childhood populations that are often much smaller than their adult population counterparts, or there are important interactive effects of early growth on the expression of certain genotypes, which could have important relevance not only to childhood growth and development, but also for adult disease risks. Very large childhood cohort studies, or multicenter collaborations such as those that have been set up between adult studies [20], are urgently needed in pediatric genetic epidemiology.

Food for thought: the human epigenome project

DNA methylation profiling of human chromosomes 6, 20 and 22

Eckhardt F, Lewin J, Cortese R, Rakyan VK, Attwood J, Burger M, Burton J, Cox TV, Davies R, Down TA, Haefliger C, Horton R, Howe K, Jackson DK, Kunde J, Koenig C, Liddle J, Niblett D, Otto T, Pettett R, Seemann S, Thompson C, West T, Rogers J, Olek A, Berlin K, Beck S
Epigenomics AG, Berlin, Germany
florian.eckhardt@epigenomics.com
Nat Genet 2006;38:1378–1385

Background: DNA methylation is the most stable type of epigenetic modification modulating the transcriptional plasticity of mammalian genomes.

Methods: This study reports the high-resolution methylation profiles of human chromosomes 6, 20 and 22, using bisulfite DNA sequencing. The data provide a resource of around 1.9 million CpG methylation values derived from 43 samples from 12 different tissues.

Results: Analysis of six annotation categories showed that evolutionarily conserved regions are the predominant sites for differential DNA methylation and that a core region surrounding the transcriptional start site is an informative surrogate for promoter methylation. 17% of the 873 analyzed genes were differentially methylated in their 5′ UTRs, and around one-third of the differentially methylated 5′ UTRs are inversely correlated with levels of transcription. Despite the fact that this study included factors reported to affect DNA methylation such as sex and age, no significant attributable effects were found.

Conclusions: These data suggest DNA methylation to be ontogenetically more stable than previously thought.

Completion of the Human Genome Project gave us the blueprint of the genetic sequence. However, many processes that regulate gene expression are governed by additional layers of epigenetic information that are not directly encoded in the DNA sequence itself but take the form of chemical modifications such as DNA methylation. The Human Epigenome Project aims to identify, catalogue and interpret genome-wide DNA methylation profiles of all human genes in all major tissues.

The current study reports the results of that project for chromosomes 6, 20 and 22 based on 43 samples derived from 12 different healthy tissues. Almost 25% of all amplicons showed tissue-specific methylation. Most genetic epidemiology studies are based on DNA samples derived from peripheral lymphocytes or buccal cells. Future studies should therefore consider the possibility of collecting other tissue samples. Recent developments in epigenetics are also described in other chapters this year [21].

References

1. Heude B, Ong KK: Population genetics and pharmacogenetics; in Carel J-C, Hochberg Z (eds): Yearbook of Pediatric Endocrinology 2006. Basel, Karger, 2006, pp 117–130.
2. Chiarelli F: Type 1 diabetes: clinical and experimental; in Carel J-C, Hochberg Z (eds): Yearbook of Pediatric Endocrinology 2007. Basel, Karger, 2007.
3. Simmons RA: Developmental origins of β-Cell failure in type 2 diabetes: the role of epigenetic mechanisms. Pediatr Res 2007 Mar 15 [Epub ahead of print].
4. Grant SF, Thorleifsson G, Reynisdottir I, Benediktsson R, Manolescu A, Sainz J, et al: Variant of transcription factor 7-like 2 (TCF7L2) gene confers risk of type 2 diabetes. Nat Genet 2006;38:320–323.
5. Loos RJ, Franks PW, Francis RW, Barroso I, Gribble FM, Savage DB, et al: TCF7L2 polymorphisms modulate proinsulin levels and β-cell function in a British Europid population. Diabetes 2007 Apr 6 [Epub ahead of print].
6. Pearson ER, Flechtner I, Njolstad PR, Malecki MT, Flanagan SE, Larkin B, et al: Switching from insulin to oral sulfonylureas in patients with diabetes due to Kir6.2 mutations. N Engl J Med 2006;355:467–477.
7. Loos RJ, Barroso I, O'Rahilly S, Wareham NJ: Comment on 'A common genetic variant is associated with adult and childhood obesity'. Science 2007;315:187.
8. Dina C, Meyre D, Samson C, Tichet J, Marre M, Jouret B, et al: Comment on 'A common genetic variant is associated with adult and childhood obesity'. Science 2007;12;315:187.
9. Rosskopf D, Bornhorst A, Rimmbach C, Schwahn C, Kayser A, Kruger A, et al: Comment on 'A common genetic variant is associated with adult and childhood obesity'. Science 2007;315:187.
10. Weedon MN, Shields B, Hitman G, Walker M, McCarthy MI, Hattersley AT, et al: No evidence of association of ENPP1 variants with type 2 diabetes or obesity in a study of 8,089 UK Caucasians. Diabetes 2006;55:3175–3179.
11. Lyon HN, Florez JC, Bersaglieri T, Saxena R, Winckler W, Almgren P, et al: Common variants in the ENPP1 gene are not reproducibly associated with diabetes or obesity. Diabetes 2006;55:3180–3184.
12. Prudente S, Trischitta V: Editorial: The pleiotropic effect of the ENPP1 (PC-1) gene on insulin resistance, obesity, and type 2 diabetes. J Clin Endocrinol Metab 2006;91:4767–4768.
13. Meyre D, Bouatia-Naji N, Tounian A, Samson C, Lecoeur C, Vatin V, et al: Variants of ENPP1 are associated with childhood and adult obesity and increase the risk of glucose intolerance and type 2 diabetes. Nat Genet 2005;37:863–867.
14. Hattersley AT, Tooke JE: The fetal insulin hypothesis: an alternative explanation of the association of low birthweight with diabetes and vascular disease. Lancet 1999;353:1789–1792.
15. Bellanne-Chantelot C, Clauin S, Chauveau D, Collin P, Daumont M, Douillard C, et al: Large genomic rearrangements in the hepatocyte nuclear factor-1β (TCF2) gene are the most frequent cause of maturity-onset diabetes of the young type 5. Diabetes 2005;54:3126–3132.
16. Stefansson H, Helgason A, Thorleifsson G, Steinthorsdottir V, Masson G, Barnard J, et al: A common inversion under selection in Europeans. Nat Genet 2005;37:129–137.
17. Heude B, Petry CJ, Pembrey M, Dunger DB, Ong KK: The insulin gene variable number of tandem repeat: associations and interactions with childhood body fat mass and insulin secretion in normal children. J Clin Endocrinol Metab 2006;91:2770–2775.
18. Le Stunff C, Fallin D, Schork NJ, Bougneres P: The insulin gene VNTR is associated with fasting insulin levels and development of juvenile obesity. Nat Genet 2000;26:444–446.
19. Dos Santos C, Fallin D, Le Stunff C, LeFur S, Bougneres P: INS VNTR is a QTL for the insulin response to oral glucose in obese children. Physiol Genomics 2004;16:309–313.
20. Ioannidis JP, Gwinn M, Little J, Higgins JP, Bernstein JL, Boffetta P, et al: A road map for efficient and reliable human genome epidemiology. Nat Genet 2006;38:3–5.
21. Hochberg Z, Carel J-C: The year in science and medicine; in Carel J-C, Hochberg Z (eds): Yearbook of Pediatric Endocrinology 2007. Basel, Karger, 2007.

Evidence-Based Medicine in Pediatric Endocrinology

Gary E Butler

Department of Paediatrics and Growth, Institute of Health Sciences, University of Reading, Surrey, UK

Evidence-based pediatric endocrinology? How does one start to define it? Where are the boundaries and what does this term encompass? These are some of the challenges with this new chapter in the Yearbook. What about the typical evidence base hierarchy; does it really hold the truth about the quality and applicability of clinical research? Are all other forms of evidence really inferior to the classical double-blind randomized controlled clinical trial? Well, this chapter reflects a selection of what has been published in the past year in pediatric endocrinology, based on searches far and wide. Includes are classic randomized controlled trials in addition to well-conducted longitudinal studies where these provide the best evidence to solve a clinical conundrum. It has been more difficult deciding what to leave out rather than what to include. Overviews from drug company's databases and consensus statements (including those of ESPE) are widely consulted sources of evidence. Therefore, this chapter has concentrated on seeking out sources which we do not always come across. As the intention has been to aid decision-making in daily clinical practice, in deciding what topics to include and what not to include, the following parameter has been used: Is the subject likely to fall within the remit of a clinical pediatrician or pediatric endocrinologist? Is this something worthwhile knowing about? Is it a subject your colleagues from other disciplines might consult you about?

There are two points which come to the fore in this review: firstly the important marriage between basic science and therapeutic clinical practice which is only just beginning to flourish, for example GH responsiveness and genotyping, and the concepts revisited section where new and important clinical findings are emerging based on revisiting well-conducted studies of the previous generation, for example the apparently protective effect of childhood GH treatment on the development of cardiovascular problems in adult women with Turner syndrome. This all bodes very well for the future.

Mechanism of the year: genotype-therapeutic links in growth hormone treatment

The d3/fl-growth hormone (GH) receptor polymorphism does not influence the effect of GH treatment (66 μg/kg/day) or the spontaneous growth in short non-GH-deficient small-for-gestational-age children: results from a 2-year controlled prospective study in 170 Spanish patients

Carrascosa A, Esteban C, Espadero R, Fernandez-Cancio M, Andaluz P, Clemente M, Audi L, Wollmann H, Fryklund L, Parodi L
Servicio de Pediatria, Unidad de Endocrinologia, Hospital Maternoinfantil Vall d'Hebron, Barcelona, Spain
ancarrascosa@vhebron.net

J Clin Endocrinol Metab 2006;91:3281–3286

Background: The d3/fl-GH receptor polymorphism has been associated with increased GH responsiveness in short SGA and ISS French children, Turner syndrome in Germany and GH deficiency in Brazil, but not in SGA children in Germany nor in Italian children with GHD. This study aimed to look at GH responsiveness and spontaneous growth in SGA children in Spain.
Methods: This prospective randomized controlled trial was of 2 years' duration. 170 short ($-2\,\text{SD}$) non-GHD SGA children (BW/BL $< -2\,\text{SD}$), 84 boys mean age 8.0 years, and 86 girls mean age 7.4 years, were recruited from 30 Spanish hospitals. Centralized genotyping and assays of IGF-1/IGFBP-3 were performed. 86 subjects were randomized to receive GH (66 μg/kg/day) for 2 years.
Results: Similar GH responsiveness was seen during the first and second years of GH treatment irrespective of genotype. Total 2-year height gain was $18.5 \pm 2.4\,\text{cm}$ in d3/d3, $18.4 \pm 2.6\,\text{cm}$ in d3/fl, and

19.5 ± 2.3 cm in fl/fl. The genotype did not predict first year responsiveness. No differences in response were found between the subgroups which remained prepubertal or entered puberty. In the non-treated patients, similar height/height velocity changes were seen in each d3/fl GHR genotype subgroups.

Conclusions: In this study of SGA children, significant height increases were seen over 2 years of GH treatment, but were similar for each of the d3/fl GHR genotypes analyzed.

This large multicenter national study has sought not only to examine the effectiveness of GH in a defined population, but also to attempt to predict GH responsiveness and outcomes in subgroups of patients with SGA with the d3/fl GH receptor polymorphism. This study did not demonstrate differences between the genotypes analyzed. The rigorous approach using a multicenter randomized controlled trial with single-center scientific analysis has demonstrated how well a national cooperative approach can work. Why are their results different from other studies, however? Well, some authors studied different conditions, for example Turner syndrome, which can have other confounding factors. The dose of GH used in the present study was much higher than in the others, however. This throws up the possibility that there is a dose-response effect which may vary according to the genotype, but is overcome by saturation exposure to GH. This developing area of applied genetics will be very important for the direction of future therapeutic approaches.

New paradigms – using old treatments in new ways

Intermittent recombinant growth hormone treatment in short children born small for gestational age: 4-year results of a randomized trial of two different treatment regimens

Simon D, Leger J, Fjellestad-Paulsen A, Crabbe R, Czernichow P
Paediatric Endocrinology and Diabetes Unit, Hospital Robert Debré, Paris
Francedominique.simon@rdb.ap-hop-paris.fr
Horm Res 2006;66:118–123

Background: GH treatment for SGA children can increase height and height velocity, but the height velocity on standard treatment wanes in the second year. This randomized study explored the efficacy of two different discontinuous GH treatment regimens using a high GH dose schedule (67 µg/kg/day) over 4 years with the intention of avoiding this slow down in response to GH therapy.

Methods: This was a multicenter (11 centers in France) randomized open-label, parallel-group comparative study of 58 SGA children aged 2–5 years, all height $</= -3$ SDS and birth weight <10th centile. Randomization was to two groups, either of alternating years' treatment, or two treatment years followed by 2 observation years. The principal outcome measure was total height gain.

Results: Height gain over 4 years was 1.4 ± 0.1 SDS in the alternating year treatment group, and 1.6 ± 0.2 SDS in the 2 years on/2 years off treatment group (NS). Height velocity increased during the treatment years and decreased during the observation years.

Conclusions: Significant 4-year growth gains were seen in both groups, but neither discontinuous regimen produced better growth than that which could be seen over 4 years with a continuous lower dosage regimen (33 µg/kg/day).

This well-designed randomized open-label, parallel-group comparative study of discontinuous GH regimens comparing alternating years treatment with the 2 years on/2 years off treatment was aimed at exploring ways of using GH therapy more efficiently in patients with SGA, and also to see whether the natural waning effect of response to treatment in second and subsequent years could be overcome by an intermittent GH regimen. Unfortunately no improvements in GH responsiveness were seen. The most important positive findings from this trial are that use of a discontinuous regimen is not detrimental to total growth gained and does not differ from continuous treatment, although an additional factor of course is the actual GH dosage itself [1]. Although continuous high-dose treatment produces the greatest long-term increases in height, absolute gains are not double the height gains on standard dose therapy. It is this factor, together with the still unknown very long-term effects of high-dose GH treatment, which has been the basis of the European Medicines Agency (EMEA) to recommend standard dose GH treatment for SGA patients. However, the evidence so far suggests that any observed metabolic changes associated with GH therapy reverse on stopping treatment. This is reassuring, and it paves the way for even more imaginative approaches to GH therapy, based on the knowledge of how children usually respond to treatment with an initial boost to growth, followed by the slowing of the height velocity. This pattern is remarkably similar across all different conditions.

New hope for health and fertility

Growth hormone treatment improves growth and clinical status in prepubertal children with cystic fibrosis: results of a multicenter randomized controlled trial

Hardin DS, Adams-Huet B, Brown D, Chatfield B, Dyson M, Ferkol T, Howenstine M, Prestidge C, Royce F, Rice J, Seilheimer DK, Steelman J, Shepherds R
Department of Pediatrics, University of Texas Southwestern Medical School, Tex., USA
hardind@pediatrics.ohio-state.edu
J Clin Endocrinol Metab 2006;91:4925–4929

Background: GH treatment has been suggested as improving growth, weight, bone content, lung function and quality of life in prepubertal children with cystic fibrosis. This study consisted of a multicenter, randomized controlled crossover trial to examine the effect of GH.
Methods: 61 prepubertal children with height and weight <25th centile were randomized to receive GH or not in year 1, followed by a crossover in year 2. In addition to standard anthropometry, other measures included: quality of life (QoL) questionnaires, metabolic measures (blood glucose), nutritional assessment, lung function tests, bone density and recording of antibiotic usage and hospital admissions.
Results: Both groups were similar at baseline, but after 1 year, GH-treated patients (0.3 mg/kg/week) showed positive weight and height gain (irrespective of baseline measurements) together with improvements in bone density and QoL, and had fewer hospital admissions. No changes in lung function were seen. The same changes were shown in the GH-treated group after crossover. After GH treatment ceased, improvements noted were maintained.
Conclusions: This short-term trial of GH treatment has shown improved growth and weight gain and is associated with better physical and mental health. Benefits noted appear to be maintained for the year after treatment is stopped.

This is an important study, not only on account of its rigorous multicenter, randomized controlled crossover trial design, but as it explores effects of GH beyond the simple auxological into the realms of better physical and psychological wellbeing in children with cystic fibrosis where poor growth is a feature of this chronic condition. The improvements in growth and the wellbeing of the patients were both notable. The focus was on the shorter and lighter individuals (<25th centile) without adjusting for parental heights, but an equal improvement in growth was seen across the study group regardless, but this observation may not hold for a longer-term study as target height would need to be taken into account. Abnormal glucose tolerance was examined for by measuring random glucose in accord with US guidelines without abnormalities being seen, although it could be argued that this is insufficiently rigorous to examine for side effects of GH treatment on glucose metabolism. Bone mineralization increased, as did some measures of lung function, but these could be explained by the greater physical growth in the treated group. It was reassuring to see a statistical improvement in QoL and body image scores, but by far the most impressive outcome of this study is the decrease in the number of hospitalizations on account of better health, presumably due to the anticatabolic/anabolic actions of GH. Although GH is expensive, the authors argue that this is offset by the reduction of inpatient treatment costs and that the effects of GH are apparently maintained after cessation. This requires a health economic evaluation with longer-term data, but is impressive so far.

Testicular growth from birth to two years of age, and the effect of orchidopexy at age nine months: a randomized, controlled study

Kollin C, Hesser U, Ritzen EM, Karpe B
Department of Woman and Child Health, Karolinska Institut, Stockholm, Sweden
Acta Paediatr 2006;95:318–324

Background: There is much debate over the benefits of early orchidopexy in the management of undescended testes. This is the first prospective randomized controlled trial in this field. Testicular growth was assessed by ultrasonography as a marker for the prediction of fertility potential.

Methods: Boys referred with congenital unilaterally palpable undescended testes were randomized at 6 months of age to surgical orchidopexy at 9 months of age (n = 70), or surgical treatment at 3 years of age (n = 79). The volume of each testis was measured at 3 weeks of age (or at referral) then at 2, 6, 12 months and annually until 5 years.

Results: Following orchidopexy, the operated (previously undescended) testes showed catch-up growth so that by 2 years of age the mean volume was significantly greater than the non-operated testes (0.49 vs. 0.36 ml, $p < 0.001$). The mean testicular growth ratio between the previously undescended and the scrotal testes in individual boys was higher at 2 years of age in the surgically treated versus untreated groups (0.84 vs. 0.63, $p < 0.001$).

Conclusions: Orchidopexy at 9 months of age is associated with catch-up growth of the operated testes by 2 years of age.

Undescended testis is a common clinical condition and a review of the existing literature by the authors in this paper highlights the lack of evidence base for the timing of orchidopexy. Concerns lie in two areas, namely risk of testicular cancer which is slightly higher, but principally on fertility outcomes as biopsies show reduction in gem cell and spermatogenesis in undescended testes. Testicular volume measured by ultrasound has previously been shown to equate with function, thus was used as the principal outcome measure for the prediction of fertility potential in this study. This large randomized controlled trial of appropriately simple design has already, in its first paper, demonstrated clear benefits of the early intervention with catch-up growth in the operated testis (although by 2 years of age this is not complete). The outcome of the later intervention is yet to be reported. This is part of a long-term longitudinal follow-up study which in due course on account of its design, should provide the definitive evidence base for this intervention.

New concerns – growth and asthma medication again

Long-term inhaled corticosteroids in preschool children at high risk for asthma

Guilbert TW, Morgan WJ, Zeiger RS, Mauger DT, Boehmer SJ, Szefler SJ, Bacharier LB, Lemanske RF Jr, Strunk RC, Allen DB, Bloomberg GR, Heldt G, Krawiec M, Larsen G, Liu AH, Chinchilli VM, Sorkness CA, Taussig LM, Martinez FD
Division of Pediatric Pulmonary Medicine, Arizona Respiratory Center, University of Arizona, Tucson, Ariz., USA
guilbert@arc.arizona.edu
N Engl J Med 2006;354:1985–1997

Background: This paper's primary aim was to determine whether inhaled corticosteroids for preschool children with a positive predictive index for asthma can modify the disease progression. The effects on growth were one of the secondary outcome measures of this study.

Methods: This was a multicenter, double-blind randomized, placebo-controlled parallel-group trial of 285 2- to 3-year-old children who either received inhaled fluticasone dipropionate 88 µg twice daily or masked placebo for 2 years, followed by a 1-year no intervention observation period for both groups. The primary outcome measure was the proportion of asthma-free days during this observation period.

Results: The study revealed no significant differences in proportion of episode-free days. This differed from during the treatment period where the steroid-receiving group had a lower number of exacerbations, less need of supplementary medication and more disease-free days. The fluticasone-treated group

Gary E Butler

grew 1.1 cm less over the 24-month treatment period (p < 0.001), but exhibited a small degree of catch-up during the observation year, so that at the end of the trial the mean reduction in height was 0.7 cm compared with the controls (total 3-year growth 19.2 ± 2.2 vs. 19.9 ± 2.2 cm, p = 0.008).

Conclusions: The primary intention of the trial was to investigate the disease-modifying effect of inhaled corticosteroids. This could not be demonstrated during an observation year following 2 years of active intervention. The findings do not provide evidence for a disease-modifying effect of inhaled corticosteroids. Two years of treatment leaves a significant deficit in growth which is only partly restored 1 year later when treatment is withdrawn.

Much has been written about growth and asthma, and whether growth deficits arise from the condition itself or from treatments such as inhaled corticosteroids. The discussion about the relationship between chronic childhood diseases, their treatment and growth continues, and the evidence here from a large multicenter, double-blind randomized, placebo-controlled parallel-group trial on the effect of inhaled steroids for asthma on growth is important, and important for two reasons: firstly, that as pediatricians, a frequently prescribed treatment for a common condition such as asthma is and remains suitable for control of symptoms only, and has no effect on altering the long-term disease process, and secondly, inappropriate use of an apparently innocuous treatment may have prolonged growth-restrictive effects, even though the overall effect is small and is controversial [2]. Height velocity was lower in the treated group (6.6 ± 1.0 cm/year) compared with the placebo group (7.3 ± 1.0 cm/year), but catch-up in the third observation year (6.4 ± 0.90 vs. 7.0 ± 0.8 cm/year in the controls) was insufficient to restore the height loss. Children in the inhaled corticosteroid group's average height centile was 51.5 ± 29.2 after treatment, recovering to centile 54.4 ± 27.9 during the observation period compared with centile 56.4 ± 26.9 in the controls. Although there were no significant differences in mean centile position between the groups, the SD in the treated group was broader. This statistical observation, together with the slightly lower mean height centile position of the treated patients, would produce, in absolute terms, a greater number of children in the lower centile bands in whom concerns over their growth may be expressed. This could be one explanation why we would see more referrals for short stature in children with asthma on inhaled corticosteroids and one reason why we as pediatric endocrinologists are involved in the asthma treatment debate.

Concepts revisited – good clinical science today is the foundation for the future

Aortic distensibility and dimensions and the effects of growth hormone treatment in the Turner syndrome

Van den Berg J, Bannink EM, Wielopolski PA, Pattynama PM, de Muinck Keizer-Schrama SM, Helbing WA
Department of Pediatrics, Erasmus MC-Sophia Children's Hospital, Rotterdam, The Netherlands
Am J Cardiol 2006;97:1644–1649

Background: Turner syndrome (TS) is associated with cardiovascular malformations, one of which is aortic dilatation, which although idiopathic, may be associated within increases in aortic size and distensibility. This study aimed to investigate the biophysical aspects and size of the aorta in TS.

Methods: 38 girls with TS who had previously been included in a randomized trial of different GH doses were included, and on this occasion an additional control group of 27 women aged 21 ± 2 years was recruited. The TS girls had been started at a mean age of 12 ± 2 years on either 0.045, 0.067 or 0.09 mg/kg/day. All had cardiac MRI imaging ±6 months after stopping GH determining aortic dimensions and distensibility in four areas: (1) the ascending aorta, (2) the descending aorta, (3) at the level of the diaphragm, and (4) the abdominal aorta.

Results: TS girls demonstrated larger aortic dimensions at all sites except within the abdomen (level 4), and tended to have reduced distensibility at the level of the diaphragm. TS patients in the lowest GH dosage group had larger aortic diameters at the diaphragm and above (levels 1–3) and reduced abdominal aortic distensibility. In patients in the two higher GH dose groups, measurements did not differ from the controls.

Conclusions: The severity of cardiac and aortic abnormalities seems to be inversely related to the dose of GH used. This would suggest larger doses of GH are beneficial to cardiac health.

The longer-term surveillance for side effects of GH treatment continues, especially when high-dose regimens are used and in conditions such as TS with known cardiovascular morbidities. The outcome of different doses of GH on the cardiovascular system in TS patients has revealed some interesting results. An important feature of this study is that this extension was possible on account of careful design and recording of clinical data in the initial randomized controlled trial. Additional investigation of outcomes together with the recruitment of an additional control group has extended the observations still further. The finding of a potentially positive benefit to high-dose GH preventing cardiovascular degeneration in TS is novel. It is encouraging therefore that sometimes we get unexpected positive benefits from treatment as in this study where the higher doses of GH seem to be beneficial. Careful monitoring of clinical practice must be done to seek to ensure that no harm is done by treatments offered, and the lack of a harmful effect of GH had been confirmed by a retrospective cross-sectional volunteer study of TS girls receiving conventional GH treatment (0.03–0.05 mg/kg/day) or no treatment by the US National Institute for Health [3]. It's back to the laboratory bench to sort this one out.

Reproductive outcome in patients treated and not treated for idiopathic early puberty: long-term results of a randomized trial in adults

Cassio A, Bal MO, Orsini LF, Balsamo A, Sansavini S, Gennari M, De Cristofaro E, Cicognani A
Department of Gynecology, Obstetrics and Pediatrics, University of Bologna, Bologna, Italy
cassio@med.unibo.it
J Pediatr 2006;149:532–536

Background: This study was conceived as outcome follow-up to assess reproductive outcome in girls who had previously received triptorelin treatment for early puberty.

Methods: 22 girls and 18 controls who had participated in 1991 in a randomized controlled trial to assess efficacy and outcomes of triptorelin treatment were recalled at a mean age of 20 years, and underwent physical examination, pelvic ultrasound and endocrine evaluation in comparison with a new control group of 22 age-matched controls.

Results: All three groups showed no significant changes in reproductive hormone levels, ultrasound results including ovarian volume and menstrual histories. The untreated group of early puberty girls showed slightly but non-significantly larger ovaries. Sexual activity was greater in those initially presenting with early puberty whether treated (76%) or not (72%) compared with the current controls (59%).

Conclusions: Triptorelin treatment for early puberty seems to have no long-term adverse effect on reproductive functioning.

This randomized controlled trial reported the effects of GnRH analogue treatment in girls with early normal treatment 15 years ago and demonstrated that there was no additional height advantage gained by this treatment, despite altering the tempo of puberty. The longer-term outcomes of suppressing puberty, especially on fertility, had yet to be determined at that stage. Although we may be more circumspect nowadays about treatment of early normal, as opposed to pathological precocious puberty, it is reassuring to know that triptorelin treatment in girls presenting with early puberty has no long-term adverse sequelae, nor does there seem to be a link with polycystic ovaries which had been reported previously. An early onset of puberty, whether or not progress is delayed with GnRH analogues, was associated with higher levels of sexual activity in early adulthood. The methodology of this paper deserves a comment. The initial randomized controlled trial was of good quality design. This permitted a follow-up study, which with the recruitment of a new control group has led to the current conclusions.

Bilateral anorchia in infancy: occurrence of micropenis and the effect of testosterone treatment

Zenaty D, Dijoud F, Morel Y, Cabrol S, Mouriquand P, Nicolino M, Bouvatier C, Pinto G, Lecointre C, Pienkowski C, Soskin S, Bost M, Bertrand AM, El-Ghoneimi A, Nihoul-Fekete C, Leger J
Assistance Publique-Hôpitaux de Paris, Robert Debré Hospital, Pediatric Endocrinology Unit, and Inserm U457, Paris, France
J Pediatr 2006;149:687–691

Background: Bilateral anorchia in infancy is rare; the etiology and its timing remains unclear. This study aimed to review clinical and histological findings and compare these with the growth of the penis in response to testosterone treatment.

Methods: This was a French multicenter retrospective study collecting clinical and histological data on 55 boys with congenital bilateral anorchia born between 1975 and 2004. The patients were divided into two groups depending on the absence (29) or presence (26) of a palpable intrascrotal or inguinal mass at first examination.

Results: 24 boys (46%) had micropenis, equal numbers in each group. Testosterone treatment produced a gain of penis length of 1.9 ± 1.3 SDS with no response in 6 patients. Histology of removed tissue showed absent testicular structures except in 3 where a hemorrhagic testis was found, possibly as a result of torsion during descent.

Conclusions: As half of the patients with congenital anorchia in this study had micropenis, but with normal male sex differentiation, this suggests that testicular damage occurs during the second half of gestation. The majority of boys responded to exogenous testosterone. Although this is a condition of heterogeneous etiology, boys with congenital anorchia are likely to have had functionally normal testes before their disappearance, although some may have an intrinsic endocrine disorder.

This was a longitudinal retrospective case study analyzing the clinical and histological findings in boys with bilateral anorchia and the response to testosterone treatment on penis length, and merits inclusion in this chapter as it represents the best way of gathering good clinical evidence in rare conditions. Data were gathered over a 30-year period, beyond the feasibility of most prospective clinical studies, but were of sufficient detail for retrospective analysis having been managed in designated pediatric endocrine units as they included histological confirmation of anorchia or testicular torsion. Evidence from this type of study is more reassuring than ground-breaking, nevertheless, with such large case series, patterns emerge. Although the majority of cases of anorchia seem to arise as a result of a testicular 'accident', a significant proportion did not show good androgen responsiveness. This suggests either a failure of testosterone secretion following on from sex differentiation, or else a degree of partial androgen resistance. Here's where prospective longitudinal studies may be of help.

Insulin pumps in pediatric routine care improve long-term metabolic control without increasing the risk of hypoglycemia

Hanas R, Adolfsson P
Department of Pediatrics, Uddevalla Hospital, Uddevalla, Sweden
ragnar.hanas@vregion.se
Pediatr Diabetes 2006;7:25–31

Background: This paper is the first 5-year pure longitudinal report of a non-randomized population-based study evaluating continuous subcutaneous insulin infusion pumps in routine care. The baseline was a detailed cross-sectional study in the first year.

Methods: 27/89 patients aged 7–21 years were transferred to insulin pumps compared with conventional treatment of 4–6 injections/day. Pump treatment was generally started to improve control when HbA1c $>8.5\%$ (HbA1c 8.9 ± 1.0 vs. $8.2 \pm 1.6\%$, p = 0.04), often due to diabetes duration >2 years. Reports of HbA1c change and frequency of adverse events were studied.

Results: In the first year using pumps, insulin dosage was lower (0.9 ± 0.1 vs. 1.0 ± 0.2 U/kg/day, p = 0.002). The incidence of severe hypoglycemia was lower with pump therapy (11.1 vs. 40.3/100 patient-years, NS) and no pump patients experienced severe hypoglycemia with unconsciousness or seizures. No admissions were seen in either group for ketoacidosis. Over the 5 years, for the patients with poor control as the main indication for starting with pump therapy, mean HbA1c fell from 9.5 to 8.9% after 1 year (p = 0.019), 8.6% in year 2 (p = 0.017), 8.6% in year 3 (p = 0.012), and then rose to 8.7% in year 4 (p = 0.062), and 8.9% in year 5 (p = 0.28). Six pump patients had ketoacidosis (4.7/100 patient-years).

Conclusions: The authors found some long-term lowering of HbA1c in a poorly controlled pediatric population even though the initial fall was not maintained. Pump therapy was associated with a decreased frequency of severe hypoglycemia and a low risk of ketoacidosis.

> Use of insulin pumps in children with diabetes may make emotions run high, so although this is not a randomized trial, it is the first objective report of 5-year longitudinal outcomes in children and adolescents using pump therapy in a single center. Five-year reductions in HbA1c of 0.6% in the poorly controlled group and of 0.2% in all patients seemed poor in comparison with the much greater initial fall, but may need to be evaluated in comparison with lifestyle convenience and a lower reported incidence of severe complications, even though there is a higher administrative cost. The debate continues.

Clinical trials, new treatments: 1 – new wine, old skins

Median nerve conduction velocity and central conduction time measured with somatosensory-evoked potentials in thyroxine-treated infants with Down syndrome

Van Trotsenburg AS, Smit BJ, Koelman JH, Dekker-van der Sloot M, Ridder JC, Tijssen JG, de Vijlder JJ, Vulsma T
Department of Pediatric Endocrinology, Emma Children's Hospital Academic Medical Center, University of Amsterdam, Amsterdam, The Netherlands
a.s.vantrotsenburg@amc.uva.nl
Pediatrics 2006;118:e825–e832

Background: Down syndrome is a common cause of developmental delay, with a predisposition to autoimmune thyroid disease. Plasma T_4 levels are usually lower in neonates with Down's. This study was conducted to ascertain whether supplementation could improve the developmental outcome in this condition using median nerve conduction velocity and central conduction time measured by somatosensory-evoked potentials which have established associations with developmental variability.

Methods: A double-blind randomized controlled trial was carried out in a single center over 4 years. Neonates with Down syndrome received either T_4 (n = 99) or placebo (n = 97) treatment for 2 years. Dosages were adjusted to keep T_4 levels in the high normal range and TSH in the normal range. Outcome measures were nerve conduction velocity and somatosensory-evoked potential recording changes ascertained at age 24 months.

Results: Peripheral nerve conduction velocity and central conduction time did not show any significant differences between the 81 T_4-treated and 84 placebo-treated subjects (nerve conduction velocity 51.0 vs. 50.1 m/s; central conduction time 8.83 vs. 8.73 ms).

Conclusions: Supplementation of Down syndrome infants with T_4 to 'normalize' levels was not associated with improvement in nerve conduction velocity and somatosensory-evoked potentials. Therefore it is likely that the impaired nerve conduction in Down syndrome is due to alternative explanations. No adverse effects were seen suggesting that high-normal T_4 levels are not harmful to nerve maturation.

> Nothing ventured, nothing gained. Down syndrome is associated with developmental delay and lesser degrees of thyroid activity. The working hypothesis was that supplementation with T_4 to normalize levels would lessen the degree of developmental delay by accelerating nerve maturation. Although this study produced negative results, they are conclusively negative on account of the quality of the study design, rigorous methodology and large sample size, and the use of a reproducible methodology which had previously been shown to accurately reflect developmental variation. Although a causal association between mild hypothyroxinemia and developmental delay cannot be ruled out [4], a treatment protocol similar to that used in true congenital hypothyroidism was not successful in accelerating neurological maturation in this condition.

Gary E Butler

The effects of oxandrolone and exercise on muscle mass and function in children with severe burns

Przkora R, Herndon DN, Suman OE
Shriners Hospitals for Children, Galveston, Tex., USA
Pediatrics 2007;119:e109–e116

Background: A structured exercise programme is standard treatment in the rehabilitation of children with severe burns to prevent muscle wasting and to improve lean body mass. This study hypothesized that the combination of the anabolic steroid oxandrolone together with the exercise programme would be superior in accelerating muscle strength and lean mass accrual, thus accelerating rehabilitation.
Methods: 51 children with severe burns (>40% total body surface area) were entered into a four-way randomized placebo-controlled trial receiving oxandrolone alone (0.1 mg/kg/day); oxandrolone + exercise; placebo alone, and placebo + exercise. Oxandrolone was started at discharge for 1 year. The exercise programme started at 6 months after the burn injury and ran for 12 weeks. Assessments at 6 and 9 months included muscle strength, lean body mass assessments by DEXA, cardiopulmonary capacity, and serum hormones.
Results: Body weight increased significantly in the oxandrolone + exercise group (14%) compared with the other subgroups (2.5–8.6%). Lean body mass increased in all three active intervention groups (mostly in the oxandrolone + exercise group) in contrast with a small reduction in the placebo group showing that children are still in a catabolic state 6 months after severe burns. Peak cardiopulmonary capacity improved in both exercise groups. Oxandrolone alone produced the most significant increase in IGF-1 levels, whereas both groups with an exercise component showed equal increments in IGFBP-3.
Conclusions: Oxandrolone in addition to a planned exercise training programme improves rehabilitation in severely burned patients.

This study has demonstrated the positive benefit from adding oxandrolone to an active rehabilitation programme aiding recovery in children who had suffered severe burn injuries in whom a continued catabolic state is the norm without intervention. The mechanism of action is still not clear for this enigmatic hormone treatment. Although significant increases in IGF-1 were seen (greater even without the exercise component, interestingly), attempts to reproduce the anabolic effect in a similar study using GH alone were unsuccessful [5]. The answer may arise from its direct anabolic effect on muscle mass, hence increased strength and lean body mass, although this paper does not address the mechanisms in any more detail. This effect, however, is similar to that seen in studies of oxandrolone in AIDS/HIV wasting and catabolic states given together with active rehabilitation. One useful practice point relates to economic costings. Exercise programmes such as used here are very resource-dependent and thus expensive, and therefore may not be available in all localities. Oxandrolone, on the other hand, is cheap, and if available on its own can produce as good an improvement in muscle mass and strength as the exercise programme. If only we knew how it worked!

Clinical trials, new treatments: 2 – pediatric endocrinology reaching outwards

Randomised, double-blind trial of oxytocin nasal spray in mothers expressing breast milk for preterm infants

Fewtrell MS, Loh KL, Blake A, Ridout DA, Hawdon J
Childhood Nutrition Research Centre, Institute of Child Health, London, UK
m.fewtrell@ich.ucl.ac.uk
Arch Dis Child Fetal Neonatal Ed 2006;91:F169–F174

Background: Oxytocin had previously been advocated for initiating and increasing human lactation as breast milk conveys advantages, especially in sick preterm infants. Whether with current early feeding practices would maternal oxytocin treatment improve milk production.
Methods: Both the total amount and pattern of milk production were measured following a double-blind randomized controlled trial of oxytocin nasal spray (100 µl/dose) for the first 5 postnatal days prior to

milk expression using a portable electric pump. The study power was calculated to detect >1 SD difference between groups.

Results: 27 mothers received oxytocin spray compared with 24 controls. The total milk production was greater in the first 2 days with oxytocin (analysis of variance p < 0.001) but then patterns of milk production converged although eventually placebo-treated mothers overtook oxytocin-treated mothers, producing more milk by weight (though not significantly more). Neither the milk production rate, parity, nor milk content differed between groups.

Conclusions: Although there was an early improvement in breast milk weight produced during the first 2 days, the use of oxytocin did not produce overall benefits to lactation stimulation. Breastfeeding support as experienced by the mothers in the control group of this trial may also have a positive benefit on lactation.

This paper of classic double-blind randomized controlled trial design has helped to clarify further some of the functions of the mysterious hormone oxytocin and whether it has any influence on the time to establish lactation and whether it can increase total milk production. Although there may be some improvement of efficiency of breast milk expression with additional oxytocin, there is no evidence for the augmentation of milk production, suggesting this is more dependent on other factors such as prolactin secretion and as yet other undetermined facets of exocrine breast gland secretory function.

Sleep hygiene and melatonin treatment for children and adolescents with ADHD and initial insomnia

Weiss MD, Wasdell MB, Bomben MM, Rea KJ, Freeman RD
Division of Child Psychiatry, University of British Columbia, Vancouver, B.C., Canada
mweiss@cw.bc.ca
J Am Acad Child Adolesc Psychiatry 2006;45:512–519

Background: Children with attention deficit hyperactivity disorder (ADHD) may show disordered patterns of sleep as part of their general behavioral disturbance. This study aimed to evaluate the efficacy of both sleep hygiene interventions and melatonin treatment in ADHD children.

Methods: 27 children aged 6–14 years with initial insomnia (sleep delay >60 min) were given advice and practical help with sleep hygiene improvement. Those who failed to respond were entered into a double-blind crossover randomized controlled trial of melatonin 5 mg or placebo for 10 days each followed by a 5-day washout period. The whole trial lasted for 90 days. The principal outcome measure was time from putting to bed to sleep onset recorded by the parents.

Results: Behavioral modification advice on sleep hygiene was successful in 5 cases only reducing time to sleep onset <60 min, with an overall effect size of 0.67. The addition of melatonin relative to placebo reduced initial insomnia by 16 min. These interventions in combination increased the effect size to 1.7 over the full 90-day trial period, with a mean decrease of initial insomnia of 60 min. ADHD symptoms did not demonstrate any beneficial effect as a result of improved sleep patterns.

Conclusions: The combination of sleep hygiene advice and melatonin is safe and effective intervention in the management of abnormal sleep patterns in children with ADHD.

Although the subject of this double-blind crossover randomized controlled trial to evaluate the efficacy of sleep hygiene and melatonin treatment for initial insomnia in children with ADHD is on the borderline of pediatric endocrine practice, it demonstrates how it is possible to plan a successful project combining a behavioral and an endocrine intervention using a robust study design. It looked specifically at one behavioral facet, namely delayed sleep onset, and so the results are not generalizable to other sleep problems, and it does not explore the effect of melatonin alone, although one could argue that this design accurately reflects a standard approach in clinical practice. Although melatonin is pivotal in defining the reproductive cycle in most mammals, its true role in human endocrine function is still unclear, and even in the control of sleep onset is not of greater importance than behavioral interventions.

Effects of calcium supplementation on bone density in healthy children: meta-analysis of randomized controlled trials

Winzenberg T, Shaw K, Fryer J, Jones G
Menzies Research Institute, Hobart, Tas., Australia
tania.winzenberg@utas.edu.au
BMJ 2006;333:775

Background: The development of osteoporosis later in life is a major public health problem, so preventative interventions are important. This paper describes a meta-analysis of studies of calcium supplementation in children to determine whether if any benefit persists after treatment stops or whether the effect is modified by any other factors.

Methods: Two reviewers independently searched electronic databases, conference proceedings and contacted authors for unpublished results. Studies included were of calcium supplementation in healthy children of at least 3 months and had bone outcome measures given as standardized mean differences as an endpoint to the study after a minimum of 6 months' follow-up.

Results: 19 studies met the selection criteria (2,859 children participants). No changes in bone density were seen at the femoral neck or lumbar spine with calcium supplementation. A small positive effect on total body bone mineral content (standardized mean difference 0.14; 95% CI 0.01–0.27) and upper limb bone mineral density (standardized mean difference 0.14; 95% CI 0.04–0.24) was identified. Negative factors were sex, pubertal stage, ethnicity, physical activity levels or baseline calcium intake.

Conclusions: Although outcome effects were non-significantly greater in females than males, and slightly more so in the upper limb, there is insufficient evidence to suggest that routine calcium supplementation improves bone density enough to reduce fracture risk later on in life to a degree of major public health importance.

Although bone density is much studied, only 19 randomized controlled trials of calcium supplementation in children with a view to prevent osteoporosis risk out of a total of 233 references were of sufficient quality of evidence to be considered in this systematic review. Additionally, with the known difficulties in adjusting bone density for body size, the authors conducted a sub-analysis comparing reports where this was done or not, but there were no differences found which would alter the overall conclusions. Calcium needed to be given as an active treatment supplement (300–1,200 mg/day) and not as dairy products to qualify for inclusion. Although the authors report a negative conclusion, maximum length of follow-up was only 7 years and equating this with absolute fracture risk is problematical. However, as an overall positive effect could be detected in the upper limbs (perhaps surprisingly) upholding the rationale behind additional calcium intake, the conclusions of the meta-analysis were upheld and called into question the public health benefits of routine calcium supplementation. What this study does not address is supplementation in children with low calcium intakes and other possible ways of increasing bone density through better fruit and vegetable intake and vitamin D supplementation.

Food for thought – diet and exercise, so don't think for too long!

Diet and sex hormones in boys: findings from the dietary intervention study in children

Dorgan JF, McMahon RP, Friedman LA, Van Horn L, Snetselaar LG, Kwiterovich PO Jr, Lauer RM, Lasser NL, Stevens VJ, Robson A, Cooper SF, Chandler DW, Franklin FA, Barton BA, Patterson BH, Taylor PR, Schatzkin A
Fox Chase Cancer Center, Philadelphia, Pa., USA
joanne.dorgan@fccc.edu
J Clin Endocrinol Metab 2006;91:3992–3996

Background: Adults who diet may show alterations in sex hormone levels, but little is known what happens in puberty. This study is ancillary to the Dietary Intervention Study in Children which is a multicenter randomized controlled trial aimed at lowering cholesterol by dietary intervention in children.

Methods: 354 healthy 8- to 10-year-old boys with elevated low-density lipoprotein were randomized to a trial diet of 28% energy from total fat (<8% from unsaturated fat and cholesterol, 75 mg/1,000 kcal) and were followed up for median 7.1 years. Outcome measures were non-SHBG-bound testosterone, total testosterone, dihydrotestosterone, androstenedione, estradiol, estrone, SHBG and Tanner puberty stage.

Results: Longitudinal analysis did not show differences in any clinical or biochemical parameter over the study period between the randomized groups.

Conclusions: When a dietary intervention which uses modest total fat, saturated fat and energy intake restriction is undertaken, no clinical or sex-hormone changes are seen in adolescent boys.

Although this was primarily conceived as a dietary intervention study in children with raised lipid levels, this randomized controlled trial also allowed the possibility of observing the effect of varying the energy intake on pubertal onset and progression. The study group before randomization was identified as having elevated low-density lipoprotein so it is not a true fully-representative population study. The trial was terminated prematurely on account of no treatment effect being observed. Nevertheless, some useful conclusions can be drawn. Boys of increased BMI (+0.86 to +1.06 SDS at baseline) did not differ from population norms or between study groups in the onset or progress through puberty. The inference is that neither modest degrees of overnutrition nor attempts to restrict this are associated with disturbances to the timing of the puberty control mechanism. However, as the trial was unsuccessful and neither lipid nor BMI reductions were seen, either more restrictive dietary parameters or a different approach should be considered, and it would be very interesting to study what degree of energy intake decrement would affect the tempo of puberty in today's overnourished adolescents.

Early determinants of physical activity in adolescence: prospective birth cohort study

Hallal PC, Wells JC, Reichert FF, Anselmi L, Victora CG
Postgraduate Program in Epidemiology, Federal University of Pelotas, Pelotas, RS, Brazil
prchallal@terra.com.br
BMJ 2006;332:1002–1007

Background: The benefits of physical activity on physical and mental health are well established, but the early social, behavioral and anthropometric variables on adolescent physical activity are unclear and the influence of 'programming' needs clarification.

Methods: 4,453 adolescents aged 10–12 years participating in the 1993 longitudinal prospective birth cohort study from Pelotas in Southern Brazil. Study measures included detailed data on levels of physical activity: sedentary classified as <300 min of physical activity/week (outside of school physical education classes).

Results: Sedentary lifestyle prevalence was 58.2% (95% CI 56.7–59.7), associated risk factors being female sex, higher maternal education and family income at birth, and lower birth order. Longitudinal measures of weight gain, or prevalence of overweight at 1 or 4 years of age, did not significantly predict adolescent physical activity levels. Sedentary lifestyle at age 10–12 years was inversely related to income and maternal reports of physical activity levels at age 4 years.

Conclusions: Factors affecting adolescent sedentary lifestyles are not programmed by infant physiological factors. Longitudinal follow-up of physical activity suggests that both genetic factors and early habit formation may be important as there was a positive association between higher birth order and greater activity in childhood and adolescence. Weight gain, whether in infancy or childhood, did not correlate with adolescent activity levels.

Physical activity to prevent obesity in young children: cluster randomised controlled trial

Reilly JJ, Kelly L, Montgomery C, Williamson A, Fisher A, McColl JH, Lo Conte R, Paton JY, Grant S
Division of Developmental Medicine, University of Glasgow, Yorkhill Hospitals, Glasgow, UK
jjr2y@clinmed.gla.ac.uk
BMJ 2006;333:1041

Background: Childhood obesity is rising in prevalence, with an earlier onset. This study was designed to assess whether an enhanced physical activity programme would reduce BMI in preschool children.

Methods: This was a cluster randomized controlled single-blind trial lasting 12 months taking place in 36 nurseries in Glasgow involving 545 children, mean age 4.2 years. The programme consisted of enhanced physical activity of three 30-minute sessions over 24 weeks, backed up by a home health education initiative to reduce sedentary behavior by encouraging play. Outcomes were BMI and evaluation of sedentary behavior by accelerometry and movement skills.

Results: This particular intervention produced no significant changes in BMI at 6 and 12 months, or on measures of physical or sedentary behavior. However, children participating in the programme performed significantly better in tests of movement skills (p = 0.0027) with adjustment for sex and baseline performance.

Conclusions: This trial showed a positive effect on improvement of motor skills with training, but no differences in overall activity levels or reduction in BMI.

Large-scale, well planned and executed longitudinal studies produce high-quality evidence for observing population changes and correlating with disease risk. Testing individual hypotheses can be done by well-planned large-scale interventional studies, but the important message here is that there must be some evidence that the proposed intervention is effective before conducting large-scale research. This is where pilot studies can be so helpful. Factors determining the onset of obesity in early childhood may have important environmental etiologies which need to be understood before successful interventions can be instigated. Active lifestyles are associated with improved cardiovascular health. Although socioeconomic factors such as higher family income and maternal education levels were predictive of lower adolescent physical activity levels, the lack of an association of early weight gain by 4 years of age with adolescent activity levels as in the paper by Hallal et al. are important and controversial findings. If promotion of an active lifestyle is desirable, then this study sends the message that it needs to start early in life, as supported by the finding of higher child and adolescent activity levels in bigger families. This study throws down the gauntlet to challenge the notion that early weight gain is a risk factor for adult metabolic and cardiovascular disease [6]. If this is really the case, have we been '*Barker'ing* up the wrong tree with the current generation thus far? The starting early with a high activity lifestyle hypothesis was put to the test in the paper by Reilly et al. which showed that using a cluster randomized trial of an enhanced physical activity programme in the preschool age group improved motor skill development, but had no overall effect on changing lifestyles or on sedentary behavior. The lack of effect on BMI (as the principal outcome measure) may have arisen from using an insufficiently rigorous exercise programme, and the lack of change in sedentary behavior was explained by the home intervention being purely educational rather than interventional. Alternatively, it could be argued that BMI per se is not the best measure of obesity in the young. This issue is clearly much more complicated than first realized and improved outcomes are going to have to depend on much more proactive family interventions, but when do we step over the line in restriction of personal liberty and where does the responsibility for this obesity problem lie?

References
1. De Zegher F, Albertsson-Wikland K, Wollmann HA, Chatelain P, Chaussain JL, Lofstrom A, et al: Growth hormone treatment of short children born small for gestational age: growth responses with continuous and discontinuous regimens over 6 years. J Clin Endocrinol Metab 2000;85:2816–2821.
2. Bisgaard H, Allen D, Milanowski J, Kalev I, Willits L, Davies P: Twelve-month efficacy and safety if inhaled fluticasone propionate in children aged 1–3 years with recurrent wheezing. Pediatrics 2004;113:e87–e94.
3. Bondy CA, Van PL, Bakalov VK, Ho VB: Growth hormone treatment and aortic dimensions in Turner syndrome. J Clin Endocrinol Metab 2006;91:1785–1788.
4. Zoeller RT, Rovet J: Timing of thyroid hormone action in the developing brain: clinical observations and experimental findings. J Neuroendocrinol 2004;16:809–818.
5. Suman J, Thomas SJ, Wilkins JP, Mlcak RP, Herndon DN: Effect of exogenous growth hormone and exercise on lean mass and muscle function in children with burns. J Appl Physiol 2003;94:2273–2281.
6. Barker DJ, Gluckman PD, Godfrey KM, Harding JF, Owens JA, Robinson JS: Fetal nutrition and cardiovascular disease in adult life. Lancet 1993;341:938–941.

Systems Biology

O. Nilsson and O. Söder

Pediatric Endocrinology Unit, Department of Woman and Child Health, Karolinska Institutet and University Hospital, Stockholm, Sweden

Systems biology is a rapidly expanding novel research discipline aiming to describe interactions in complex biological systems. This is done by collection, integration and analysis of large quantities of data from multiple experimental sources employing powerful computational and informatics tools. The 'omics' techniques are typically used to collect quantitative data to construct and validate models. Starting with genomics, proteomics and transcriptomics, these techniques are constantly expanded by addition of new tools such as metabolomics, interactomics, cytomics, etc., that add to the increasing complexity of systems biology to be incorporated into biological networks. The following original and review papers published in 5/2006–3/2007 are a selection of works employing systems biology approaches to address important questions in endocrinology and general biology of relevance for human medicine.

New genes
Angry gene identified

Molecular analysis of flies selected for aggressive behavior

Dierick HA, Greenspan RJ
The Neurosciences Institute, San Diego, Calif., USA
dierick@nsi.edu
Nat Genet 2006;38:1023–1031

Background: Aggressive behavior is common in most animals but little is known about its molecular background.

Methods: To address this problem, the authors developed a population-based selection procedure to increase aggression in *Drosophila melanogaster*. They measured changes in aggressive behavior in the selected subpopulations with a new two-male arena assay. In only 10 generations of selection, the aggressive lines became markedly more aggressive than the neutral lines.

Results: After 21 generations, the fighting index increased more than 30-fold. Using microarray analysis, the authors identified genes with differing expression levels in the aggressive and neutral lines as candidates for this strong behavioral selection response. A small set of these genes was tested through mutant analysis and found that one significantly increased fighting frequency.

Conclusion: These results suggest that selection for increases in aggression can be used to molecularly dissect this behavior.

Systems biology starts with a careful selection of the phenotypes. These investigators developed a population-based selection procedure to enhance aggression using two aggressive and two neutral fly populations derived from a single starting population and quantified the behavioral selection response with males that engaged in repeated fights over a female. After only 10 generations of selection, both aggressive selected lines were significantly more aggressive than both neutral lines, and these differences further increased under continued selection pressure. Differential expression of genes in the head (brain) of aggressive and neutral lines of flies was investigated by microarray. 28 genes showed higher expression (>25%) and 14 genes lower expression in aggressive flies. Five differentially expressed genes were mutated and aggressiveness of the offspring investigated. Two genes that produced a direct effect on aggression encode a cytochrome P_{450} (*Cyp6a20*) and an odor-binding protein. Translation of the present findings into humans is important but difficult. This study and forthcoming work using the same approach will reveal candidate genes to be explored in higher species. An appalling science fiction scenario fuelled by this work is the creation of the 'Universal

Soldier' (referring to the movie with the same name), in which selection for aggressiveness is an important tool. However, at the present stage, one must be happy that the insect species employed was small and harmless and that the studies were not conducted in wasps. Interestingly, aggressive animals were not more active than neutral ones.

More genes affected by estrogen

Sensitive ChIP-DSL technology reveals an extensive estrogen receptor α-binding program on human gene promoters

Kwon YS, Garcia-Bassets I, Hutt KR, Cheng CS, Jin M, Liu D, Benner C, Wang D, Ye Z, Bibikova M, Fan JB, Duan L, Glass CK, Rosenfeld MG, Fu XD
Department of Cellular and Molecular Medicine, University of California at San Diego School of Medicine, La Jolla, Calif., USA
Proc Natl Acad Sci USA 2007;104:4852–4857

Background: Even though transcriptional initiation is a major research focus, little is known about how many genes are direct targets for a particular nuclear receptor. However, genome-wide chromatin immunoprecipitation (ChIP) coupled with microarray, known as ChIP-on-chip, offers a strategy to address these types of questions by determining promoters bound directly by transcription factors. Surprisingly, recent promoter and tiling array analyses suggest that ER-α frequently binds to intergenic regions and relatively rarely to gene promoters http://www.pnas.org/cgi/content/full/104/12/4852 - B12#B12. In order to improve specificity and sensitivity, a new technology called ChIP-DSL, a modified ChIP-on-chip technology, was developed.
Methods: The authors developed a modified ChIP-on-chip technology using the DNA selection and ligation (DSL) strategy, thus permitting robust analysis with much reduced materials compared with standard procedures.
Results: Using the ChIP-DSL technology, general and sequence-specific DNA-binding transcription factors were profiled using a full human genome promoter, revealing approximately four times as many ER-α target promoters as were detected in previous genome-wide location studies. Gene expression profiling showed that only a fraction of these direct ER-α target genes were found to be highly responsive to estrogen. However, expression of those ER-α-bound, estrogen-inducible genes was associated with breast cancer progression in humans.
Conclusions: This study demonstrates the power of the ChIP-DSL technology in revealing regulatory gene expression programs that have been previously invisible in the human genome.

In order to map regulatory networks in mammalian cells the authors applied genome-wide chromatin immunoprecipitation (ChIP) coupled with microarray. This methodology has shown to provide a powerful tool for genome-wide detection of transcription factor binding. Aiming at improving the specificity and sensitivity of such analysis, the authors developed a new technology called ChIP-DSL using the DNA selection and ligation (DSL) strategy, permitting robust analysis with much reduced materials compared with standard procedures. The authors profiled general and sequence-specific DNA-binding transcription factors using a full human genome promoter array based on the ChIP-DSL technology, revealing an unprecedented number of the estrogen receptor-α (ER-α) target genes in MCF-7 cells. Only a small fraction of these genes are strongly regulated by estrogen. However, expression of genes that are under ER-α regulation is associated with breast cancer progression. In addition to developing a new technology and identifying novel transcriptional targets of ER-α, this study demonstrates how improvements of current technology may provide a much different answer to known biological questions. It also highlights the ever-increasing complexity of the regulatory networks induced by nuclear receptors in general and estrogen receptors in particular. Now when one knows what to look for it is easy to see translation of this work into the clinic in many disciplines including that of pediatric endocrinology.

Changes in gene expression foreshadow diet-induced obesity in genetically identical mice

Koza RA, Nikonova L, Hogan J, Rim JS, Mendoza T, Faulk C, Skaf J, Kozak LP
Pennington Biomedical Research Center, Baton Rouge, La., USA

PLoS Genet 2006;2:e81

Background: High phenotypic variation in diet-induced obesity in male inbred mice suggests a molecular model to investigate non-genetic mechanisms of obesity.

Methods and Results: Feeding mice a high-fat diet beginning at 8 weeks of age resulted in a 4-fold difference in adiposity. The phenotypes of mice characteristic of high or low gainers were evident by 6 weeks of age, when mice were still on a low-fat diet; they were amplified after being switched to the high-fat diet and persisted even after the obesogenic protocol was interrupted with a calorically restricted, low-fat chow diet. Susceptibility to diet-induced obesity in genetically identical mice is a stable phenotype that can be detected in mice shortly after weaning. Chronologically, differences in adiposity preceded those of feeding efficiency and food intake, suggesting that observed difference in leptin secretion is a factor in determining phenotypes related to food intake. Gene expression analyses of adipose tissue and hypo-thalamus from mice with low and high weight gain, by microarray and qRT-PCR, showed major changes in the expression of genes of Wnt signaling and tissue re-modeling in adipose tissue. In particular, elevated expression of SFRP5, an inhibitor of Wnt signaling, the imprinted gene MEST and BMP3 may be causally linked to fat mass expansion, since differences in gene expression observed in biopsies of epididymal fat at 7 weeks of age (before the high-fat diet) correlated with adiposity after 8 weeks on a high-fat diet.

Conclusions: It is proposed that C57BL/6J mice have the phenotypic characteristics suitable for a model to investigate epigenetic mechanisms within adipose tissue that underlie diet-induced obesity.

Obesity is a multifactorial disease in which inherited allelic variation, together with environmental variation, determines the predisposition of an individual to developing the disease. Although the evidence in support of a genetic component to the development of obesity is overwhelming, and a number of promising candidate genes are being tested as underlying causes of obesity, it remains difficult to quantify the genetic contribution to the obesity epidemic during the past 25 years, a period too short for the accumulation of additional obesogenic alleles. The authors show that regarding fat accumulation, the phenotypes among C57BL/6J mice are highly variable by 6 weeks of age, even before they are fed a high-fat diet, indicating that some mice are destined to be high gainers, while others from the same litter are to become low gainers. The microarray analysis of gene expression in adipose tissue from high and low gainers suggests that the Wnt signaling pathway and genes associated with vascularization and tissue remodeling are major regulatory points controlling differences in adipose tissue expansion and that some of these genes are differentially expressed even before mice are fed a high-fat diet.

The findings strongly suggest that variation in energy balance in an inbred strain provides a model to explore epigenetic mechanisms that are powerful in causing obesity. Although an excess over the needs of calorie intake is the main cause of obesity, it has long been appreciated that the internal fate of absorbed calories may vary substantially between individuals. Numerous studies have tried to pinpoint the mechanisms and genetic factors involved in the regulation of these processes albeit without much success. The systems biology approach taken here gives promises for more rapid advances in the field which are highly warranted.

Whole genome microarray analysis of growth hormone-induced gene expression in bone: T-box 3, a novel transcription factor, regulates osteoblast proliferation

Govoni KE, Lee SK, Chadwick RB, Yu H, Kasukawa Y, Baylink DJ, Mohan S

Musculoskeletal Disease Center (151), Jerry L. Pettis Memorial Veterans Affairs Medical Center, Loma Linda, Calif., USA

Am J Physiol Endocrinol Metab 2006;291:E128–E136

Background: Growth hormone (GH) has an important role in bone metabolism, but the IGF-dependent and -independent molecular pathways involved are still largely unknown.

Methods: Microarray analysis were used to evaluate GH signaling pathways in 4-week-old GH-deficient mice following a single injection of GH or PBS at 6 or 24 h after treatment.

Results: 6,160 genes were differentially expressed, and 17% of these genes were identified at both time points. More than half of the genes differentially expressed were previously unknown genes. Subsequent studies were focused on T-box 3 (Tbx3), a novel transcription factor, which increased more than 2-fold at both time points. Pretreatment with IGF-binding protein-4 did not block GH-induced Tbx3 expression, whereas pretreatment with TNF-α did block GH-induced Tbx3 expression. Tbx3 expression increased during osteoblast differentiation and following BMP-7 and Wnt3a treatment. Blocking Tbx3 expression by small interfering RNA decreased osteoblast proliferation and number.

Conclusions: GH caused changes in expression of several unknown genes, suggesting that several GH-induced signaling pathways and target genes remain to be discovered. Furthermore, Tbx3 expression is GH-regulated in osteoblasts and blockage of Tbx3 expression decreased cell number and DNA synthesis, thus suggesting that Tbx3 is a determinant of osteoblast cell number.

In this paper, the authors use microarray and a mouse model of GH deficiency (little mice) to explore the regulatory role of GH on bone metabolism. They identify the gene T-box 3, mutations of which causes ulnar-mammary syndrome characterized by skeletal defects, hypoplasia of mammary glands, micropenis, delayed puberty, and obesity, to be acutely regulated by GH in bone as well as an important regulator of osteoblast proliferation in vitro. The microarray analysis also identified several genes induced by GH of which little information is available, implicating novel direct actions of GH. Interestingly, several of these unknown genes include zinc finger motifs, thus indicating a potential role for these genes as transcription factors. This is good news for pediatric endocrinologists and other researchers working on GH research as the presented results open new gates to yet unexplored research fields that may be extended beyond bone.

Systems biology makes it possible to see the forest *and* the trees!

Cancer: a systems biology disease

Hornberg JJ, Bruggeman FJ, Westerhoff HV, Lankelma J

Department of Molecular Cell Physiology, Institute for Molecular Cell Biology, BioCentrum Amsterdam, Faculty of Earth and Life Sciences, Vrije Universiteit, Amsterdam, The Netherlands

jorrit.hornberg@falw.vu.nl

Biosystems 2006;83:81–90

Background: Cancer research has focused on the identification of molecular differences between cancerous and healthy cells. The emerging picture is overwhelmingly complex. Molecules out of many parallel signal transduction pathways are involved. Their activities appear to be controlled by multiple factors. The action of regulatory circuits, cross-talk between pathways and the non-linear reaction kinetics of biochemical processes complicate the understanding and prediction of the outcome of intracellular signaling. In addition, interactions between tumor and other cell types give rise to a complex supracellular communication network. If cancer is such a complex system, how can one ever predict the effect of a mutation in a particular gene on a functionality of the entire system? And, how should one go about identifying drug targets?

Methods and Results: Review paper in which the authors argue that one aspect is to recognize where the essence resides, i.e. recognize cancer as a systems biology disease. Then, more cancer biologists could become systems biologists aiming to provide answers to some of the above systemic questions. To this aim, they should integrate the available knowledge stemming from quantitative experimental results through mathematical models.

Discussion and Conclusion: Models that have contributed to the understanding of complex biological systems are discussed. It is shown that the architecture of a signaling network is important for determining the site at which an oncologist should intervene. Finally, it is discussed the possibility of applying network-based drug design to cancer treatment and how rationalized therapies, such as the application of kinase inhibitors, may benefit from systems biology.

During recent years, there has been great progress in the knowledge in the field of molecular cell biology of cancer. At the same time, the emerging complexity of the entire 'cancer system' overwhelms us, leaving an enormous gap in our understanding. In this paper, different aspects of this complexity are discussed. Molecules out of many parallel signal transduction pathways are involved in carcinogenesis. Their activities appear to be controlled by multiple factors. The action of regulatory circuits, cross-talk between pathways and the non-linear reaction kinetics of biochemical processes complicate the understanding and prediction of the outcome of intracellular signalling. This is a systems biology view on cancer adding another useful dimension to our understanding of the biology of cancer disorders. It is easy to accept the view that cancer researchers should also be system biologists. The paper gives new concepts of clinical usefulness not only for oncologists.

Mechanism of the year

Zac1 regulates an imprinted gene network critically involved in the control of embryonic growth

Varrault A, Gueydan C, Delalbre A, Bellmann A, Houssami S, Aknin C, Severac D, Chotard L, Kahli M, Le Digarcher A, Pavlidis P, Journot L
Institut de Génomique Fonctionnelle, CNRS-UMR5203, INSERM-U661, Université Montpellier 1, Université Montpellier 2, Montpellier, France
Dev Cell 2006;11:711–722

Background: Genomic imprinting is an epigenetic mechanism of regulation that restrains the expression of a small subset of mammalian genes to one parental allele. The reason for the targeting of these approximately 80 genes by imprinting remains uncertain.

Methods and Results: It is shown that inactivation of the maternally repressed Zac1 transcription factor results in intrauterine growth restriction, altered bone formation, and neonatal lethality. A meta-analysis of microarray data reveals that Zac1 is a member of a network of coregulated genes comprising other imprinted genes involved in the control of embryonic growth. Zac1 alters the expression of several of these imprinted genes, including Igf2, H19, Cdkn1c, and Dlk1, and it directly regulates the Igf2/H19 locus through binding to a shared enhancer.

Conclusion: These data identify a network of imprinted genes, including Zac1, which controls embryonic growth and which may be the basis for the implementation of a common mechanism of gene regulation during mammalian evolution.

Imprinting is understood as a mechanism aimed at controlling the amount of maternal resources allocated to the offspring from conception to weaning. Imprinted genes are members of various gene families, but a recurrent theme in the biology of imprinted genes is the control of embryonic development. Analysis of gain- and loss-of-function mouse mutants indicates that a number of imprinted genes are critically involved in the control of embryonic growth, either directly or by modulating the transport of nutrients across the placenta. The number and identity of imprinted genes involved in these processes, and the underlying gene networks, remain unclear. In order to understand the function of the maternally repressed transcription factor, Zac1, the authors inactivate the gene by homologous recombination. Next they identified the underlying network they did a meta-analysis of microarray data of genes that are co-expressed with Zac1 in different tissues and studied the regulatory effect of Zac1 on the members of the network. Zac1 was found to be critical for embryonic growth, and for gene expression of a large network of imprinted genes, including IGF2, Cdkn1c, and Dlk1.

Zac1 is identified as a central regulator of a large network of imprinted genes and may thus be part of a novel mechanism of gene regulation during mammalian development. Imprinted genes have often been observed to act in common developmental or physiological pathways. The present report exploring the function of the transcription factor *Zac1* reveals just how extensive the transcriptional network of imprinted genes may be.

New paradigms

Circadian clocks are resounding in peripheral tissues

Ptitsyn AA, Zvonic S, Conrad SA, Scott LK, Mynatt RL, Gimble JM
Experimental Obesity Laboratory, Louisiana State University Pennington Biomedical Research Center, Baton Rouge, La., USA
PLoS Comput Biol 2006;2:e16

Background: Circadian rhythms are prevalent in most organisms. Even the smallest disturbances in the orchestration of circadian gene expression patterns among different tissues can result in functional asynchrony, at the organism level, and may to contribute to a wide range of physiologic disorders. It has been reported that as many as 5–10% of transcribed genes in peripheral tissues follow a circadian expression pattern.

Methods: The authors have conducted a comprehensive study of circadian gene expression on a large dataset representing three different peripheral tissues. The data have been produced in a large-scale microarray experiment covering replicate daily cycles in murine white and brown adipose tissues as well as in liver. The authors applied three alternative algorithmic approaches to identify circadian oscillation in time series expression profiles.

Results: Analyses of our own data indicate that the expression of at least 7–21% of active genes in mouse liver, and in white and brown adipose tissues follow a daily oscillatory pattern. Indeed, analysis of data from other laboratories suggests that the percentage of genes with an oscillatory pattern may approach 50% in the liver. For the rest of the genes, oscillation appears to be obscured by stochastic noise. Phase classification and computer simulation studies based on multiple datasets indicate no detectable boundary between oscillating and non-oscillating fractions of genes.

Conclusion: Greater attention should be given to the potential influence of circadian mechanisms on any biological pathway related to metabolism and obesity.

The metabolism of living organisms changes over the 24-hour daily cycle in an oscillatory manner. This repeating pattern of 'peak' and 'trough' expression is known as a 'circadian rhythm'. We now know that the body's internal clock is controlled by a discrete group of genes. These important regulators are found in many different organs of the body, and they control expression of many other genes. In order to further understanding of the circadian rhythms of metabolism, the authors studied circadian gene expression using microarray analysis in liver, and in white and brown fat of mice using three different mathematical tests. They present data indicating that the majority of active genes fluctuate rhythmically over a 24-hour period. This work suggests that future studies should pay close attention to the influence of the circadian rhythm in obesity and in fat metabolism. Make sure in your clinical or animal studies to draw your samples at the same time each day.

O. Nilsson/O. Söder

A small step of a protein but a giant step of function

Unraveling adaptive evolution: how a single point mutation affects the protein coregulation network

Knight CG, Zitzmann N, Prabhakar S, Antrobus R, Dwek R, Hebestreit H, Rainey PB
Department of Plant Sciences, Oxford, UK
chris.knight@manchester.ac.uk
Nat Genet 2006;38:1015–1022

Background: Understanding the mechanisms of evolution requires identification of the molecular basis of the multiple (pleiotropic) effects of specific adaptive mutations.
Methods: The authors have characterized the pleiotropic effects on protein levels of an adaptive single base pair substitution in the coding sequence of a signaling pathway gene in the bacterium *Pseudomonas fluorescens* SBW25.
Results: 52 proteomic changes were found, corresponding to 46 identified proteins. None of these proteins is required for the adaptive phenotype. Instead, many are found within specific metabolic pathways associated with fitness-reducing (that is, antagonistic) effects of the mutation. The affected proteins fall within a single coregulatory network.
Conclusions: The mutation 'rewires' this network by drawing particular proteins into tighter coregulating relationships. Although these changes are specific to the mutation studied, the quantitatively altered proteins are also affected in a coordinated way in other examples of evolution to the same niche.

This work demonstrates the power of a systems biology approach to dissect the pleiotropic molecular events accompanying evolution. The simple mutation introduced into the model bacteria allowed the occupation of an environmental niche that was not available to the ancestral strain. The single base pair mutation caused 52 proteomic changes involving 46 identified proteins, none of which were required for the adaptive phenotype of the host. The affected proteins all belonged to the same single coregulatory network and were found to be associated with transport and metabolism of amino acids. The systems biology model used here will help to understand better the complex construction of integrated molecular systems and how they may be affected by evolution. The dramatic phenotypic change observed was the result of a simple mutation with profound effects on the proteome. The results demonstrate clearly that discrete mutational changes may result in dramatic effects on phenotypes, thus allowing major evolutionary steps. This challenges the view that evolution is driven by minute functional alterations of mutated proteins with negative or positive impact on their functions.

Mutations affecting gene expression may underlie common disorders

Natural selection on gene expression

Gilad Y, Oshlack A, Rifkin SA
Department of Human Genetics, University of Chicago, Chicago, Ill., USA
gilad@uchicago.edu
Trends Genet 2006;22:456–461

Background: Changes in genetic regulation contribute to adaptations in natural populations and influence susceptibility to human diseases. Despite their potential phenotypic importance, the selective pressures acting on regulatory processes in general and gene expression levels in particular are largely unknown.
Methods and Results: Review article discussing the microarray-based observations that led to disparate interpretations from studies in model organisms suggesting that (1) expression levels of most genes evolve under stabilizing selection, although a few are consistent with adaptive evolution, and (2) gene expression levels in primates evolve largely in the absence of selective constraints.
Conclusion: It is concluded that in both primates and model organisms, stabilizing selection is likely to be the dominant mode of gene expression evolution. An important implication is that mutations affecting gene expression will often be deleterious and might underlie many human diseases.

This is an important review paper using recent systems biology data to advance the discussion on the evolution biology of species including man. Data from model systems in lower species and from primates indicate that negative stabilizing selection is much more common whereas positive adaptive selection occurs more rarely. This suggests that changes in gene expression are deleterious and that they are involved in disease processes in humans. The specific sets of genes whose regulation are more commonly under adaptive pressures are yet to be defined. This paper is recommended as an up-to-date source of concepts and terminology in the field. The most interesting part is addressing novel views on the causes of common disorders in human.

Reviews
How do women choose males? (Theory)

Dissecting the complex genetic basis of mate choice

Chenoweth SF, Blows MW
School of Integrative Biology, University of Queensland, Brisbane, Qld., Australia
Nat Rev Genet 2006;7:681–692

Background and Methods: Review paper discussing the topic of mate choice. The genetic analysis of mate choice is fraught with difficulties. Males produce complex signals and displays that can consist of a combination of acoustic, visual, chemical and behavioral phenotypes. Female preferences for these male traits are notoriously difficult to quantify.

Results and Conclusions: During mate choice, genes not only affect the phenotypes of the individual they are in, but can influence the expression of traits in other individuals. How can genetic analyses be conducted to encompass this complexity? Tighter integration of classical quantitative genetic approaches with modern genomic technologies promises to advance our understanding of the complex genetic basis of mate choice.

Mate choice is thought to be one of the fundamental means of Darwinistic evolution. Males produce signals and displays that can consist of complex combinations of phenotypic expressions including ornamental and behavioral traits. Females differ in their preferences for these male traits but studies in this field have been hampered by difficulties to quantify the female responses. This review article describes the present status and challenges of this important field of evolutionary and behavioral genetics. To be successful genetic analysis of mate choice requires integrative approaches taking onboard modern systems biology technologies. The authors are hopeful that tighter integration of classical quantitative genetic approaches with modern genomic technologies will advance our understanding of the complex genetic basis of mate choice. Although direct translation of this research into human medicine may seem far-sighted basic insights into this the field are of importance for better understanding of the physiology and pathophysiology of behavioral traits and disturbances that may occur during human adolescence and early adult life.

New hope
How do women choose males II? (Practice)

Testing the genetics underlying the co-evolution of mate choice and ornament in the wild

Qvarnstrom A, Brommer JE, Gustafsson L
Animal Ecology, Department of Ecology and Evolution, Uppsala University, Uppsala, Sweden
anna.qvarnstrom@ebc.uu.se
Nature 2006;441:84–86

Background: One of the most debated questions in evolutionary biology is whether female choice of males with exaggerated sexual displays can evolve as a correlated response to selection acting on genes coding for male attractiveness or high overall viability. To date, empirical studies have provided support for parts of this scenario, but evidence for all key genetic components in a natural population is lacking.

Methods: Here the authors use animal-model quantitative genetic analysis on data from over 8,500 collared flycatchers (*Ficedula albicollis*) followed for 24 years to quantify all of the key genetic requirements of both fisherian and 'good-genes' models on sexual selection in the wild.

Results: It was found that significant additive genetic variances of all the main components: male ornament (forehead patch size), female mate choice for this ornament, male fitness and female fitness. However, when the necessary genetic correlations between these components were taken into account, the estimated strength of indirect sexual selection on female mate choice was negligible.

Conclusion: The results show that the combined effect of environmental influences on several components reduces the potential for indirect sexual selection in the wild. This study provides insight into the field of sexual selection by showing that genes coding for mate choice for an ornament probably evolve by their own pathways instead of 'hitchhiking' with genes coding for the ornament.

Current models of sexual selection (mate choice) suggest that males carry genes coding for sexual attractiveness (display of ornaments; fisherian model) and viability (good genes model) enhancing the competitiveness of their offspring. Females preferentially mate with highly ornamented males implicating a genetic correlation between the ornament and the mate choice with a linkage to good genes expressed in the offspring. The models have partial support from several studies but solid evidence covering all genetic components from a wild-life population perspective has been lacking. The authors test whether the preference of female collared flycatchers (*Ficedula albicollis*) for males with large forehead patches could have evolved as a by-product of selection acting on male patch size. They find that the crucial genetic correlation between female choice and male patch size is not significant, and conclude that preference for large patches must have been shaped directly by selection. This is good news! Lack of inherited good looks (strong ornaments) can be compensated for by hard work (environmental influence).

Mechanism of the year
Excitation by paracrine glutamate start you up

Quantitative proteomics identifies a change in glial glutamate metabolism at the time of female puberty

Roth CL, McCormack AL, Lomniczi A, Mungenast AE, Ojeda SR
Division of Neuroscience, Oregon National Primate Research Center, Oregon Health and Sciences University, Beaverton, Oreg, USA
Mol Cell Endocrinol 2006;254/255:51–59

Background: Mammalian puberty requires activation of luteinizing hormone-releasing hormone (LHRH) neurons. In turn, these neurons are controlled by transsynaptic and glia-to-neuron communication pathways, which employ diverse cellular proteins for proper function.

Methods: The authors used a high throughput relative quantitative proteomics technique to identify proteins involved in pubertal activation. They selected the method of two-dimensional liquid chromatography tandem mass spectrometry (2DLC-MS/MS) and cleavable isotope-coded affinity tags (cICAT), to both identify and quantify individual proteins within a complex protein mixture. The proteins used derived from the hypothalamus of juvenile (25-day-old) and peripubertal (first proestrus, LP) female rats, and their identity was established by analyzing their mass spectra via database searching.

Results: Five proteins involved in glutamate metabolism were detected and two of them appeared to be differentially expressed. They were selected for further analysis, because of their importance in controlling glutamate synthesis and degradation, and their preferential expression in astroglial cells. One, glutamate dehydrogenase (GDH) catalyzes glutamate synthesis; its hypothalamic content detected by 2DLC-MS/MS increases at first proestrus. The other, glutamine synthetase (GS), catalyzes the metabolism of glutamate to glutamine; its content decreases in proestrus. Western blot analysis verified these results. Because these changes suggested an increased glutamate production at puberty, we measured glutamate release from hypothalamic fragments from juvenile 29-day-old rats, and from rats treated with PMSG to induce a premature proestrus surge of luteinizing hormone (LH). To determine the net output of glutamate in the absence of re-uptake, we used the excitatory amino acid transporter (EAAT) inhibitor L-trans-pyrrolidine-2,4-dicarboxylic acid (PDC). PDC elicited significantly more glutamate and LHRH release from the proestrus hypothalamus.

Conclusion: An increase excitatory drive to the LHRH neuronal network provided by glutamatergic inputs of glial origin is an event contributing to the pubertal activation of LHRH secretion.

This study illustrates the power of a proteomics approach to study systemic time-restricted maturational events in biology, here verifying the important role of glutamate as an excitatory signal at the onset of puberty. The present study demonstrates that the onset of female puberty is accompanied by opposite changes in the hypothalamic content of glutamate dehydrogenase and glutamine synthetase, two enzymes involved in the homeostatic control of brain glutamate metabolism. The results also show that these changes in protein content are physiologically important, because they are accompanied by an increased capability of the hypothalamus to release glutamate. The relevance of these changes to the control of LHRH secretion is evidenced by the increased LHRH output that follows the peripubertal changes in glutamate release. The results thus verify that puberty starts after providing LHRH neurons an increased excitatory drive exerted by paracrine glutamate derived from local astroglial cells. The results are not exactly novel but the experimental context implicates a physiological significance. The next question is of course what comes before glutamate? Proteomics succeeded where genomics failed, suggesting that the onset of puberty is not necessarily in our gene DNA sequence but rather in gene expression, which may be regulated by the environment.

Food for thought
Males and females are more different than we think but not in the brain!

Tissue-specific expression and regulation of sexually dimorphic genes in mice

Yang X, Schadt EE, Wang S, Wang H, Arnold AP, Ingram-Drake L, Drake TA, Lusis AJ
Department of Medicine, David Geffen School of Medicine, University of California, Los Angeles, Calif., USA
Genome Res 2006;16:995–1004

Background: Sexual dimorphism in gene expression in various tissues is an important target of investigation but progress has been hampered by low-power and non-comprehensive approaches of hitherto published studies.

Methods and Results: The authors report a comprehensive analysis of gene expression differences between sexes in multiple somatic tissues of 334 mice derived from an intercross between inbred mouse strains C57BL/6J and C3H/HeJ. The analysis of a large number of individuals provided the power to detect relatively small differences in expression between sexes, and the use of an intercross allowed analysis of the genetic control of sexually dimorphic gene expression. Microarray analysis of 23,574 transcripts revealed that the extent of sexual dimorphism in gene expression was much greater than previously recognized. Thus, thousands of genes showed sexual dimorphism in liver, adipose, and muscle, and hundreds of genes were sexually dimorphic in brain. These genes exhibited highly tissue-specific patterns of expression and were enriched for distinct pathways represented in the Gene Ontology database. They also showed evidence of chromosomal enrichment, not only on the sex chromosomes, but also on several autosomes.

Conclusion: The analyses provided evidence of the global regulation of subsets of the sexually dimorphic genes, as the transcript levels of a large number of these genes were controlled by several expression quantitative trait loci (eQTL) hotspots that exhibited tissue-specific control. Many tissue-specific transcription factor binding sites were found to be enriched in the sexually dimorphic genes.

Common diseases often have a sex bias and systematic understanding of the physiological differences between sexes is therefore of great importance to advance the field. In this work the authors present a comprehensive analysis of gene expression differences between sexes in multiple somatic tissues in mice. Thousands of genes in liver, fat and muscle, and hundreds of genes in brain were found to be sexually dimorphic, defined as >1.2-fold difference in expression between sexes. These genes exhibited a highly sex-specific tissue expression pattern and had a chromosomal enrichment not only restricted to the sex chromosomes. Liver showed the greatest degree of sex difference with more than 70% of expressed genes whereas the brain showed the lowest with less than 14% of expressed genes. Most differences were small and the percentages of genes with >2-fold difference in expression between sexes were 1.1% for liver, 0.8% for fat, 0.6% for muscle and 0.1% for brain. The sexually dimorphic genes were clustered into several functional categories such as immune response, lipid metabolism, steroid hormone metabolism and polyamine metabolism dependent on tissue (liver, fat, muscle). The brain was an exception showing RNA helicase activity as an enriched dimorphic category. The widespread sex differences in gene expression observed here are most likely due to differential effects of sex steroids, which contribute to sex differences both directly and indirectly (mediated by growth hormone profile). Despite the importance of hormones, an increasing amount of evidence supports a regulatory cascade concept of sexual dimorphism in gene expression; that is, the initiating events of sexual differentiation such as *Sry* expression trigger differential expression in many mediator genes that further regulate the sexually dimorphic expression of downstream genes. These results need extension to other tissues and organs and confirmation in humans, but the findings demonstrate clearly the potential impact of transcriptomics to advance our understanding of the pathophysiology behind the gender differences in common disorders.

New methodology
Model for reproductive 'toxicotranscriptomics'

Identification of genetic networks involved in the cell injury accompanying endoplasmic reticulum stress induced by bisphenol A in testicular Sertoli cells

Tabuchi Y, Takasaki I, Kondo T
Division of Molecular Genetics Research, Life Science Research Center, University of Toyama, Toyama, Japan
ytabu@cts.u-toyama.ac.jp
Biochem Biophys Res Commun 2006;345:1044–1050

Background: The molecular mechanisms mediating cell injury by xenobiotics are virtually unknown but are important to investigate in order to develop better diagnostic and preventive measures in reproductive toxicology.
Methods: To identify detailed mechanisms by which bisphenol A (BPA), an endocrine-disrupting chemical, induces cell injury in mouse testicular Sertoli TTE3 cells, the authors performed genome-wide microarray and computational gene network analyses.
Results: BPA (200 μM) significantly decreased cell viability and simultaneously induced an increase in mRNA levels of HSPA5 and DDIT3, endoplasmic reticulum (ER) stress marker genes. Of the 22,690 probe sets analyzed, BPA downregulated 661 probe sets and upregulated 604 probe sets by >2.0-fold. Hierarchical cluster analysis demonstrated nine gene clusters. In decreased gene clusters, two significant genetic networks were associated with cell growth and proliferation and the cell cycle. In increased gene clusters, two significant genetic networks including many basic-region leucine zipper transcription factors were associated with cell death and DNA replication, recombination, and repair.
Conclusion: The results will provide additional novel insights into the detailed molecular mechanisms of cell injury accompanying ER stress induced by BPA in Sertoli cells.

The authors use genome-wide microarray and gene network analysis covering 22,690 genes to study cellular responses to exposure to the endocrine disrupting toxicant bisphenol A (BPA). This compound downregulated 661 genes and upregulated 604 genes by more than 2-fold. These genes were found to be associated with nine genetic networks. Upregulated gene clusters included two significant networks harboring several transcription factors associated with cell rescue mechanisms such as

DNA replication, recombination and repair. Downregulated gene clusters included genes important for cell growth and cell cycle control. The principles applied in this laborious cellular toxicotranscriptomics study have a potential to become a model for toxicological screening programs. In Europe this has recently become highly relevant under the new EU legislation on registration, evaluation and authorization of new chemicals (REACH).

Approaching the virtual cell

Establishing glucose- and ABA-regulated transcription networks in *Arabidopsis* by microarray analysis and promoter classification using a relevance vector machine

Li Y, Lee KK, Walsh S, Smith C, Hadingham S, Sorefan K, Cawley G, Bevan MW
Department of Cell and Developmental Biology, John Innes Centre, Norwich, UK
Genome Res 2006;16:414–427

Background: Transcriptional regulatory networks are difficult but import to delineate. Novel techniques for analysis of gene expression data and promoter sequences show great promise in this respect.

Methods: The authors developed a novel promoter classification method using a relevance vector machine (RVM) and bayesian statistical principles to identify discriminatory features in the promoter sequences of genes that can correctly classify transcriptional responses. The method was applied to microarray data obtained from *Arabidopsis* seedlings treated with glucose or abscisic acid (ABA).

Results: Of genes showing >2.5-fold changes in expression level, approximately 70% were correctly predicted as being up- or downregulated (under 10-fold cross-validation), based on the presence or absence of a small set of discriminative promoter motifs. Many of these motifs have known regulatory functions in sugar- and ABA-mediated gene expression. One promoter motif that was not known to be involved in glucose-responsive gene expression was identified as the strongest classifier of glucose upregulated gene expression. It was shown it mediated glucose-responsive gene expression in conjunction with another promoter motif, thus validating the classification method.

Conclusion: The authors were able to establish a detailed model of glucose and ABA transcriptional regulatory networks and their interactions, which will help us to understand the mechanisms linking metabolism with growth in *Arabidopsis*. This study shows that machine-learning strategies coupled to bayesian statistical methods hold significant promise for identifying functionally significant promoter sequences.

Bioinformatic methods that define relationships between gene expression levels and putative regulatory sequences in upstream regions of genes are increasingly used to establish genome-scale transcriptional regulatory networks. The authors apply and validate such techniques. Microarray data obtained from cultures of *Arabidopsis* seedlings treated with glucose, ABA or both were analyzed using a RVM and bayesian statistics in order to establish genome-scale regulatory networks. A number of regulatory elements that are responsible for ABA- and glucose-regulated gene expression was identified. Based on the presence or absence of a small number of these regulatory elements, the authors were able to predict response to treatment. Some of these regulatory elements have not previously been associated with glucose-responsive gene expression. This is complicated methodology but the paper holds promises for integrated metabolomics and proteomics models that are important and necessary building blocks for creation of the 'virtual cell'.

References

Readers who want a basic update and learn more about the methodologies employed in systems biology research are referred to the following review papers and books.

Alberghina L, Westerhoff H: Systems Biology: Definitions and Perspectives. Berlin, Springer, 2005.

Alon U: An Introduction to Systems Biology: Design Principles of Biological Circuits. London, Chapman & Hall/CRC, Taylor & Francis, 2006.

Kitano H (ed): Foundations of Systems Biology. Cambridge/MA, MIT Press, 2001.

Klipp E, Herwig R, Kowald A, Wierling C, Lehrach H: Systems Biology in Practice. London, Wiley, 2005.

Schnell S, Grima R, Maini PK: Multiscale modeling in biology. Am Sci 2007;95:134–142.

Editor's Choice

Jean-Claude Carel and Ze'ev Hochberg

Linked to grow

Genetic linkage of human height is confirmed to 9q22 and Xq24

Liu YZ, Xiao P, Guo YF, Xiong DH, Zhao LJ, Shen H, Liu YJ, Dvornyk V, Long JR, Deng HY, Li JL, Recker RR, Deng HW
Osteoporosis Research Center, Creighton University Medical Center, Omaha, Nebr., USA
Hum Genet 2006;119:295–304

Background: Human height is an important and heritable trait. The author's previous two genome-wide linkage studies using 630 (WG1 study) and an extended sample of 1,816 Caucasians (WG2 study) identified 9q22 [maximum LOD score (MLS) = 2.74 in the WG2 study] and preliminarily confirmed Xq24 (two-point LOD score = 1.91 in the WG1 study, 2.64 in the WG2 study) linked to height.
Methods: Here, with a much further extended large sample containing 3,726 Caucasians, a new genome-wide linkage scan was performed and confirmed, in high significance, the two regions' linkage to height.
Results: A MLS of 4.34 was detected on 9q22 and a two-point LOD score of 5.63 was attained for Xq24. In an independent sub-sample (i.e., the subjects not involved in the WG1 and WG2 studies), the two regions also achieved significant empirical p values (0.002 and 0.004, respectively) for 'region-wise' linkage confirmation. Importantly, the two regions were replicated on a genotyping platform different from the WG1 and WG2 studies (i.e., a different set of markers and different genotyping instruments). Interestingly, 9q22 harbors the ROR2 gene, which is required for growth plate development, and Xq24 was linked to short stature.
Conclusions: With the largest sample from a single population of the same ethnicity in the field of linkage studies for complex traits, the current study, together with the two previous ones, provided overwhelming evidence substantiating 9q22 and Xq24 for height variation. In particular, the three consecutive whole genome studies are uniquely valuable as they represent the first practical (rather than simulated) example of how significant increase in sample size may improve linkage detection for human complex traits.

Genetic studies using association or whole genome linkage approaches have suggested quite a few genes and genomic regions associated with or linked to human height. However, few such genes and genomic regions have been replicated across studies. This may be attributed to the relatively small sample sizes for most of the studies and the modest significance levels for the majority of the reported findings. As a result, genuine genetic effects could be missed or a reported linkage or association could be a false positive. The present study was performed on 3,726 subjects of the same ethnicity. With a MLS of 4.34, 9q22 can now be regarded to have a strong link to growth, and with a two-point LOD score of 5.63 Xq24 (didn't we expect Xp to be the major growth region?) is now open to hunt. Admittedly, Xp22 also achieved very significant linkage signals. Our growth plate investigators will be delighted to hear of 9q22-ROR2 gene, which is required for growth plate development. Linked to the Xq24 region were several syndromes characterized by short stature, including the mental retardation, x-linked, with short stature syndrome (MIM 300360), the mental retardation, x-linked, with short stature, small testes, muscle wasting, and tremor syndrome (MIM 300354) and the mental retardation, x-linked, with isolated growth hormone deficiency syndrome (MIM 300123). On a similar topic, the same group with the same cohort aimed to search for potential genomic regions that harbor interactive genes underlying human height [1]. Performing variance component linkage analyses of height based on a two-locus epistatic model, they found significant genetic interaction between 6p21 and 2q21. Interestingly, 6p21 contains a cluster of candidate genes for skeletal growth, suggesting a mechanism whereby 2q21 regulates height through 6p21.

Estrogen deficiency and bone loss: an inflammatory tale

Weitzmann MN, Pacifici R
Division of Endocrinology, Metabolism, and Lipids and Molecular Pathogenesis Program, Emory University, Atlanta, Ga., USA
J Clin Invest 2006;116:1186–1194

Background: Estrogen plays a fundamental role in skeletal growth and bone homeostasis in both men and women. Although remarkable progress has been made in our understanding of how estrogen deficiency causes bone loss, the mechanisms involved have proven to be complex and multifaceted.

New concepts involving the immune system: Although estrogen is established to have direct effects on bone cells, recent animal studies have identified additional unexpected regulatory effects of estrogen centered at the level of the adaptive immune response. Furthermore, a potential role for reactive oxygen species has now been identified in both humans and animals.

Challenge: The integration of a multitude of redundant pathways and cytokines, each apparently capable of playing a relevant role, into a comprehensive model of postmenopausal osteoporosis.

This review presents the current understanding of the process of estrogen deficiency-mediated bone destruction and explores some recent findings and hypotheses to explain estrogen action in bone. Due to the inherent difficulties associated with human investigation, many of the lessons learned have been in animal models. Consequently, many of these principles await further validation in humans. Estrogen receptors (ER) α and β are expressed in multiple organs, and the industry is in a race to develop a selective estrogen receptor modulator (SERM) that would activate the ER in bone but not in the breast. In 2002, a synthetic ligand, named estren, was reported to have increased bone mass and strength in gonadectomized mice but had no effects on uterine breast cancer cells [2]. The effect of estren was attributed to non-genomic activation of transcription factors by several kinase cascades. PubMed shows 96 entries for estrens. While everyone expected the results of their use in humans, a few reports have questioned the non-genomic mechanism of estrens. We now learn that while estrens were able to prevent gonadectomy-induced bone loss, they showed no bone anabolic effects when given at the same doses and in the same manner as originally reported. Moreover, they increased uterine weight and enhanced the proliferation of human breast cancer cells. The paper shows that estrens bind more strongly to androgen receptor than ER and suggests that they act more as androgens than estrogens.

Klotho converts canonical FGF receptor into a specific receptor for FGF23

Urakawa I, Yamazaki Y, Shimada T, Iijima K, Hasegawa H, Okawa K, Fujita T, Fukumoto S, Yamashita T
Pharmaceutical Research Laboratories, Kirin Brewery Co., Ltd, Takasaki, Gunma, Japan
iurakawa@kirin.co.jp
Nature 2006;444:770–774

Context: FGF23 is a unique member of the fibroblast growth factor (FGF) family because it acts as a hormone that derives from bone and regulates kidney functions, whereas most other family members are thought to regulate various cell functions at a local level. The renotropic activity of circulating FGF23 indicates the possible presence of an FGF23-specific receptor in the kidney.

Results: A previously undescribed receptor conversion by Klotho, a senescence-related molecule, generates the FGF23 receptor. Using a renal homogenate, the authors found that Klotho binds to FGF23. Forced expression of Klotho enabled the high-affinity binding of FGF23 to the cell surface and restored the ability of a renal cell line to respond to FGF23 treatment. Moreover, FGF23 incompetence was induced by injecting wild-type mice with an anti-Klotho monoclonal antibody.

Conclusions: Klotho is essential for endogenous FGF23 function. Because Klotho alone seemed to be incapable of intracellular signaling, they searched for other components of the FGF23 receptor and found FGFR1(IIIc), which was directly converted by Klotho into the FGF23 receptor. Thus, the concerted action of Klotho and FGFR1(IIIc) reconstitutes the FGF23 receptor. These findings provide insights into the diversity and specificity of interactions between FGF and FGF receptors.

Last year, the *Yearbook* described the new hormone Klotho (daughter of Zeus and Themis, etc.), and how it suppresses tyrosine phosphorylation of insulin and IGF-1 receptors, which result in reduced activity of IRS proteins and their association with PI_3-kinase, thereby inhibiting insulin and IGF-1 signaling, and suppressing aging [3]. This year, Klotho gets closer to pediatric endocrinology. It converts FGF receptor-1, a canonical receptor for various FGFs, into a specific receptor for FGF23, the bone-derived phosphaturic hormone that has been implicated in three different varieties of hypophosphatemic rickets [4].

Eflornithine cream combined with laser therapy in the management of unwanted facial hair growth in women: a randomized trial

Smith SR, Piacquadio DJ, Beger B, Littler C
Therapeutics, Inc., San Diego, Calif., USA
ssmith@therapeuticsresearch.com
Dermatol Surg 2006;32:1237–1243

Background: Eflornithine cream is approved for the reduction of unwanted facial hair in women. The mechanism of action for eflornithine is reduction in follicular cell growth rate, while laser photoepilation heats hair and adjacent tissues to suspend growth. The objective was to assess the efficacy and safety of eflornithine or vehicle with laser therapy in the treatment of unwanted facial hair in women.
Methods: Subjects were randomized to treatment with eflornithine on one side of the face and vehicle on the contralateral side for 34 weeks. Subjects received Nd:YAG or alexandrite laser therapy to both sides of the face at weeks 2 and 10. Blinded evaluations included left to right comparisons and appearance relative to baseline.
Results: Fifty-four women completed the trial. From weeks 6 through 22, eflornithine-treated sides showed significant reduction in hair growth. By week 34, no significant differences were seen. Subject grading showed significant and persistent hair reduction through week 34 for eflornithine-treated sides. The safety profile for combination therapy is similar to eflornithine alone.
Conclusion: Eflornithine is safely used in conjunction with laser hair removal treatments and promotes more rapid hair removal when combined with laser treatment. Patients demonstrate a clear preference for treatment with laser and eflornithine.

You will recognize that this isn't one of the journals we usually cite, but it seems that this new drug went unnoticed by the pediatric endocrine community, and its story is really fascinating. African sleeping sickness affects 300,000 new cases every year, and is caused by *Trypanosoma brucei*, which is transmitted by the bite of an infected tsetse fly. Eflornithine (difluoromethylornithine, DFMO, 1970s), which was developed as a potential anticancer drug by inhibiting ornithine decarboxylase (polyamine biosynthesis) and impairing cellular division, was evaluated for its efficacy in a mouse model of trypanosomiasis. Following dramatic results in mice, clinical trials showed revitalization of comatose sleeping sickness, and was named 'the resurrection drug'. The problem was that with parenteral administration, and costing USD 600/year, it wasn't practical or profitable for the industry to pursue and it was decided to discontinue production. At the end of 2000, the remaining vials were 1 year past expiration; the entire stockpile was projected to be depleted in another 6–9 months. Clinical observations in sleeping sickness showed for eflornithine side effects of hair loss and hearing loss (loss of hair cells in organ of Corti). It was tested and shown that when topically applied, DFMO inhibits DNA synthesis and hair follicular function. The topical formulation received FDA approval in July 2005. The happy end: Bristol-Myers Squibb, Dow Chemical Co., Akorn Manufacturing Inc., and Aventis, who are to make a fortune, have agreed to supply WHO with adequate supplies of parenteral eflornithine to last for the next 3 years.

Identification of a hormonal basis for gallbladder filling

Choi M, Moschetta A, Bookout AL, Peng L, Umetani M, Holmstrom SR, Suino-Powell K, Xu HE, Richardson JA, Gerard RD, Mangelsdorf DJ, Kliewer SA
Department of Molecular Biology, University of Texas Southwestern Medical Center, Dallas, Tex., USA
Nat Med 2006;12:1253–1255

Context: The cycle of gallbladder filling and emptying controls the flow of bile into the intestine for digestion.
Results: Here the authors show that fibroblast growth factor-15, a hormone made by the distal small intestine in response to bile acids, is required for gallbladder filling.
Conclusions: These studies demonstrate that gallbladder filling is actively regulated by an endocrine pathway and suggest a postprandial timing mechanism that controls gallbladder motility.

The hormone cholecystokinin (CCK), which is secreted from the proximal duodenum, is the major determinant of gallbladder emptying. Fibroblast growth factor-19 (FGF15 in the mouse) is a hormone that has a central role in the feedback regulation of bile acid synthesis in the liver. It is made by the ileum, where its expression is induced by bile acids acting through the farnesoid X receptor. Mice lacking FGF15 have gallbladders that are almost devoid of bile and providing this new hormone stimulates gallbladder filling. Interestingly, all four FGF receptor mRNAs were detected in the gallbladder, with Fgfr3 mRNA levels being the highest, suggesting a role for Fgfr3. Here is how this new endocrine loop works in the temporal regulation of gallbladder motility. During feeding, CCK secreted from the duodenum causes gallbladder contraction and the release of bile into the duodenum, which facilitates digestion and suppresses further CCK secretion. After traversing the small intestine, bile acids induce FGF19 synthesis in the ileum, which stimulates gallbladder refilling. It remains to be seen whether FGF19 will inhibit the effects of CCK on other physiological processes including gastric emptying, pancreatic enzyme secretion and food intake.

Family composition and menarcheal age: anti-inbreeding strategies

Matchock RL, Susman EJ
Department of Psychology, Pennsylvania State University, Altoona, Pa., USA
rlm191@psu.edu
Am J Hum Biol 2006;18:481–491

Background: Family composition (e.g., the absence of a father) is associated with pubertal timing in women, although the socioendocrinology of the human primate is poorly understood.
Methods: To better understand social influences on sexual maturation, retrospective data were collected on menarcheal age and family composition from a sample of approximately 1,938 participants from a college population.
Results: Absence of a biological father, the presence of half- and stepbrothers, and living in an urban environment were associated with earlier menarche. The presence of sisters in the household while growing up, especially older sisters, was associated with delayed menarche. Menarcheal age was not affected by the number of brothers in the household, nor was there an effect of birth order. Body weight and race were also associated with menarche.
Conclusions: The present findings advance the literature as they are suggestive of putative human pheromones that modulate sexual maturation to promote gene survival and prevent inbreeding, as occurs in rodents and non-human primates.

Prevention of inbreeding is so crucial to successfully spread healthy genes that anti-inbreeding strategies are conserved across species. As part of an evolutionary strategy to prevent inbreeding, chemical cues from fathers may be delaying the onset of sexual maturity in daughters. If the biological father is removed from rodent families, the daughters tend to mature faster. In the human olfactory system a little-known pheromone receptor gene may link the role of pheromones to menarche. Menarcheal data collected from 1,938 college students indicate that girls without fathers matured approximately 3 months before girls whose fathers were present; the earlier the absence, the earlier the menarche. The presence of half- and stepbrothers was also linked to earlier menarche. Girls living in an urban environment also had earlier menarche compared to girls in a rural environment, even when fathers were present for both groups, and had similar levels of education. The authors speculate that urban environments provide greater opportunities to get away from parents' inhibitory pheromones, and encounter attracting pheromones from unrelated members of the opposite sex.

Evolution of hormone-receptor complexity by molecular exploitation

Bridgham JT, Carroll SM, Thornton JW
Center for Ecology and Evolutionary Biology, University of Oregon, Eugene, Oreg., USA
Science 2006;312:97–101

Background: According to Darwinian theory, complexity evolves by a stepwise process of elaboration and optimization under natural selection. Biological systems composed of tightly integrated parts seem to challenge this view, because it is not obvious how any element's function can be selected for unless the partners with which it interacts are already present.
Aim: To demonstrate how an integrated molecular system, the specific functional interaction between the steroid hormone aldosterone and its partner the mineralocorticoid receptor evolved by a stepwise Darwinian process.
Results: Using ancestral gene resurrection, this paper shows that, long before the hormone evolved, the receptor's affinity for aldosterone was present as a structural by-product of its partnership with chemically similar, more ancient ligands. Introducing two amino acid changes into the ancestral sequence recapitulates the evolution of present-day receptor specificity.
Conclusions: Tight interactions can evolve by molecular exploitation-recruitment of an older molecule, previously constrained for a different role, into a new functional complex.

Were hormones constructed to fit given receptors? Or did the latter evolve to fit existing ligands? Is it possible that the pair evolved together? The existence of orphan receptors suggested that receptors came first. This paper takes a closer look at this mystery and discovers a different answer in the molecular evolution of hormone-receptor interactions. Charles Darwin famously remarked that 'if it could be demonstrated that any complex organ existed which could not possibly have been formed by numerous successive slight modifications, my theory would absolutely break down'. I will not keep you suspended; there is no 'intelligent design' behind the endocrine pair. Luckily, it is now possible to reconstruct the ancestral genes of an existing species so that we can now study a gene's evolution. You recall that cortisol activates not only the glucocorticoid receptor but also the mineralocorticoid receptor if it wasn't for 11β-HSD-2. Phylogeny tells us that an ancestral corticoid receptor gave rise to the glucocorticoid receptor and the mineralocorticoid receptor in a gene-duplication event more than 450 million years ago. Aldosterone evolved much later. Without aldosterone present, how could the mineralocorticoid receptor evolve to be activated by it? What the authors find is a surprise: Not only is the ancestral corticoid receptor sensitive to cortisol as expected, it is also activated by 11-deoxycorticosterone (DOC) and aldosterone. Because aldosterone was not present at the time, this sensitivity must be a by-product of sensitivity to another steroid, a promiscuity that has been exploited by evolution.

Effects of psychosocial stimulation and dietary supplementation in early childhood on psychosocial functioning in late adolescence: follow-up of randomized controlled trial

Walker SP, Chang SM, Powell CA, Simonoff E, Grantham-McGregor SM
Epidemiology Research Unit, Tropical Medicine Research Institute, University of the West Indies, Kingston, Jamaica
susan.walker@uwimona.edu.jm
BMJ 2006;333:472

Background: To determine whether dietary supplementation or psychosocial stimulation given to growth-retarded (stunted) children aged 9–24 months has long-term benefits for their psychosocial functioning in late adolescence.

Design: Sixteen-year follow-up study of a randomized controlled trial.

Methods: The study was set in poor neighborhoods in Kingston, Jamaica. The participants were 129 stunted children identified at age 9–24 months of whom 103 adolescents aged 17–18 were followed up. Intervention consisted in supplementation with 1 kg milk-based formula each week or psychosocial stimulation (weekly play sessions with mother and child), or both, for 2 years. The outcome measures included anxiety, depression, self-esteem, and antisocial behavior assessed by questionnaires administered by interviewers; attention deficit, hyperactivity, and oppositional behavior assessed by interviews with parents.

Results: Primary analysis indicated that participants who received stimulation had significantly different overall scores from those who did not (F = 2.047, p = 0.049). Supplementation had no significant effect (F = 1.505, p = 0.17). Participants who received stimulation reported less anxiety (mean difference −2.81), less depression (−0.43), and higher self-esteem (1.55) and parents reported fewer attention problems (−3.34). These differences are equivalent to effect sizes of 0.40–0.49 standard deviations.

Conclusions: Stimulation in early childhood has sustained benefits to stunted children's emotional outcomes and attention.

The reactive response to stunted growth in a poor neighborhood is to provide food supplementation. Whereas the importance of food cannot be overestimated, this paper shows that in the long run, psychosocial stimulation was a better investment than food was. Walker and colleagues show that in this group of poor Jamaican growth-retarded (stunted) children, aged 9–24 months, interventions to stimulate children and expose them to more positive parenting reduce the risks of antisocial behavior, pregnancy, substance misuse, delinquency, and emotional and behavioral disorders in adolescence, whereas food supplementation had no sustained effect on any of these crucial parameters. For us, in the field of growth promotion of stunted children, it may be high time to shift emphasis from reactive intervention to prevention and health promotion.

Toward a therapy for Marfan syndrome

Losartan, an AT1 antagonist, prevents aortic aneurysm in a mouse model of Marfan syndrome

Habashi JP, Judge DP, Holm TM, Cohn RD, Loeys BL, Cooper TK, Myers L, Klein EC, Liu G, Calvi C, Podowski M, Neptune ER, Halushka MK, Bedja D, Gabrielson K, Rifkin DB, Carta L, Ramirez F, Huso DL, Dietz HC
Howard Hughes Medical Institute and Department of Pediatrics, Johns Hopkins University School of Medicine, Baltimore, Md., USA
Science 2006;312:117–121

Background: Aortic aneurysm and dissection are manifestations of Marfan syndrome, a disorder caused by mutations in the gene that encodes fibrillin-1. Selected manifestations of Marfan syndrome reflect excessive signaling by the transforming growth factor-β (TGF-β) family of cytokines.

Results: In a mouse model of Marfan syndrome, aortic aneurysm is associated with increased TGF-β signaling and can be prevented by TGF-β antagonists such as TGF-β-neutralizing antibody or the angiotensin II type 1 receptor (AT1) blocker, losartan. AT1 antagonism also partially reversed noncardiovascular manifestations of Marfan syndrome, including impaired alveolar septation.

Conclusions: These data suggest that losartan, a drug already in clinical use for hypertension, merits investigation as a therapeutic strategy for patients with Marfan syndrome and has the potential to prevent the major life-threatening manifestation of this disorder.

Marfan syndrome is caused by mutations in the gene encoding fibrillin-1, a component of the extracellular matrix that regulates TGF-β. This paper reports that losartan, an FDA-approved angiotensinogen II type 1 receptor antagonist that also antagonizes TGF-β, prevents aortic aneurysm in a mouse model of Marfan syndrome. Treatment of pregnant mice with losartan in the drinking water, or of postnatal mice by intraperitoneal injection, either prevented or resulted in a complete reversion of these major, life-threatening manifestations of the syndrome. Treated mice also showed a reduction in distal airspace of the lung. A clinical trial is planned to test the drug in individuals with Marfan syndrome.

Repression of smoothened by patched-dependent (pro-)vitamin D₃ secretion

Bijlsma MF, Spek CA, Zivkovic D, van de Water S, Rezaee F, Peppelenbosch MP
Center for Experimental and Molecular Medicine, Academic Medical Center, University of Amsterdam, Amsterdam, The Netherlands
m.f.bijlsma@amc.uva.nl
PLoS Biol 2006;4:e232

Context: The developmentally important hedgehog pathway is activated by binding of hedgehog to patched (Ptch1), releasing smoothened (Smo) and the downstream transcription factor glioma associated (Gli) from inhibition. The mechanism behind Ptch1-dependent Smo inhibition remains unresolved. *Results:* The authors now show that by mixing Ptch1-transfected and Ptch1 small interfering RNA-transfected cells with Gli reporter cells, Ptch1 is capable of non-cell autonomous repression of Smo. The magnitude of this non-cell autonomous repression of Smo activity was comparable to the fusion of Ptch1-transfected cell lines and Gli reporter cell lines, suggesting that it is the predominant mode of action. CHOD-PAP analysis of medium conditioned by Ptch1-transfected cells showed an elevated 3β-hydroxysteroid content, which was hypothesized to mediate the Smo inhibition. Indeed, the inhibition of 3β-hydroxysteroid synthesis impaired Ptch1 action on Smo, whereas adding the 3β-hydroxysteroid (pro-)vitamin D₃ to the medium effectively inhibited Gli activity. Vitamin D₃ bound to Smo with high affinity in a cyclopamine-sensitive manner. Treating zebrafish embryos with vitamin D₃ mimicked the smo(−/−) phenotype, confirming the inhibitory action in vivo. Hh activates its signaling cascade by inhibiting Ptch1-dependent secretion of the 3β-hydroxysteroid (pro-)vitamin D₃. *Conclusions:* This action not only explains the seemingly contradictory cause of Smith-Lemli-Opitz syndrome, but also establishes hedgehog as a unique morphogen, because binding of Hh on one cell is capable of activating hedgehog-dependent signaling cascades on other cells.

We are used to think of vitamin D in terms of calcium metabolism, but a large volume of recent evidence links it to cancer. This paper makes an interesting connection through the hedgehog (Hh) pathway whose signaling mechanism is poorly understood. It suggests that vitamin D₃ (or its precursor) keeps the pathway silenced in the absence of the hedgehog ligand. Individuals who suffer from decreased hedgehog signaling have high levels of 7-dehydrocholesterol (provitamin D₃ or 7-DHC which accumulates in Smith-Lemli-Opitz syndrome). 7-DHC inhibits the Hh receptor SMO, and the other Hh receptor PTCH1 normally pumps out vitamin D₃ (or its precursor) from the cell, which then inhibits SMO in cells nearby. When hedgehog comes along and binds to PTCH1, the pump shuts down, and SMO is free to activate the intracellular hedgehog pathway.

Concepts revised: born to run (2)

Physical activity and clustered cardiovascular risk in children: a cross-sectional study (The European Youth Heart Study)

Andersen LB, Harro M, Sardinha LB, Froberg K, Ekelund U, Brage S, Anderssen SA
Department of Sports Medicine, Norwegian School of Sport Sciences, Oslo, Norway
lars.bo.andersen@nih.no
Lancet 2006;368:299–304

Background: Atherosclerosis develops from early childhood; physical activity could positively affect this process. The aim of the study was to assess the associations of objectively measured physical activity with clustering of cardiovascular disease risk factors in children and derive guidelines on the basis of this analysis. *Methods:* Cross-sectional study of 1,732 randomly selected 9- and 15-year-old schoolchildren from Denmark, Estonia, and Portugal. Risk factors included in the composite risk factor score (mean of z scores) were systolic blood pressure, triglyceride, total cholesterol/HDL ratio, insulin resistance, sum of four skinfolds, and aerobic fitness. Individuals with a risk score >1 SD of the composite variable were defined as being at risk. Physical activity was assessed by accelerometry.

Results: Odds ratios for having clustered risk for ascending quintiles of physical activity (counts per min; cpm) were 3 • 29, 3 • 13, 2 • 51, and 2 • 03, respectively, compared with the most active quintile. The first to the third quintile of physical activity had a raised risk in all analyses. The mean time spent >2,000 cpm (equivalent to walking about 4 km/h) in the fourth quintile was 116 min/day in 9-year-old children and 88 min/day in 15-year-old children.

Conclusion: Physical activity levels should be higher than the current international guidelines of at least 1 h/day of physical activity of at least moderate intensity to prevent clustering of cardiovascular disease risk factors.

Objectively measured physical activity and fat mass in a large cohort of children

Ness AR, Leary SD, Mattocks C, Blair SN, Reilly JJ, Wells J, Ingle S, Tilling K, Smith GD, Riddoch C
Departments of Oral and Dental Science and Social Medicine, University of Bristol, UK; Arnold School of Public Health, University of South Carolina, Columbia, S.C., USA, and Division of Developmental Medicine, University of Glasgow; Medical Research Council Childhood Nutrition Research Centre, Institute of Child Health, University College London, and London Sport Institute, Middlesex University, London, UK
PLoS Med 2007;4:e97

Background: Previous studies have been unable to characterize the association between physical activity and obesity, possibly because most relied on inaccurate measures of physical activity and obesity.

Methods: A cross-sectional analysis on 5,500 12-year-old children enrolled in the Avon Longitudinal Study of Parents and Children was carried out. Total physical activity and minutes of moderate and vigorous physical activity were measured using the Actigraph accelerometer. Fat mass and obesity (defined as the top decile of fat mass) were measured using the Lunar Prodigy dual x-ray emission absorptiometry scanner.

Results: There were strong negative associations between moderate and vigorous physical activity and fat mass that were unaltered after adjustment for total physical activity. There was also a strong negative dose-response association between moderate and vigorous physical activity and obesity. The odds ratio for obesity in adjusted models between top and the bottom quintiles of minutes of moderate and vigorous physical activity was 0.03 (p value for trend <0.0001) in boys and 0.36 (p value for trend = 0.006) in girls.

Conclusions: There was a strong graded inverse association between physical activity and obesity that was stronger in boys. The data suggest that higher intensity physical activity may be more important than total activity.

Body weight is related to the balance of two essential components, food intake and energy expenditure, modulated by the genetic background and epigenetic influences. Physical activity is an essential component of energy expenditure and has received less attention than diet as the cause of the obesity epidemic. One of the reasons for this might have been the difficulty in measuring physical activity which was so far mostly based on questionnaires. The use of accelerometers has allowed a relatively precise evaluation of physical activity and its importance is illustrated in these two studies, evaluating the components of fat mass or cardiovascular risks in community-based samples of European children. In the study by Andersen et al., there was a more than 3-fold increased risk of having a cardiovascular risk profile in children with the lowest vs. highest activity. In the Avon Longitudinal Study, the relationship was demonstrated with fat mass, with special effect of moderate and vigorous physical activity. These studies remind us that during the past half century, the drastic change in food intake that occurred in developed countries was associated with a similarly drastic change in daily physical activities. *Homo sapiens* was selected to be the best endurance runner of all mammalians [5]. These new data remind us that we have to pay a tribute to this selection process in the form of regular exercise. From a clinical point of view, it is likely that accelerometers will become a useful tool to evaluate obese patients in the clinical setting.

Awakening from sleep and hypoglycemia in type 1 diabetes mellitus

Gabriely I, Shamoon H
Department of Medicine and Diabetes Research Center, Albert Einstein College of Medicine, Bronx, N.Y., USA
gabriely@aecom.yu.edu
PLoS Med 2007;4:e99

Background: Nocturnal hypoglycemia frequently occurs in patients with type 1 diabetes mellitus. It can be fatal and is believed to promote the development of the hypoglycemia unawareness syndrome. Whether hypoglycemia normally provokes awakening from sleep in individuals who do not have diabetes, and whether this awakening response is impaired in type 1 diabetic patients, is unknown.

Methods: Two groups of 16 type 1 diabetic patients and 16 healthy control participants were tested. They had comparable distributions of gender, age, and body mass index. In one night, a linear fall in plasma glucose to nadir levels of 2.2 mmol/l was induced by infusing insulin over a 1-hour period starting as soon as polysomnographic recordings indicated that stage 2 sleep had been reached. In another night (control), euglycemia was maintained.

Results: Only 1 of the 16 type 1 diabetic patients, as compared to 10 healthy control participants, awakened upon hypoglycemia (p = 0.001). In the control nights, none of the study participants in either of the two groups awakened during the corresponding time. Awakening during hypoglycemia was associated with increased hormonal counterregulation. In all the study participants (from both groups) who woke up, and in 5 of the study participants who did not awaken (3 type 1 diabetic patients and 2 healthy control participants), plasma epinephrine concentration increased with hypoglycemia by at least 100% (p < 0.001). A temporal pattern was revealed such that increases in epinephrine in all participants who awakened started always before polysomnographic signs of wakefulness (7.5 ± 1.6 min).

Conclusions: A fall in plasma glucose to 2.2 mmol/l provokes an awakening response in most healthy control participants, but this response is impaired in type 1 diabetic patients. The counterregulatory increase in plasma epinephrine that we observed to precede awakening suggests that awakening forms part of a central nervous system response launched in parallel with hormonal counterregulation. Failure to awaken increases the risk for type 1 diabetic patients to suffer prolonged and potentially fatal hypoglycemia.

Corticotrophin-releasing factor receptors within the ventromedial hypothalamus regulate hypoglycemia-induced hormonal counterregulation

McCrimmon RJ, Song Z, Cheng H, McNay EC, Weikart-Yeckel C, Fan X, Routh VH, Sherwin RS
Department of Internal Medicine, Yale University School of Medicine, New Haven, Conn., USA
rory.mccrimmon@yale.edu
J Clin Invest 2006;116:1723–1730

Background: Recurrent episodes of hypoglycemia impair sympathoadrenal counterregulatory responses to a subsequent episode of hypoglycemia. For individuals with type 1 diabetes, this markedly increases (by 25-fold) the risk of severe hypoglycemia and is a major limitation to optimal insulin therapy. The mechanisms through which this maladaptive response occurs remain unknown. The corticotrophin-releasing factor (CRF) family of neuropeptides and their receptors (CRFR1 and CRFR2) play a critical role in regulating the neuroendocrine stress response.

Methods: Direct in vivo application to the ventromedial hypothalamus (VMH) of Sprague-Dawley rats, a key glucose-sensing region.

Results: Urocortin I, an endogenous CRFR2 agonist, suppressed (~55–60%), whereas CRF, a predominantly CRFR1 agonist, amplified (~50–70%) counterregulatory responses to hypoglycemia. Urocortin I was shown to directly alter the glucose sensitivity of VMH glucose-sensing neurons in whole cell current clamp recordings in brain slices. The suppressive effect of urocortin I-mediated CRFR2 activation persisted for at least 24 h after in vivo VMH microinjection.

Conclusion: The data suggest that regulation of the CRR is largely determined by the interaction between CRFR2-mediated suppression and CRFR1-mediated activation in the VMH.

Hypoglycemia is one of the main limiting factors to metabolic control in diabetic patients. Several decades of clinical research initiated by Phil Cryer who writes a thoughtful editorial with the *JCI* paper of McCrimmon et al. [6] who have evaluated its clinical importance and mechanisms. In the first study selected this year, diabetic patients submitted to a graded nocturnal hypoglycemia did not wake up, as compared to unaffected controls. This was associated with a decreased epinephrine, norepinephrine, ACTH and cortisol secretion in response to hypoglycemia in diabetic patients and with altered sleep structure during hypoglycemia. The patients had a wide range of HbA1c and the correlation between awakening response and HbA1c was not evaluated but it is likely that the pattern of defective awakening response to hypoglycemia is more pronounced in those with lower HbA1c (and therefore higher risk of previous hypoglycemia). The second paper tackles the same issue from a very different approach and analyses the influence of hypothalamic CRF signaling on counterregulatory hormones' response to hypoglycemia, hypoglycemia, a topic which we discussed previously [7]. CRF signals through two receptors that play important roles not only in the regulation of the corticotropic axis but also in the behavioral response to stress. The two types of receptors have specific ligands and can be manipulated separately and allowed to dissect there respective roles in hypoglycemia. Urocortin I, a CRF type 2 receptor agonist, suppressed the response to hypoglycemia with a persistent action. These observations provide a mechanistic substratum for hypoglycemia-associated autonomic failure in type 1 diabetes, by suggesting that hypoglycemia elicits urocortin I release during antecedent hypoglycemia that could explain a decreased sympathoadrenal response to subsequent hypoglycemia. However, that causal connection was not demonstrated and, therefore, remains a possibility.

Clinical trials. The missing hormone: androgens in hypopituitary women

Effects of testosterone therapy on cardiovascular risk markers in androgen-deficient women with hypopituitarism

Miller KK, Biller BM, Schaub A, Pulaski-Liebert K, Bradwin G, Rifai N, Klibanski A
Neuroendocrine Unit, Massachusetts General Hospital and Department of Laboratory Medicine, Children's Hospital, Harvard Medical School, Boston, Mass., USA
J Clin Endocrinol Metab 2007 [Epub ahead of print]

Background: Hypopituitarism in women is characterized by profound androgen deficiency due to a loss of adrenal and/or ovarian function. The effects of testosterone replacement in this population have not been reported. The objective of the study was to determine whether physiologic testosterone replacement improves bone density, body composition, and/or neurobehavioral function in women with severe androgen deficiency secondary to hypopituitarism.

Methods: This was a 12-month randomized, placebo-controlled study, conducted at a general clinical research center. 51 women of reproductive age with androgen deficiency due to hypopituitarism participated. Physiologic testosterone administration using a patch that delivers 300 µg daily or placebo was administered. Bone density, fat-free mass, and fat mass were measured by dual x-ray absorptiometry. Thigh muscle and abdominal cross-sectional area were measured by computed tomography scan. Mood, sexual function, quality of life, and cognitive function were assessed using self-administered questionnaires.

Results: Mean free testosterone increased into the normal range during testosterone administration. Mean hip (p = 0.023) and radius (p = 0.007), but not posteroanterior spine, bone mineral density increased in the group receiving testosterone, compared with placebo, as did mean fat-free mass (p = 0.040) and thigh muscle area (p = 0.038), but there was no change in fat mass. Mood (p = 0.029) and sexual function (p = 0.044) improved, as did some aspects of quality of life, but not cognitive function. Testosterone at physiologic replacement levels was well tolerated, with few side effects.

Conclusions: This is the first randomized, double-blind, placebo-controlled study to show a positive effect of testosterone on bone density, body composition, and neurobehavioral function in women with severe androgen deficiency due to hypopituitarism.

Clinical endocrinology is based on the principle of exogenously restoring a defective hormonal milieu and all clinical endocrinologists know that this is better said than done. Hypopituitarism is one of the most challenging endocrine disorders due to the multiplicity of interacting hormonal systems that need replacement. Androgen deficiency in women has been associated with decreased bone mass, lean mass and sexual function. This is the first study to address the question in women with hypopituitarism and confirms a positive influence of testosterone on bone, mood, quality of life and sexual function. With a dose of 300 µg daily, the treatment was well tolerated and did not induce androgenic signs. A similar study was published also this year with similar findings using DHEA which is converted to testosterone [8] and an ESPE 2007 abstract suggests a beneficial effect of testosterone in Turner syndrome [9]. These studies performed in adult women raise the question of the replacement of adrenarche and of testosterone secretion during pubertal development in female. Innovative clinical trials with relevant endpoint should be organized to address these questions in adolescents with hypopituitarism. A recent consensus summary suggested that androgen therapy in women remains investigational [10].

New concerns

Growth hormone treatment and risk of second neoplasms in the childhood cancer survivor

Ergun-Longmire B, Mertens AC, Mitby P, Qin J, Heller G, Shi W, Yasui Y, Robison LL, Sklar CA
Department of Pediatrics, Memorial Sloan-Kettering Cancer Center, New York, N.Y., USA
J Clin Endocrinol Metab 2006;91:3494–3498

Background: GH deficiency is common in childhood cancer survivors. In a previous report, although no increase in the risk of disease recurrence in survivors treated with GH was detected, GH-treated survivors did have an increased risk of developing a second neoplasm (rate ratio 3.21).
Methods: In this analysis, the risk of GH-treated survivors developing a second neoplasm after an additional 32 months of follow-up was reassessed. This was a retrospective cohort multicenter study. Among a total of 14,108 survivors who were enrolled in the Childhood Cancer Survivor Study, a retrospective cohort of 5-year survivors of childhood cancer, 361 who were treated with GH were identified. The risk of developing a second neoplasm was assessed.
Results: During the extended follow-up, 5 new second neoplasms developed in survivors treated with GH, for a total of 20 second neoplasms, all solid tumors. Using a time-dependent Cox model, the rate ratio of GH-treated survivors developing a second neoplasm, compared with non-GH-treated survivors, was 2.15 (95% confidence interval, 1.3–3.5; p = 0.002). Meningiomas were the most common second neoplasm (n = 9) among the GH-treated group.
Conclusion: Although cancer survivors treated with GH appear to have an increased risk of developing a second neoplasm compared with survivors not so treated, the elevation of risk due to GH use appears to diminish with increasing length of follow-up. Continued surveillance is essential.

The question of long-term risks of any chronic treatment is always very difficult to address given the fact that small increases of rare adverse events are very difficult to detect. Several reviews have been written on GH treatment and the risk of cancer including the very thoughtful paper by the team of Steve Shalet [11]. Cancer survivors can become GH-deficient as a result of their neoplasm or its treatment raising the question whether GH treatment increases the risk of a second neoplasm in this population. Cancer survivors are a particularly difficult group where to assess this risk, given that, as a group, they are at increased risk of developing a second neoplasm. Large observational databases comprising GH-exposed and non-exposed individuals can help answer this question, although multivariate analysis after adjustment on covariates always raises the question of undetected confounding factors. The very powerful Childhood Cancer Survivor Study comprises ≈14,000 patients of whom 361 had received GH. After adjustment on covariates, a significant 2.1-fold increase of the risk of developing a second neoplasm was detected in GH-treated patients. A second neoplasm occurred in 20/361 GH-treated patients, on average 6.3 ± 4.1 years after initiation of GH treatment. Meningiomas, associated with radiotherapy, were the most common second neoplasm. These worrisome data raise several important points. First they call for an assessment of the risk-benefit balance in this population of patients, who often have severe GH deficiency, with its intrinsic morbidity. Second they put the pediatric endocrinologist in a difficult position where detailed information is needed on a particularly sensitive issue in families who have already gone through the ordeal of oncology treatments. Last, they need to be replicated, to have a more definitive answer on this particularly sensitive issue.

New mechanisms: Gnas regulation unraveled

Identification of an imprinting control region affecting the expression of all transcripts in the Gnas cluster

Williamson CM, Turner MD, Ball ST, Nottingham WT, Glenister P, Fray M, Tymowska-Lalanne Z, Plagge A, Powles-Glover N, Kelsey G, Maconochie M, Peters J
MRC Mammalian Genetics Unit, Harwell, Oxon, UK
Nat Genet 2006;38:350–355

Background: Genomic imprinting results in allele-specific silencing according to parental origin. Silencing is brought about by imprinting control regions that are differentially marked in gametogenesis. The group of imprinted transcripts in the mouse Gnas cluster (Nesp, Nespas, Gnasxl, Exon 1A and Gnas) provides a model for analyzing the mechanisms of imprint regulation. The authors have previously identified an imprinting control region that specifically regulates the tissue-specific imprinted expression of the Gnas gene.

Results: A second imprinting control region at the Gnas cluster is identified here. A paternally derived targeted deletion of the germline differentially methylated region (DMR) associated with the antisense Nespas transcript unexpectedly affects both the expression of all transcripts in the cluster and methylation of two imprinting control regions.

Conclusions: These results establish that the Nespas DMR is the principal imprinting control region at the Gnas cluster and functions bidirectionally as a switch for modulating expression of the antagonistically acting genes Gnasxl and Gnas. Uniquely, the Nespas DMR acts on the downstream imprinting control region at exon 1A to regulate tissue-specific imprinting of the Gnas gene.

The Gnas gene is of interest to pediatric endocrinologists for its involvement in several diseases including pseudohypoparathyroidism type Ia and Ib, acromegaly and McCune-Albright syndrome. Old textbooks clearly had trouble defining the mode of transmission of pseudohypoparathyroidism quoting it as dominant, recessive or sex-linked. Indeed, Mendel had not foreseen imprinting mechanisms and we now know that the Gnas gene is imprinted and that parental origin affects the clinical expression of these diseases. However, the mechanisms behind the differential expression of paternal and maternal alleles of this particularly complex gene are still being worked up. Here, in a mouse model, several lines were created with deletions of promoters within the Gnas gene, associated with point mutations in the Gnas coding sequence, similar to those of pseudohypoparathyroidism type Ia. An imprinting control region is identified that is affects the methylation of other control regions in the gene and the expression of key transcripts from the gene. Deletion of this imprinting control region rescues the phenotype due to a point mutation in the Gnas transcript (a therapeutic approach for pseudohypoparathyroidism type Ia?). Importantly, this imprinting control region behaves in accordance with the parental-conflict theory where it is the interest of paternal genes in the offspring to acquire resources from the mother and the interest of maternal genes to spare these resources. As Gnas transcript $Xl\alpha$ is involved in the postnatal adaptation to breast feeding [12], it is of the 'interest' of the father to promote its expression. Since $Xl\alpha$ and $Gs\alpha$ act antagonistically, it is also of the 'interest' of the father to repress Gnas. Altogether, the complex puzzle of the regulation of the Gnas gene is progressively solved and shows the complexity of gene regulation and its implication in human diseases.

A single IGF1 allele is a major determinant of small size in dogs

Sutter NB, Bustamante CD, Chase K, Gray MM, Zhao K, Zhu L, Padhukasahasram B, Karlins E, Davis S, Jones PG, Quignon P, Johnson GS, Parker HG, Fretwell N, Mosher DS, Lawler DF, Satyaraj E, Nordborg M, Lark KG, Wayne RK, Ostrander EA
National Human Genome Research Institute, Bethesda, Md., USA

Science 2007;316:112–115

The domestic dog exhibits greater diversity in body size than any other terrestrial vertebrate. We used a strategy that exploits the breed structure of dogs to investigate the genetic basis of size. First, through a genome-wide scan, we identified a major quantitative trait locus (QTL) on chromosome 15 influencing size variation within a single breed. Second, we examined genetic variation in the 15-megabase interval surrounding the QTL in small and giant breeds and found marked evidence for a selective sweep spanning a single gene (*IGF1*), encoding insulin-like growth factor 1. A single *IGF1* single-nucleotide polymorphism haplotype is common to all small breeds and nearly absent from giant breeds, suggesting that the same causal sequence variant is a major contributor to body size in all small dogs.

The evolution of dogs is mostly man-made, and the vast majority of dog breeds originate from enforced breeding over the past few hundred years. This resulted in size variation in the domestic dog that is extreme and surpasses that of most other living and extinct species. These authors show that sequence variation in the *IGF-1* gene plays a causal role in dog size: a single allele of the (IGF-1) gene is shared by all small dog breeds that have significantly lower serum levels of IGF-1, but is nearly absent from giant dog breeds, which carry one or both of two distinct haplotypes. This explanation is different from the dogma of phenotypic diversity due to elevated mutation or recombination rates. Rather, intense artificial selection has left a signature in the proximity of IGF-1. The ability to identify a gene contributing to morphology without doing a genetic cross, provides a precedent for future studies aimed at identifying the genetic basis for complex traits in dogs and other species with small populations that have experienced strong artificial or natural selection.

References

1. Liu YZ, Guo YF, Xiao P, Xiong DH, Zhao LJ, Shen H, et al: Epistasis between loci on chromosomes 2 and 6 influences human height. J Clin Endocrinol Metab 2006;91:3821–3825.
2. Kousteni S, Chen JR, Bellido T, Han L, Ali AA, O'Brien CA, et al: Reversal of bone loss in mice by non-genotropic signaling of sex steroids. Science 2002;298:843–846.
3. Hochberg Z, Carel JC: The year in science and medicine; in Carel JC, Hochberg Z (eds): Yearbook of Pediatric Endocrinology 2006. Basel, Karger, 2006, pp 175–192.
4. Tiosano D: Calcium metabolism; in Carel JC, Hochberg Z (eds): Yearbook of Pediatric Endocrinology 2005. Basel, Karger, 2005, pp 63–80.
5. Hochberg Z, Carel JC: The year in science and medicine; in Carel JC, Hochberg Z (eds): Yearbook of Pediatric Endocrinology 2005. Basel, Karger, 2005, pp 175–194.
6. Cryer PE: Mechanisms of sympathoadrenal failure and hypoglycemia in diabetes. J Clin Invest 2006;116:1470–1473.
7. Carel JC, Hochberg Z: Editor's choice; in Carel JC, Hochberg Z (eds): Yearbook of Pediatric Endocrinology 2006. Basel, Karger, 2006, pp 193–206.
8. Brooke AM, Kalingag LA, Miraki-Moud F, Camacho-Hubner C, Maher KT, Walker DM, et al: Dehydroepiandrosterone improves psychological well-being in male and female hypopituitary patients on maintenance growth hormone replacement. J Clin Endocrinol Metab 2006;91:3773–3779.
9. Zuckerman-Levin N, Hochberg Z, et al: Androgen replacement therapy in Turner syndrome. Horm Res 2007; in press.
10. Wierman ME, Basson R, Davis SR, Khosla S, Miller KK, Rosner W, et al: Androgen therapy in women: an Endocrine Society Clinical Practice guideline. J Clin Endocrinol Metab 2006;91:3697–3710.
11. Jenkins PJ, Mukherjee A, Shalet SM: Does growth hormone cause cancer? Clin Endocrinol (Oxf) 2006;64:115–121.
12. Coutant R: Growth and growth factors; in Carel JC, Hochberg Z (eds): Yearbook of Pediatric Endocrinology 2005. Basel, Karger, 2005, pp 33–46.

The Year in Science and Medicine

Ze'ev Hochberg and Jean-Claude Carel

Mechanism of the year: epigenetics; it ain't new, but the progress it has made in the last year is astounding

Genome-wide high-resolution mapping and functional analysis of DNA methylation in *Arabidopsis*

Zhang X, Yazaki J, Sundaresan A, Cokus S, Chan SW, Chen H, Henderson IR, Shinn P, Pellegrini M, Jacobsen SE, Ecker JR
Department of Molecular, Cell and Developmental Biology, University of California, Los Angeles, Calif., USA
http://epigenomics.mcdb.ucla.edu/DNAmeth/
Cell 2006;126:1189–1201

Background: Cytosine methylation is important for transposon silencing and epigenetic regulation of endogenous genes although the extent to which this DNA modification functions to regulate the genome is still unknown.

Methods: Using a tiling microarray with 35 bp resolution, the authors carried out the first comprehensive mapping of DNA methylation in the entire genome of the flowering plant *Arabidopsis thaliana*.

Results: Pericentromeric heterochromatin, repetitive sequences and regions producing small interfering RNAs were heavily methylated. Unexpectedly, over one third of expressed genes contained methylation within transcribed regions, whereas only ~5% of genes contained methylation within promoter regions. Interestingly, genes methylated in transcribed regions were highly expressed and constitutively active, whereas promoter-methylated genes showed a greater degree of tissue-specific expression.

Conclusions: Whole genome tiling array transcriptional profiling of DNA methyltransferase null mutants identified hundreds of genes and intergenic non-coding RNAs with altered expression levels, many of which may be epigenetically controlled by DNA methylation.

The first genome-wide DNA methylation map has been published and provided important insights into how this DNA modification regulates gene expression. It turns out that almost 19% of the *Arabidopsis* genome is methylated. As expected, much of this methylation occurs in heterochromatin, including centromeres, which harbors transposons and repetitive elements, but a considerable amount of methylation is also found in euchromatin. Unsurprisingly, the highest levels are seen in pseudogenes and unexpressed genes, but around 5% of expressed genes have methylated promoters and 33% are methylated within a transcribed region (the body-methylated genes). A comparison of DNA methylation sites with microarray expression data from a number of tissues and conditions revealed that body-methylated genes are more highly expressed than unmethylated genes, with promoter-methylated genes showing the lowest levels of expression. Promoter-methylated genes tend to be expressed in a tissue-specific manner, whereas body-methylated genes tend to be constitutively expressed. The stage is set for other methylome analyses.

RNA-mediated non-Mendelian inheritance of an epigenetic change in the mouse

Rassoulzadegan M, Grandjean V, Gounon P, Vincent S, Gillot I, Cuzin F
INSERM, U636, Nice, France
minoo@unice.fr
Nature 2006;441:469–474

Background: Paramutation is a heritable epigenetic modification induced in plants by cross-talk between allelic loci.

Results: The authors found a similar modification of the mouse *Kit* gene in the progeny of heterozygotes with the null mutant Kit[tm1Alf] (a *lacZ* insertion). In spite of a homozygous wild-type genotype, their off-spring maintain, to a variable extent, the white spots characteristic of *Kit* mutant animals. Efficiently inherited from either male or female parents, the modified phenotype results from a decrease in *Kit* messenger RNA levels with the accumulation of non-polyadenylated RNA molecules of abnormal sizes. Sustained transcriptional activity at the postmeiotic stages – at which time the gene is normally silent – leads to the accumulation of RNA in spermatozoa. Microinjection into fertilized eggs either of total RNA from *Kit[tm1Alf/+]* heterozygotes or of *Kit*-specific microRNAs induced a heritable white tail phenotype.
Conclusions: This paper identifies an unexpected mode of epigenetic inheritance associated with the zygotic transfer of RNA molecules.

Paramutation, which was described 50 years ago, is inconsistent with Mendelian laws: an allele interacts with its homologue and somehow instigates a heritable change. In this era of epigenetics we aren't shocked any more [1]. But there is now evidence that one instance of paramutation in mice is mediated by RNA; a mutant RNA transcript seems to alter the expression of the wild-type allele and transmits the modified phenotype to future generations of offspring. The mouse proto-oncogene Kit encodes a transmembrane tyrosine kinase, with a strong structural homology to the colony-stimulating factor-1 receptor and the platelet-derived growth factor receptor. Kit mutations in the mouse produce spots of white fur on otherwise dark-colored mice, sterility, and anemia, attributable to failure of stem cell populations to migrate and proliferate effectively during development. The null allele of Kit that gives rise this phenotype (*Kit[tm1Alf]*) is dominant; however, most offspring of a Kit heterozygous mouse and a WT one had white spots, even when they carried two copies of the WT Kit allele. The explanation for this unusual inheritance was suggested by the fact that the WT Kit allele produces many oddly sized RNA transcripts. When RNA from Kit mutant cells was injected into wild-type fertilized eggs, mice developed white spots. The involvement of microRNAs in all this seems likely given their recognized association with paramutation and other epigenetic phenomena: the regulatory RNAs might degrade the normal Kit message, or modify the WT allele itself. The fitness benefits of an RNA-based inheritance system are easy to imagine: any advantage that a mutated allele conferred in one generation could be passed on to offspring, without the need to rely on mutation and selection to increase the representation of the fitter allele. If that sounds to you like Lamarckism inheritance of acquired traits, you may be right.

Fine-tune a flower power

Variation in the epigenetic silencing of FLC contributes to natural variation in *Arabidopsis* vernalization response

Shindo C, Lister C, Crevillen P, Nordborg M, Dean C
Cell and Developmental Biology, John Innes Centre, Norwich, UK
Genes Dev 2006;20:3079–3083

Background: Vernalization, the cold-induced acceleration of flowering, involves the epigenetic silencing of the floral repressor gene *flowering locus c* (FLC).
Methods: This group investigated the molecular basis for variation in vernalization in *Arabidopsis* natural accessions adapted to different climates.
Results: A major variable was the degree to which different periods of cold caused stable FLC silencing. In accessions requiring long vernalization, FLC expression was reactivated following non-saturating vernalization, but this reactivation was progressively attenuated with increasing cold exposure. This response was correlated with the rate of accumulation of FLC histone H3 Lys 27 trimethylation (H3K27me3).
Conclusions: Variation in epigenetic silencing of FLC appears to have contributed to *Arabidopsis* adaptation.

Plant scientists introduced epigenetics and still teach us a lesson: epigenetic silencing controls variation in flowering time – a key adaptive trait. Like many other plants, *Arabidopsis thaliana* (thale cress, or mouse-ear cress, a small flowering plant related to cabbage and mustard) need to be exposed to a period of cold before they can flower – a response called vernalization. Growing in a wide range of environments, they show considerable differences in flowering times and vernalization responses. Initially thought to be genetic, this paper shows that there was no correlation between RNA levels of specific markers and the length of exposure to the cold. Rather, cold period quantitatively enhanced the stability of gene repression by differential accumulation of histone methylation. They propose that vernalization occurs in three phases: an insensitive phase is followed by a phase in which silencing occurs; when the levels of histone modification are sufficient, the third phase begins, in which the gene is fully silenced. The time taken to accumulate sufficient histone methylation levels determines the speed of the response to vernalization. Children respond to the environment in many ways, and for pediatric endocrinologists the secular trend of growth and puberty is an obvious analogue to vernalization. Epigenetics is here to stay and we will not be surprised when it eventually explains the secular trend.

Gene body-specific methylation on the active X chromosome

Hellman A, Chess A
Center for Human Genetic Research and Department of Medicine, Massachusetts General Hospital, Harvard Medical School, Boston, Mass., USA
hellman@chgr.mgh.harvard.edu
Science 2007;315:1141–1143

Background: Differential DNA methylation is important for the epigenetic regulation of gene expression. Allele-specific methylation of the inactive X chromosome has been demonstrated at promoter CpG islands, but the overall pattern of methylation on the active X (Xa) and inactive X (Xi) chromosomes is unknown.
Methods: An allele-specific analysis of more than 1,000 informative loci along the human X chromosome was performed.
Results: The Xa displays more than two times as much allele-specific methylation as Xi. This methylation is concentrated at gene bodies, affecting multiple neighboring CpGs. Before X inactivation, all of these Xa gene body-methylated sites are biallelically methylated. Thus, a bipartite methylation-demethylation program results in Xa-specific hypomethylation at gene promoters and hypermethylation at gene bodies.
Conclusion: These results suggest a relationship between global methylation and expression potentiality.

If you thought that methylation silences genes, this paper used a genome-wide analysis of DNA methylation to show, surprisingly, that the transcribed regions of genes on the active human X chromosome (Xa) are hypermethylated, both in females and males. Equivalent regions on the Xi are hypomethylated. Prior to X inactivation, both X chromosomes are methylated, which suggests that methylation was lost. Paramutations were reported more than 50 years ago. They may be the oldest form of epigenetics, but they are probably not the most common; we are now almost friendly with imprinting. See the next article.

An RNA gene expressed during cortical development evolved rapidly in humans

Pollard KS, Salama SR, Lambert N, Lambot MA, Coppens S, Pedersen JS, Katzman S, King B, Onodera C, Siepel A, Kern AD, Dehay C, Igel H, Ares M Jr, Vanderhaeghen P, Haussler D
Center for Biomolecular Science and Engineering, Department of Molecular, Cell and Developmental Biology, University of California, Santa Cruz, Calif., USA
Nature 2006;443:167–172

Background: The developmental and evolutionary mechanisms behind the emergence of human-specific brain features remain largely unknown. However, the recent ability to compare our genome to that of our closest relative, the chimpanzee, provides new avenues to link genetic and phenotypic changes in the evolution of the human brain.
Methods: A ranking of regions in the human genome that show significant evolutionary acceleration was devised.

Results: The most dramatic of these 'human accelerated regions', HAR1, is part of a novel RNA gene (*HAR1F*) that is expressed specifically in Cajal-Retzius neurons in the developing human neocortex from 7 to 19 gestational weeks, a crucial period for cortical neuron specification and migration. *HAR1F* is co-expressed with reelin, a product of Cajal-Retzius neurons that is of fundamental importance in specifying the six-layer structure of the human cortex.

Conclusions: HAR1 and the other human accelerated regions provide new candidates in the search for uniquely human biology.

The brains of humans and chimpanzees are anatomically not so different, except in scale. About 2 million years ago, the hominin brain began to enlarge until, in modern times, it has become about three times larger than that of chimpanzees, contributing to the cognitive differences between the two species. This is followed now by a study of the speed at which various human genome regions have changed in recent times, and 49 Highly Accelerated Regions include the HAR1-HAR49. HAR1 is part of an RNA gene that is expressed in the embryonic neocortex, associated with higher cognitive functions, and influences the migration of neurons. It has accrued 18 changes in sequence in this time, when only one or no substitutions would be expected to occur by chance. Interestingly, all but two of the most-accelerated regions lie outside protein-coding sequences – in the enigmatic 'dark matter' of the human genome (*Yearbook 2006*). HAR1F is also expressed in the ovary and testis of adult humans; indeed, sexual selection of genes expressed in these tissues has often driven unusual sequence changes. Rapid human-specific evolution, and particularly the evolution of behavioral traits, may thus be associated more with epigenetic fine-tuning of gene expression than with altering the molecular functions of their encoded proteins.

Central role of p53 in the suntan response and pathologic hyperpigmentation

Cui R, Widlund HR, Feige E, Lin JY, Wilensky DL, Igras VE, D'Orazio J, Fung CY, Schanbacher CF, Granter SR, Fisher DE
Melanoma Program in Medical Oncology, Dana-Farber Cancer Institute, Harvard Medical School, Boston, Mass., USA
Cell 2007;128:853–864

Background: UV-induced pigmentation (suntanning) requires induction of α-melanocyte-stimulating hormone (α-MSH) secretion by keratinocytes. α-MSH and other bioactive peptides are cleavage products of pro-opiomelanocortin (POMC).

Results: The authors provide biochemical and genetic evidence demonstrating that UV induction of POMC/MSH in skin is directly controlled by p53. Whereas p53 potently stimulates the POMC promoter in response to UV, the absence of p53, as in knockout mice, is associated with absence of the UV-tanning response. The same pathway produces β-endorphin, another POMC derivative, which potentially contributes to sun-seeking behaviors. Furthermore, several instances of UV-independent pathologic pigmentation are shown to involve p53 'mimicking' the tanning response. p53 thus functions as a sensor/effector for UV pigmentation, which is a nearly constant environmental exposure. Moreover, this pathway is activated in numerous conditions of pathologic pigmentation and thus mimics the tanning response.

Pigmentation of the skin results from the synthesis of melanin in the melanocyte, followed by distribution and transport of pigment granules to neighboring keratinocytes. Melanin is crucial for absorption of free radicals that have been generated within the cytoplasm by UV, and it acts as a direct shield protecting the DNA from UV and visible light radiation. It also prevents UV from its target vitamin D photosynthesis, and hence black-skin children are prone to develop rickets. This paper shows that the tumor suppressor gene p53, which ensures that DNA damage is detected early on and is mutated in 50% of human cancers, plays an important role in melanin generation, and that p53 absence ablates the tanning response, which endocrinologists call hyperpigmentation. UV light activates p53 in skin keratinocyte, which among others activates POMC, α-MSH and ACTH expression in the keratinocyte, which might involve primarily local paracrine, or perhaps autocrine, effects within the epidermis. The authors suggest that one of POMC end-products β-endorphin might contribute to sun-seeking behavior. We can at the time only speculate that multiple instances of clinical hyperpigmentation may arise due to such p53-mediated mimicking of the UV-pigmentation pathway. Previous dogma claimed that the entire spectrum of skin color is caused by polymorphism of the

MC4R to provide selective advantages at distinct latitudes based upon regulation of the UV-induced pigmentation response. It is possible that polymorphisms in p53 or p53-related pathways may also play a role.

Of drivers and passengers in a cancer cell

Patterns of somatic mutation in human cancer genomes

Greenman C, Stephens P, Smith R, Dalgliesh GL, Hunter C, Bignell G, Davies H, Teague J, Butler A, Stevens C, Edkins S, O'Meara S, Vastrik I, Schmidt EE, Avis T, Barthorpe S, Bhamra G, Buck G, Choudhury B, Clements J, Cole J, Dicks E, Forbes S, Gray K, Halliday K, Harrison R, Hills K, Hinton J, Jenkinson A, Jones D, Menzies A, Mironenko T, Perry J, Raine K, Richardson D, Shepherd R, Small A, Tofts C, Varian J, Webb T, West S, Widaa S, Yates A, Cahill DP, Louis DN, Goldstraw P, Nicholson AG, Brasseur F, Looijenga L, Weber BL, Chiew YE, DeFazio A, Greaves MF, Green AR, Campbell P, Birney E, Easton DF, Chenevix-Trench G, Tan MH, Khoo SK, Teh BT, Yuen ST, Leung SY, Wooster R, Futreal PA, Stratton MR
Cancer Genome Project, Wellcome Trust Sanger Institute, Wellcome Trust Genome Campus, Hinxton, Cambridge, UK
Nature 2007;446:153–158

Context: Cancers arise owing to mutations in a subset of genes that confer growth advantage. The availability of the human genome sequence led the authors to propose that systematic resequencing of cancer genomes for mutations would lead to the discovery of many additional cancer genes.

Results: More than 1,000 somatic mutations found in 274 Mb of DNA corresponding to the coding exons of 518 protein kinase genes in 210 diverse human cancers are reported. There was substantial variation in the number and pattern of mutations in individual cancers reflecting different exposures, DNA repair defects and cellular origins. Most somatic mutations are likely to be 'passengers' that do not contribute to oncogenesis. However, there was evidence for 'driver' mutations contributing to the development of the cancers studied in approximately 120 genes.

Conclusions: Systematic sequencing of cancer genomes therefore reveals the evolutionary diversity of cancers and implicates a larger repertoire of cancer genes than previously anticipated.

The Human Cancer Genome Project starts to provide us with important data. This paper reports mutations in the genes encoding all 518 protein kinases in 210 cancers, identifying 1,000 mutations, most of them novel. Mutations were relatively common in cancers of the lung, stomach, ovary, colon and kidney, and rare in cancers of the testis and breast, and in carcinoid tumors. Cancer provides an amazing evolutionary laboratory; by the time it is diagnosed, it comprises billions of cells carrying the DNA abnormalities that initiated malignant proliferation, but also many additional genetic lesions acquired along the way. Some of these secondary mutations emerge owing to selective pressure during tumorigenesis (drivers); others may be incidental (passengers), resulting from mutational exposures, genome instability or simply the large number of cell doublings that leads from a single transformed cell to a clinically detectable cancer. Using a statistical model, 158 predicted driver mutations were identified in 120 kinase genes. It is likely that the full range of somatic mutation patterns will not be apparent until thousands of cancer samples have been sequenced, each one yielding several dozen mutations each. For some cancers this may require sequencing of hundreds of megabases. This information will ultimately provide new opportunities for molecular diagnosis and therapeutics.

Sequencing and analysis of Neanderthal genomic DNA

Noonan JP, Coop G, Kudaravalli S, Smith D, Krause J, Alessi J, Chen F, Platt D, Paabo S, Pritchard JK, Rubin EM
US Department of Energy Joint Genome Institute, Walnut Creek, Calif., USA
Science 2006;314:1113–1118

Background: Our knowledge of Neanderthals is based on a limited number of remains and artifacts from which we must make inferences about their biology, behavior, and relationship to ourselves.
Results: The authors describe the characterization of these extinct hominids from a new perspective, based on the development of a Neanderthal metagenomic library and its high-throughput sequencing and analysis. Several lines of evidence indicate that the 65,250 base pairs of hominid sequence so far identified in the library are of Neanderthal origin, the strongest being the ascertainment of sequence identities between Neanderthal and chimpanzee at sites where the human genomic sequence is different. These results enabled to calculate the human-Neanderthal divergence time based on multiple randomly distributed autosomal loci. These analyses suggest that on average the Neanderthal genomic sequence obtained and the reference human genome sequence share a most recent common ancestor approximately 706,000 years ago, and that the human and Neanderthal ancestral populations split approximately 370,000 years ago, before the emergence of anatomically modern humans. The finding that the Neanderthal and human genomes are at least 99.5% identical led to develop and successfully implement a targeted method for recovering specific ancient DNA sequences from metagenomic libraries.
Conclusion: This initial analysis of the Neanderthal genome advances our understanding of the evolutionary relationship of *Homo sapiens* and *Homo neanderthalensis* and signifies the dawn of Neanderthal genomics.

Modern humans and Neanderthals overlapped in Europe and West Asia for at least a few thousand years, and perhaps up to 10,000 years as of ~35,000 years ago; some researchers continue to argue that the two species interbred. We now get a genomic support for the view that Neanderthals are a separate branch of the hominid family tree that diverged from our own ancestors some 450,000 years ago or more. Ancient DNA is problematic, and the divergence between living people and Neanderthals is so small compared to the DNA damage and the sequencing error that it's still hard to be confident of any results. Comparing the new sequences to the modern human genome and to the chimpanzee genome and tallied the sequence differences between each pair of species, the two humans are signposts to changes that were key to their individual evolution. Eventually those changes could lead researchers to the genetic basis of *Homo sapiens* speciation. As expected, the Neanderthal and human genomes proved more than 99.5% identical, 27 bases varied between modern humans and Neanderthals, indicating sites where evolution occurred after the two species diverged. They conclude that the most recent common ancestor of the two human species lived 468,000 to 1 million years ago. As to the question of admixture, there were no sites where the Neanderthal possessed a rare SN found only in Europeans, which one would expect had interbreeding occurred. In parallel, a Leipzig group identified a 38,000-year-old Neanderthal fossil that was exceptionally free of contamination from modern human DNA [2]. Comparing with the human and chimpanzee genomes, they suggest that modern human and Neanderthal DNA sequences diverged on average about 500,000 years ago, even though evidence still suggests that modern human males might have invaded the Neanderthal gene pool by sometimes fathering children with Neanderthal females, but not necessarily vice versa. Because the extinct Neanderthals are our closest relatives, comparing their DNA to ours may one day reveal the mutations that set *Homo sapiens* apart from all other species, as well as the timing of key evolutionary changes.

Comparative genome sequencing of *Escherichia coli* allows observation of bacterial evolution on a laboratory timescale

Herring CD, Raghunathan A, Honisch C, Patel T, Applebee MK, Joyce AR, Albert TJ, Blattner FR, van den Boom D, Cantor CR, Palsson BO
Department of Bioengineering, University of California, San Diego, Calif., USA
Nat Genet 2006;38:1406–1412

Methods: Whole-genome resequencing of *Escherichia coli* was used to monitor the acquisition and fixation of mutations that conveyed a selective growth advantage during adaptation to a glycerol-based growth medium.
Results: Thirteen different de novo mutations in five different *E. coli* strains were identified and their fixation was monitored over a 44-day period of adaptation. The observed spontaneous mutations were responsible for improved fitness by creating single, double and triple site-directed mutants that had growth rates matching those of the evolved strains.
Conclusions: The success of this new genome-scale approach indicates that real-time evolution studies will now be practical in a wide variety of contexts.

Paleontologists look at the fossil record to study how evolution of dinosaurs and other animals occurred over millions of years, but in the case of the *E. coli*, new technology provides the ability to observe evolution as it is occurring over a matter of days. Using comparative genome sequencing technology, they grew *E. coli* in an environment that favored the emergence of mutants: the organism was fed glycerol, a poorly metabolized carbon and energy source. After 6 days of growth, mutations appeared in the glycerol kinase gene, which initiates the process of metabolizing glycerol. Cells with mutations grew 20–60% faster. Surprisingly, mutations also appeared in a second, unrelated gene for RNA polymerase, and these bacteria grew 150% faster than the starting strain. All the mutants arose in the experiments presumably as the result of naturally occurring errors in copying DNA into daughter cells during cell division. 'Experimental evolution' may refine the theory of evolution and the related process of natural selection of individuals with traits that convey a selective survival advantage. It may also be used as a tool for discovery and analysis, and could even be used to design bacteria to do useful jobs. A month later, and a second team developed a model for experimental evolution on a chip 'fitness landscape' [3]. They made a row of microscopic chambers on a silicon chip in which *E. coli* may grow. The bacteria can move between the chambers along narrow corridors. Adjusting the nutrient supply to each of these patches creates gradients in habitability, representing a fitness landscape that can be made arbitrarily 'smooth' or 'rugged'.

Designed to kill

The second most prestigious scientific prize, the *Albert Lasker Award for Basic Medical Research*, was shared in 2006 by Elizabeth H. Blackburn, Carol W. Greider and Jack W. Szostak 'for the prediction and discovery of telomerase, a remarkable RNA-containing enzyme that synthesizes the ends of chromosomes, protecting them and maintaining the integrity of the genome'.
Telomeres and telomerase are critical regulators of genomic stability and replicative lifespan in mammalian cells. Here is a shortlist of where to expect the utilization of telomeres and telomerase in pediatric endocrinology? Growth plate senescence and fusion: in vitro studies showed that chronic oxidative stress caused by repeated exposure to peroxide, or superphysiologic oxygen tension caused growth plate chondrocytes to senesce prematurely and before extensive telomere erosion occurred [4]. The presence of telomerase activity within primary endocrine tumors was shown to indicate a malignant tumor and might suggest the need for an attentive search for concomitant metastases. Quantification of human telomerase reverse transcriptase protein subunit mRNA could be used in clinical practice to exclude malignancy in most endocrine tumors [5]. Telomerase may soon become a drug and drug target for the treatment of thyroid cancer.

Transforming the architecture of compound eyes

Zelhof AC, Hardy RW, Becker A, Zuker CS
Howard Hughes Medical Institute and Department of Neurobiology, University of California at San Diego,
La Jolla, Calif., USA
charles@flyeye.ucsd.edu
Nature 2006;443:696–699

Background: Eyes differ markedly in the animal kingdom, and are an extreme example of the evolution of multiple anatomical solutions to light detection and image formation. A salient feature of all photoreceptor cells is the presence of a specialized compartment (disc outer segments in vertebrates, and microvillar rhabdomeres in insects), whose primary role is to accommodate the millions of light receptor molecules required for efficient photon collection. In insects, compound eyes can have very different inner architectures. Fruitflies and houseflies have an open rhabdom system, in which the seven rhabdomeres of each ommatidium are separated from each other and function as independent light guides. In contrast, bees and various mosquitoes and beetle species have a closed system, in which rhabdomeres within each ommatidium are fused to each other, thus sharing the same visual axis.

Methods: To understand the transition between open and closed rhabdom systems, the role of *Drosophila* genes involved in rhabdomere assembly were isolated and characterized.

Results: Spacemaker, a secreted protein expressed only in the eyes of insects with open rhabdom systems, acts together with prominin and the cell adhesion molecule chaoptin to choreograph the partitioning of rhabdomeres into an open system. Furthermore, the complete loss of spacemaker converts an open rhabdom system to a closed one, whereas its targeted expression to photoreceptors of a closed system markedly reorganizes the architecture of the compound eyes to resemble an open system.

Conclusions: These results provide a molecular atlas for the construction of microvillar assemblies and illustrate the critical effect of differences in a single structural protein in morphogenesis.

When evolution skeptics want to attack Darwin's theory, they often point to the human eye. How could something so complex, they argue, have developed through random mutations and natural selection, even over millions of years? If evolution occurs through gradations, how could it have created the separate parts of the eye – the lens, the retina, the pupil, and so forth – since none of these structures by themselves would make vision possible? Darwin acknowledged from the start that the eye would be a difficult case for his new theory to explain. Building on this enigma, Richard Dawkins' *The Blind Watchmaker* has been acclaimed as the most influential work on evolution written in the last hundred years, and is highly recommended and enjoyable reading. It is not often that we get such a clear glimpse of the blind watchmaker at work as in this article. We learn that contemporary flies see better than their ancestors. Those ancestral flies that did not see well contributed more to the evolution of frogs than to the fly lineage. Zelhof et al. reveal how flies improved the resolution of their eyes by evolving a specific modification to how their photoreceptor cells stick together. You may be interested to know that the mechanism utilized in insect vision has very little to do with the mechanism we operate.

Organization of interphase microtubules in fission yeast analyzed by electron tomography

Hoog JL, Schwartz C, Noon AT, O'Toole ET, Mastronarde DN, McIntosh JR, Antony C
European Molecular Biology Laboratory, Cell Biology and Biophysics Program, Heidelberg, Germany
Dev Cell 2007;12:349–361

Background: Polarized cells, such as neuronal, epithelial, and fungal cells, all display a specialized organization of their microtubules. The interphase microtubule cytoskeleton of the rod-shaped fission yeast, *Schizosaccharomyces pombe*, has been extensively described by fluorescence microscopy.

Methods: A large-scale, electron tomography investigation of *S. pombe* is described, including a 3D reconstruction of a complete eukaryotic cell volume at sufficient resolution to show both how many microtubules there are in a bundle and their detailed architecture.

Results: Most cytoplasmic microtubules are open at one end and capped at the other, providing evidence about their polarity. Electron-dense bridges between the microtubules themselves and between microtubules and the nuclear envelope were frequently observed. Finally, we have investigated structure/function relationships between microtubules and both mitochondria and vesicles.

Conclusions: Our analysis shows that electron tomography of well-preserved cells is ideally suited for describing fine ultrastructural details that were not visible with previous techniques.

In your future teaching, you will probably use these high-resolution, three-dimensional images of a cell developed this year by electron tomography. They scanned 250-nm-thick slices of frozen budding yeast, and assembled the scans into a computer-generated three-dimensional image. Save the spectacular photos. For more on far-field fluorescence microscopy with a focal-plane resolution of 15–20 nm in biological samples, see Donnert et al. [6].

Three boat lengths to the line

Increased App expression in a mouse model of Down's syndrome disrupts NGF transport and causes cholinergic neuron degeneration

Salehi A, Delcroix JD, Belichenko PV, Zhan K, Wu C, Valletta JS, Takimoto-Kimura R, Kleschevnikov AM, Sambamurti K, Chung PP, Xia W, Villar A, Campbell WA, Kulnane LS, Nixon RA, Lamb BT, Epstein CJ, Stokin GB, Goldstein LS, Mobley WC
Department of Neurology and Neurological Sciences, Stanford University, Stanford, Calif., USA
asalehi@stanford.edu
Neuron 2006;51:29–42

Background: Degeneration of basal forebrain cholinergic neurons (BFCNs) contributes to cognitive dysfunction in Alzheimer's disease and Down's syndrome.

Methods: This paper used Ts65Dn and Ts1Cje mouse models of Down's syndrome.

Results: The increased dose of the amyloid precursor protein gene, App, acts to markedly decrease NGF retrograde transport and cause degeneration of BFCNs. NGF transport was also decreased in mice expressing wild-type human APP or a familial Alzheimer-linked mutant APP; while significant, the decreases were less marked and there was no evident degeneration of BFCNs. Because of evidence suggesting that the NGF transport defect was intra-axonal, they explored within cholinergic axons the status of early endosomes. NGF-containing early endosomes were enlarged in Ts65Dn mice and their App content was increased.

Conclusion: This study provides evidence for a pathogenic mechanism for Down's syndrome in which increased expression of App, in the context of trisomy, causes abnormal transport of NGF and cholinergic neurodegeneration.

Intensive efforts over the last 3 years may finally lead to understanding of the enigma how a triple dose of chromosome 21 leads to the mental retardation of Down's syndrome. The neurotrophin, nerve growth factor (NGF), needs to be transported from the axon terminal to the neuronal cell body in order to promote cell survival. Following the development of an animal model of Down syndrome (*Yearbook 2006*), this paper shows that the retrograde transport of NGF malfunctions in a mouse model of Down syndrome results in neuronal death. The factor responsible for this deficit in NGF transport is amyloid precursor protein (APP), which is encoded by one of the genes triplicated in Down syndrome. A second article in the same journal [7] reports defects in the neurotrophin BDNF (brain-derived neurotrophic factor), which may prevent BDNF from driving neuronal survival in the cortex and hippocampus. Downregulation of the truncated BDNF receptor in the Down syndrome model restores BDNF signaling and reverses neuronal loss. Mechanisms provide promises for therapy; restoration of the neurotrophin signaling in the brain may be a promising therapeutic approach in

Down syndrome. From a pediatric endocrine angle, the abnormal thyroid functions seem to be an inherent feature of the trisomy rather than a problem in a subset of patients [8].

Fair trade-offs

Costs of encephalization: the energy trade-off hypothesis tested on birds

Isler K, van Schaik C
Anthropologisches Institut und Museum, Universität Zürich Irchel, Zürich, Switzerland
kisler@aim.unizh.ch
J Hum Evol 2006;51:228–243

Background: Costs and benefits of encephalization are a major topic of debate in the study of primate and human evolution. Comparative studies provide an opportunity to test the validity of a hypothesis as a general principle, rather than it being a special case in primate or hominid evolution. If a population evolves a larger brain, the metabolic costs of doing so must be paid for by either an increased energy turnover (direct metabolic constraint) or by a trade-off with other energetically expensive costs of body maintenance, locomotion, or reproduction, here referred to as the energy trade-off hypothesis, an extension of the influential *Expensive Tissue Hypothesis* of Aiello and Wheeler [Curr Anthropol 1995;36:199–221].

Methods: The authors tested these hypotheses on birds using raw species values, family means, and independent contrasts analysis to account for phylogenetic influences. First, we tested whether basal metabolic rates are correlated with brain mass or any other variable of interest.

Results: This not being the case, we examined various trade-offs between brain mass and the mass of other expensive tissues such as gut mass, which is approximated by gut length or diet quality. Only weak support was found for this original *Expensive Tissue Hypothesis* in birds. However, other energy allocations such as locomotor mode and reproductive strategy may also be reduced to shunt energy to an enlarged brain. There was a significantly negative correlation between brain mass and pectoral muscle mass, which averages 18% of body mass in birds and is indicative of their relative costs of flight. Reproductive costs, on the other hand, are positively correlated with brain mass in birds. An increase in brain mass may allow birds to devote more energy to reproduction, although not through an increase in their own energy budget as in mammals, but through direct provisioning of their offspring.

Conclusions: The trade-off between locomotor costs and brain mass in birds lets the authors conclude that an analogous effect could have played a role in the evolution of a larger brain in human evolution.

Ever since Darwin, anthropologists have been intrigued by the dramatic contrast in relative brain size between humans and our great ape relatives. As it goes for evolutionary theory, the costs of an enlarged brain, as ultimately only net benefit, i.e., benefits minus costs, will determine the selective advantage of a trait. The 1980s hypothesis that stressed the energetic costs of increased brain size rather than its adaptive benefits was the direct metabolic constraints hypothesis. A direct link between basal metabolic rate and brain size was postulated based on a similarity of scaling exponents of these parameters to body size. In the 1990s it was the dietary shift toward meat eating in hominins, which is likely to have occurred roughly at the same time as the major enlargement in brain size. As proposed by the *Expensive Tissue Hypothesis,* an animal is able to meet the high metabolic cost of a large brain without incurring a compensatory increase in basal metabolic rate by decreasing the amount of other metabolically expensive tissues (i.e., heart, lung, kidney, liver, and gastrointestinal tract). We now learn of a significantly negative correlation between brain mass and pectoral muscle mass, which averages 18% of body mass in birds and is indicative of their relative costs of flight. This is birds, but the trade-off between locomotor costs and brain mass suggests that an analogous effect could have played a role in the evolution of a larger brain in human evolution.

Compensatory growth impairs adult cognitive performance

Fisher MO, Nager RG, Monaghan P
Division of Environmental Evolutionary Biology, Institute of Biomedical and Life Sciences, University of Glasgow, Glasgow, UK
PLoS Biol 2006;4:e251

Background: Several studies have demonstrated that poor early nutrition, followed by growth compensation, can have negative consequences later in life. However, it remains unclear whether this is attributable to the nutritional deficit itself or a cost of compensatory growth. This distinction is important to understand both of the proximate and ultimate factors that shape growth trajectories and of how best to manage growth in humans and other species following low birth weight.

Methods: Sibling pairs of zebra finches were reared on different quality nutrition for the first 20 days of life only and their learning performance examined in adulthood.

Results: Final body size was not affected. However, the speed of learning a simple task in adulthood, which involved associating a screen color with the presence of a food reward, was negatively related to the amount of growth compensation that had occurred. Learning speed was not related to the early diet itself or the amount of early growth depression.

Conclusions: The results show that the level of compensatory growth that occurs following a period of poor nutrition is associated with long-term negative consequences for cognitive function and suggest that a growth-performance trade-off may determine optimal growth trajectories.

Although we are all familiar with the concept of catch-up growth, we have to realize that its mechanisms and regulators are poorly understood. The recognition that a growing organism can transiently grow much more rapidly to catch-up implies that the mean growth of a population is not maximized but selected by evolution as a trade-off between too fast and too slow. We knew of the negative role of early catch-up on subsequent cardiovascular risk. We also knew that poor development in early life affected subsequent intelligence. This paper addresses the influence of catch-up itself on cognitive performances in birds. Pairs of birds received either a normal diet or a deficient diet during the 20 days after hatching, resulting in a mean weight deficit of 14%. By day 70, all birds were fully grown and the deficient ones had caught up vs. their normally fed pairs. The influence of the marked individual variability of catch-down and catch-up growth on adult cognition was analyzed. There was no influence of the rate of catch-down, but a marked influence of catch-up growth with the animals growing more rapidly performing more poorly in adulthood. This suggests that the prioritization of central nervous system during development is variable between individuals. Some individuals might commit more energy into somatic growth, therefore compromising central nervous system development further. The mechanisms involved are unknown but could involve behavioral, endocrine or neurological changes. Although this is an experimental study in birds that does not apply to humans, it would be interesting to revisit the studies linking birth weight and cognition in the light of these findings. These data suggest that rapid catch-up might not be the best option in the long term.

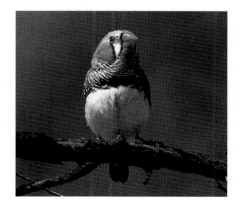

Lipoprotein genotype and conserved pathway for exceptional longevity in humans

Atzmon G, Rincon M, Schechter CB, Shuldiner AR, Lipton RB, Bergman A, Barzilai N
Institute for Aging Research, Albert Einstein College of Medicine, Bronx, New York, N.Y., USA
PLoS Biol 2006;4:e113

Background: Alteration of single genes involved in nutrient and lipoprotein metabolism increases longevity in several animal models. Because exceptional longevity in humans is familial, it is likely that polymorphisms in genes favorably influence certain phenotypes and increase the likelihood of exceptional longevity.

Methods: A group of Ashkenazi Jewish centenarians (n = 213), their offspring (n = 216), and an age-matched Ashkenazi control group (n = 258) were genotyped for 66 polymorphisms in 36 candidate genes related to cardiovascular disease. These genes were tested for association with serum lipoprotein levels and particle sizes, apolipoprotein A1, B, and C-3 levels and with outcomes of hypertension, insulin resistance, and mortality.

Results: The prevalence of homozygosity for the 641C allele in the APOC3 promoter (rs2542052) was higher in centenarians (25%) and their offspring (20%) than in controls (10%) (p = 0.0001 and p = 0.001, respectively). This genotype was associated with significantly lower serum levels of APOC3 and a favorable pattern of lipoprotein levels and sizes. There was a lower prevalence of hypertension and greater insulin sensitivity in the 641C homozygotes, suggesting a protective effect against cardiovascular disease and the metabolic syndrome. Finally, in a prospectively studied cohort, a significant survival advantage was demonstrated in those with the favorable 641C homozygote (p < 0.0001).

Conclusion: Homozygosity for the APOC3 641C allele is associated with a favorable lipoprotein profile, cardiovascular health, insulin sensitivity, and longevity. Because modulation of lipoproteins is also seen in genetically altered longevity models, it may be a common pathway influencing lifespan from nematodes to humans.

Resveratrol improves health and survival of mice on a high-calorie diet

Baur JA, Pearson KJ, Price NL, Jamieson HA, Lerin C, Kalra A, Prabhu VV, Allard JS, Lopez-Lluch G, Lewis K, Pistell PJ, Poosala S, Becker KG, Boss O, Gwinn D, Wang M, Ramaswamy S, Fishbein KW, Spencer RG, Lakatta EG, Le Couteur D, Shaw RJ, Navas P, Puigserver P, Ingram DK, de Cabo R, Sinclair DA
Department of Pathology, Paul F. Glenn Laboratories for the Biological Mechanisms of Aging, Harvard Medical School, Boston, Mass., USA
Nature 2006;444:337–342

Background: Resveratrol (3,5,49-trihydroxystilbene) extends the lifespan of diverse species including *Saccharomyces cerevisiae*, *Caenorhabditis elegans* and *Drosophila melanogaster*. In these organisms, lifespan extension is dependent on Sir2, a conserved deacetylase proposed to underlie the beneficial effects of caloric restriction.

Results: The authors show that resveratrol shifts the physiology of middle-aged mice on a high-calorie diet towards that of mice on a standard diet and significantly increases their survival. Resveratrol produces changes associated with longer lifespan, including increased insulin sensitivity, reduced insulin-like growth factor-1 levels, increased AMP-activated protein kinase and peroxisome proliferator-activated receptor-c coactivator 1a activity, increased mitochondrial number, and improved motor function. Parametric analysis of gene set enrichment revealed that resveratrol opposed the effects of the high-calorie diet in 144 out of 153 significantly altered pathways.

Conclusion: These data show that improving general health in mammals using small molecules is an attainable goal, and point to new approaches for treating obesity-related disorders and diseases of aging.

Longevity research is a hot topic these days and uses several approaches with two examples here, using classical genetic association studies and high throughput screening of chemicals affecting relevant pathways. In the paper by Atzmon et al., relevant gene variants were compared in a population of centenarians from the Ashkenazi Jewish community and in relevant controls. 25% of the centenarians vs. 10% of the control were homozygous for the 641C allele in the APOC3 promoter, associated with lower APOC3 levels and more favorable lipoprotein profiles. The frequency of homozygosity for the 641C allele increased with age from 65 to 100 years and survival after the age of 75 was associated with the genotype. The APOC3 is a major component of very low density lipoproteins and chylomicron remnants and this study confirms the influence of lipoprotein metabolism on longevity in humans. Although the association does not prove causality and the data needs to be replicated in other ethnic groups, there is a strong case for the role of APOC3 in the factors affecting longevity.

The second paper suggests a pharmacological approach to longevity and illustrates how new drugs are discovered, based on systematic targeting of relevant pathways. The sirtuin pathway has been identified as a mediator of diet-induced increased longevity in several species. Of the 7 sirtuin genes in mammals, SIRT1 regulates metabolism and cell survival and was the target of a systematic search of 20,000 molecules that enhance its activity. Resveratrol, a molecule produced by plants in response to stress, emerged as the most potent and was evaluated in simple organisms. The present paper reports its use in mice fed a high-fat diet. Resveratrol prevented body weight gain, increased survival and insulin sensitivity. Microarray analysis was used to identify the pathways targeted by the drug and identified Cidea, a regulator of energy balance in brown fat as a downregulated gene. Remarkably, resveratrol is a small molecule that can be administered orally that did not seem to prove toxicity during the limited studies represented here. Whether this is the next wonder drug capable of alleviating the negative effect of overfeeding in western societies will become apparent in the years to come.

New hopes. Prolactin, a heartbreaking hormone

A cathepsin D-cleaved 16 kDa form of prolactin mediates postpartum cardiomyopathy

Hilfiker-Kleiner D, Kaminski K, Podewski E, Bonda T, Schaefer A, Sliwa K, Forster O, Quint A, Landmesser U, Doerries C, Luchtefeld M, Poli V, Schneider MD, Balligand JL, Desjardins F, Ansari A, Struman I, Nguyen NQ, Zschemisch NH, Klein G, Heusch G, Schulz R, Hilfiker A, Drexler H
Department of Cardiology and Angiology, MHH, Hannover, Germany
hilfiker.denise@mh-hannover.de
Cell 2007;128:589–600

Background: Postpartum cardiomyopathy is a disease of unknown etiology and exposes women to a high risk of mortality after delivery.

Results: Female mice with a cardiomyocyte-specific deletion of STAT3 develop postpartum cardiomyopathy. In these mice, cardiac cathepsin D expression and activity is enhanced and associated with the generation of a cleaved antiangiogenic and proapoptotic 16 kDa form of the nursing hormone prolactin. Treatment with bromocriptine, an inhibitor of prolactin secretion, prevents the development of postpartum cardiomyopathy, whereas forced myocardial generation of 16 kDa prolactin impairs the cardiac capillary network and function, thereby recapitulating the cardiac phenotype of postpartum cardiomyopathy. Myocardial STAT3 protein levels are reduced and serum levels of activated cathepsin D and 16 kDa prolactin are elevated in postpartum cardiomyopathy patients.

Conclusion: A biologically active derivative of the pregnancy hormone prolactin mediates postpartum cardiomyopathy, implying that inhibition of prolactin release may represent a novel therapeutic strategy for postpartum cardiomyopathy.

This paper not only provides the mechanistic basis and the hope for an effective disease of a deadly disease, but is a great example of how careful hypothesis-driven observations can lead to important discoveries. The investigators made the hypothesis that oxidative stress and apoptosis were involved in postpartum cardiomyopathy and that STAT3 was involved in heart protection. This proved correct using a mouse model with targeted deletion of stat3 in the heart. The role of prolactin in pregnancy and postpartum as well as its angiogenic properties made this hormone an interesting candidate in the disease. Indeed, 23 kDa prolactin (the one we know as endocrinologists) is cleaved into a 16 kDa fragment which exerts antiangiogenic properties. Several experiments led to identify this 16 kDa prolactin as a key player in postpartum cardiomyopathy. Moreover, a preliminary trial of bromocriptine to reduce prolactin levels in 6 women at high risk of postpartum cardiomyopathy improved heart function, as compared to 6 untreated women of whom 3 died within a few months after delivery. Whether prolactin is the only mediator and whether defective STAT3 function is associated with postpartum cardiomyopathy in humans remains to be determined. Large-scale trials of dopaminergic agents will represent hope for women who were so far counseled not to have additional pregnancies when they had survived postpartum cardiomyopathy [9].

New hopes. The origins of thymic epithelial cells

Clonal analysis reveals a common progenitor for thymic cortical and medullary epithelium

Rossi SW, Jenkinson WE, Anderson G, Jenkinson EJ
MRC Centre for Immune Regulation, Division of Immunity and Infection, Institute for Biomedical Research, Medical School, University of Birmingham, Birmingham, UK
Nature 2006;441:988–991

Background: The thymus provides an essential environment for the development of T cells from hemopoietic progenitors. This environment is separated into cortical and medullary regions, each containing functionally distinct epithelial populations that are important at successive stages of T-cell development and selection. However, the developmental origin and lineage relationships between cortical and medullary epithelial cell types remain controversial.

Results: The authors describe a clonal assay to investigate the developmental potential of single, individually selected, thymic epithelial progenitors (marked with enhanced yellow fluorescent protein) developing within the normal architecture of the thymus. Using this approach, it is shown that cortical and medullary epithelial cells share a common origin in bipotent precursors, providing definitive evidence that they have a single rather than dual germ layer origin during embryogenesis.

Conclusions: These findings resolve a long-standing issue in thymus development, and are important in relation to the development of cell-based strategies for thymus disorders and the possibility of restoring function of the atrophied adult thymus.

Formation of a functional thymus initiated by a postnatal epithelial progenitor cell

Bleul CC, Corbeaux T, Reuter A, Fisch P, Monting JS, Boehm T
Department of Developmental Immunology, Max Planck Institute of Immunobiology, Freiburg, Germany
Nature 2006;441:992–996

Background: The thymus is essential for the generation of self-tolerant effector and regulatory T cells. Intrathymic T-cell development requires an intact stromal microenvironment, of which thymic epithelial cells constitute a major part. For instance, cell-autonomous genetic defects of forkhead box N1 (Foxn1) and autoimmune regulator (Aire) in thymic epithelial cells cause primary immunodeficiency and autoimmunity, respectively. During development, the thymic epithelial rudiment gives rise to two major compartments, the cortex and medulla. Cortical thymic epithelial cells positively select T cells, whereas medullary thymic epithelial cells are involved in negative selection of potentially autoreactive T cells. It has long been unclear whether these two morphologically and functionally distinct types of epithelial cells arise from a common bipotent progenitor cell and whether such progenitors are still present in the postnatal period.

Results: Using in vivo cell lineage analysis in mice, the presence of a common progenitor of cortical and medullary thymic epithelial cells after birth is demonstrated. To probe the function of postnatal progenitors, a conditional mutant allele of Foxn1 was reverted to wild-type function in single epithelial cells in vivo. This led to the formation of small thymic lobules containing both cortical and medullary areas that supported normal thymopoiesis.

Conclusions: Thus, single epithelial progenitor cells can give rise to a complete and functional thymic microenvironment, suggesting that cell-based therapies could be developed for thymus disorders.

The thymus is the central organ of the immune system and the source of mature T cells that fight infections. It is composed of developing thymocytes derived from the bone marrow and of a backbone thymic epithelium. This epithelium is subdivided into the cortex and the medulla whose function are well identified and distinct. The cortex is responsible for the positive selection of T cells (i.e. the capacity to function in a major histocompatibility complex restricted fashion) and the medulla is in charge of purging the forming T cells from those that are autoreactive to self. The Aire gene is involved in the expression of peripheral self antigens in medullary thymic epithelial cells [10] and a defect in medullary thymic epithelial cells proinsulin expression plays a role in type 1 diabetes [11]. Although the functions and morphological characteristics of thymic epithelial cells are well known, their developmental pattern was unclear, with some believing that they had different (endodermal and ectodermal) origin and others that both types came from the endoderm. The two studies discussed here show that a single progenitor cell can give rise to both types of epithelial cells and that these cells exist in the adult thymus. The importance of these findings is not only theoretical since several human diseases result from thymic dysfunction. Rare immunodeficiencies can result from a loss of function of the FOXN1 gene, known in the mouse to result in the 'nude' phenotype (alopecia and deficient T cells). The data suggest that expressing FOXN1 in thymic precursors of affected patients will result in immune reconstitution. Beyond this rare disease, these findings open the way to manipulation of the thymus in autoimmune diseases, currently the only hope of re-establishing self tolerance.

Concerns. Drug safety monitoring

The FDA and drug safety: a proposal for sweeping changes

Furberg CD, Levin AA, Gross PA, Shapiro RS, Strom BL
Department of Public Health Sciences, Wake Forest University School of Medicine, Winston-Salem, N.C., USA
cfurberg@wfubmc.edu
Arch Intern Med 2006;166:1938–1942

Background: The current Food and Drug Administration (FDA) system of regulating drug safety has serious limitations and is in need of changes. The major problems include the following: the design of initial preapproval studies lets uncommon, serious adverse events go undetected; massive underreporting of adverse events to the FDA postmarketing surveillance system reduces the ability to quantify risk accurately; manufacturers do not fulfill the majority of their postmarketing safety study commitments; the FDA lacks authority to pursue sponsors who violate regulations and ignore postmarketing safety study commitments; the public increasingly perceives the FDA as having become too close to the regulated pharmaceutical industry; the FDA's safety oversight structure is suboptimal, and the FDA's expertise and resources in drug safety and public health are limited.
Conclusions: To address these problems, we urge Congress, which is ultimately responsible for the FDA's performance, to implement the following five recommendations: (1) give the FDA more direct legal authority to pursue violations, (2) authorize the adoption of a conditional drug approval policy, at least for selected drugs, (3) provide additional financial resources to support the safety operations, (4) mandate a reorganization of the agency with emphasis on strengthening the evaluation and proactive monitoring of drug safety, and (5) require broader representation of safety experts on the FDA's advisory committees.

Although this paper deals with US mechanisms of drug approval and safety surveillance, the issues discussed are valid worldwide and reflect the intrinsic difficulty of improving the health of the population with active drugs while avoiding adverse events due to these drugs. There is therefore a difficult balance between releasing a potentially lifesaving or useful drug and the data needed to have a full assessment of the risks of this drug. This is particularly true for rare events occurring late after the drug is started. The paper lists six major problems with the current system of drug safety surveillance, including (1) that serious adverse events can be undetected during the approval process, (2) that only 10% of serious adverse events are reported, (3) that the threshold for action when an adverse event is detected is subjective and therefore variable, (4) that the FDA does not control the performance of postmarketing studies, (5) that the FDA (and other agencies) have a conflict of interest since it is both involved in drug approval and in safety actions if adverse events arise, and (6) that the FDA has a shortage of expertise in drug safety. The authors make several recommendations indicated above. This report reminds us that we have to balance our actions in the best interest of our patients and that we have to stay vigilant for adverse events in our daily practice.

Food for thought

A non-invasive test for prenatal diagnosis based on fetal DNA present in maternal blood: a preliminary study

Dhallan R, Guo X, Emche S, Damewood M, Bayliss P, Cronin M, Barry J, Betz J, Franz K, Gold K, Vallecillo B, Varney J
Ravgen Inc., Columbia, Md., USA
rdhallan@ravgen.com
Lancet 2007;369:474–481

Background: Use of free fetal DNA to diagnose fetal chromosomal abnormalities has been hindered by the inability to distinguish fetal DNA from maternal DNA. The aim of this study was to establish whether single nucleotide polymorphisms (SNPs) can be used to distinguish fetal DNA from maternal DNA – and to determine the number of fetal chromosomes – in maternal blood samples.
Methods: Formaldehyde-treated blood samples from 60 pregnant women and the stated biological fathers were analyzed. Maternal plasma fractions were quantified at multiple SNPs, and the ratio of the unique fetal allele signal to the combined maternal and fetal allele signal calculated. The mean ratios of SNPs on chromosomes 13 and 21 were compared to test for potential fetal chromosomal abnormalities.
Results: The mean proportion of free fetal DNA was 34.0% (median 32.5%, range 17.0–93.8). Three samples with significant differences in the fetal DNA ratios for chromosome 13 and chromosome 21, indicative of trisomy 21, were identified; the remaining 57 samples were deemed to be normal. Amniocentesis or newborn reports from the clinical sites confirmed that the copy number of fetal chromosomes 13 and 21 was established correctly for 58 of the 60 samples, identifying 56 of the 57 normal samples, and two of the three trisomy-21 samples. Of the incorrectly identified samples, one was a false negative and one was a false positive. The sensitivity and positive predictive value were both 66.7% and the specificity and negative predictive values were both 98.2%.
Conclusions: The copy number of chromosomes of interest can be directly established from maternal plasma. Such a non-invasive prenatal test could provide a useful complement to currently used screening tests.

Non-invasive techniques are the Holy Grail of prenatal diagnosis and are already used for the diagnosis of sex in specialized laboratories and for specific indications (for instance for fetuses are risk of congenital adrenal hyperplasia). Non-invasive techniques for the diagnosis of fetal aneuploidies would alleviate the risk associated with amniocentesis and would pave the way for non-invasive techniques for the diagnosis of monogenic disorders. This study is based on the isolation of free fetal DNA in the maternal plasma and uses the ratio of the paternal fetal allele to the maternal alleles as an indicator of the number of chromosomes 21 and 13. As such the study is preliminary and only 2 of 3 fetuses with abnormalities were detected. In another study, based on the analysis of circulating placental RNA, fetal trisomy 21 was detected non-invasively in 90% of cases and excluded in 96.5% of controls [12]. Parents and health providers will be faced with more ethical problems as technology progresses in the future and will have to adapt to these new challenges.

References

1. Hochberg Z, Carel JC: The year in science and medicine; in Carel JC, Hochberg Z (eds): Yearbook of Pediatric Endocrinology 2006. Basel, Karger, 2006, pp 175–192.
2. Green RE, Krause J, Ptak SE, Briggs AW, Ronan MT, Simons JF, et al: Analysis of one million base pairs of Neanderthal DNA. Nature 2006;444:330–336.
3. Keymer JE, Galajda P, Muldoon C, Park S, Austin RH: Bacterial metapopulations in nanofabricated landscapes. Proc Natl Acad Sci USA 2006;103:17290–17295.
4. Martin JA, Brown TD, Heiner AD, Buckwalter JA: Chondrocyte senescence, joint loading and osteoarthritis. Clin Orthop Relat Res 2004;(suppl):S96–S103.
5. Vezzosi D, Bouisson M, Escourrou G, Laurell H, Selves J, Seguin P, et al: Clinical utility of telomerase for the diagnosis of malignant well-differentiated endocrine tumours. Clin Endocrinol (Oxf) 2006;64:63–67.
6. Donnert G, Keller J, Medda R, Andrei MA, Rizzoli SO, Luhrmann R, et al: Macromolecular-scale resolution in biological fluorescence microscopy. Proc Natl Acad Sci USA 2006;103:11440–11445.
7. Dorsey SG, Renn CL, Carim-Todd L, Barrick CA, Bambrick L, Krueger BK, et al: In vivo restoration of physiological levels of truncated TrkB.T1 receptor rescues neuronal cell death in a trisomic mouse model. Neuron 2006;51:21–28.
8. Meyerovitch J, Sherf M, Antebi F, Hochberg Z: Loss of TSH set points in Down syndrome. ESPE Annual Meeting. Horm Res 2007, in press.
9. Leinwand LA: Molecular events underlying pregnancy-induced cardiomyopathy. Cell 2007;128:437–438.
10. Anderson MS, Venanzi ES, Klein L, Chen Z, Berzins SP, Turley SJ, et al: Projection of an immunological self-shadow within the thymus by the aire protein. Science 2002;298:1395–1401.
11. Faideau B, Lotton C, Lucas B, Tardivel I, Elliott JF, Boitard C, et al: Tolerance to proinsulin-2 is due to radioresistant thymic cells. J Immunol 2006;177:53–60.
12. Lo YM, Tsui NB, Chiu RW, Lau TK, Leung TN, Heung MM, et al: Plasma placental RNA allelic ratio permits noninvasive prenatal chromosomal aneuploidy detection. Nat Med 2007;13:218–223.

Author Index

Bignell, G. 205
Bijlsma, M.F. 193
Biller, B.M. 196
Binoux, M. 39
Birney, E. 3, 205
Bisello, A. 134
Bistritzer, T. 78
Bitner-Glindzicz, M. 12
Blair, E. 120
Blair, H.C. 54, 55
Blair, S.N. 194
Blake, A. 169
Blanc, H. 26
Blangero, J. 155
Blasi, P. 102
Blattner, F.R. 207
Bleul, C.C. 214
Bloch, C.A. 84
Bloomberg, G.R. 164
Blows, M.W. 182
Blum, W.F. 45, 50
Bo, W. 54
Boehm, B.O. 31
Boehm, T. 214
Boehmer, S.J. 164
Boehnke, M. 150
Boepple, P. 72
Bognetti, E. 106
Boileau, P. 26
Bolk, N. 19
Boll, S. 33
Bollag, G. 33
Bomben, M.M. 170
Bona, G. 30
Bonda, T. 213
Bondeson, A.G. 122
Bondy, C.A. 76
Bonewald, L.F. 53
Bonfanti, R. 106
Bonjour, J.-P. 61
Bonnycastle, L.L. 150
Bookout, A.L. 17, 190
Borch-Johnsen, K. 149
Bornstein, S.R. 94
Borson-Chazot, C. 6
Boss, O. 212
Bost, M. 167
Bottcher, Y. 152
Bottomley, B. 125
Bouchard, P. 81
Bougneres, P. 26
Bouillon, R. 64
Bouloux, P. 72
Bousquet-Melou, A. 89
Boutin, P. 147, 157
Bouvatier, C. 167
Bowles, J. 71
Boye, K.R. 94
Boyle, M. 43
Brabant, G. 23

Bradley, R.H. 44
Bradshaw, B. 155
Bradwin, G. 196
Brage, S. 144, 193
Brasseur, F. 205
Brauer, V.F. 28
Braun, J. 54
Braun, L. 45
Brauner, R. 3, 77
Bredow, M. 44
Bresnick, E.H. 12
Breuning, M.H. 48
Bridgham, J.T. 191
Brillante, B. 8
Bristow, J. 34
Britton, O.L. 42
Brommer, J.E. 182
Brooks, A.G. 104
Brown, C.J. 156
Brown, D. 163
Brown, R.S. 25
Brue, T. 4, 6
Bruggeman, F.J. 178
Brunham, L.R. 133
Bryant, H.U. 57
Bucciarelli, T. 115
Buchanan, T.A. 150
Büchler, C. 123
Buck, G. 205
Buj-Bello, A. 81
Bulsara, M. 120
Burger, M. 158
Burren, O. 112
Burrill, C.P. 150
Burton, J. 158
Bustamante, C.D. 199
Butcher, S.K. 87
Butler, A. 205
Butler, G.E. 161
Butler, P.C. 100
Butman, J.A. 8
Butts, D.L. 13
Buyukgebiz, A. 78
Byrne, S. 120

Cabral, W.A. 65
Cabrol, S. 77, 167
Cahill, D.P. 205
Cai, H. 134
Caillou, B. 27
Calabresi, P.A. 99
Calafiore, R. 102
Calender, A. 6
Calori, G. 106
Calvi, C. 192
Calvo, E. 91
Camerino, G. 80, 81
Cameron, I.T. 91

Campbell, P. 205
Campbell, W.A. 209
Camper, S.A. 10, 13
Cantor, C.R. 207
Cao, D. 45
Cappa, M. 5
Cardon, L.R. 148
Cardoso-Landa, L. 54
Carel, J.-C. 187, 201
Carel, J.C. 77
Carley, W. 96
Carlsson, B. 121
Carlsson, E. 122
Carlsson, L.M.S. 121
Carmeliet, G. 64
Carmeliet, P. 64
Carmignac, D. 12
Carmina, E. 76
Carpenter, M.K. 101
Carr, B.R. 79
Carrascosa, A. 161
Carre, A. 27
Carroll, S.M. 191
Carson, A.R. 156
Carson, S.A. 79
Carta, C. 34
Carta, L. 192
Carvalho, L.R. 4, 49
Casey, P.H. 44
Cassio, A. 166
Castano, J.P. 9
Cataldo, N.A. 79
Catteeuw, D. 47
Cavagnini, F. 6
Cavener, D.R. 26
Cawley, M. 186
Cha, J.Y. 134
Chaboissier, M.C. 80
Chadwick, R.B. 178
Chan, S.W. 201
Chan, Y. 111
Chandarana, K. 125
Chandler, D.W. 171
Chandy, K.G. 99
Chang, S.M. 191
Chang, W. 65
Chanson, P. 8
Charon, C. 26
Charpentier, G. 147
Chase, H.P. 107
Chase, K. 199
Chatfield, B. 163
Chaudhuri, T.R. 38
Chaussain, J.L. 77
Chawengsaksophak, K. 71
Chelala, C. 26
Chen, F. 206
Chen, G. 149
Chen, H. 66, 201

Chen, H.L. 37
Chen, K. 134
Chen, W. 37, 156
Chen, Y. 29, 149
Chenevix-Trench, G. 205
Cheng, C.S. 176
Cheng, C.Y. 79
Cheng, G. 74
Cheng, H. 195
Cheng, Y.Z. 72
Cheng, Z. 156
Chenoweth, S.F. 182
Cherman, N. 8
Chernomoretz, A. 91
Chess, A. 203
Chevenne, D. 106, 157
Chiarelli, F. 99, 112, 115
Chiew, Y.E. 205
Chinchilli, V.M. 164
Chines, P.S. 150
Chiumello, G. 5, 62, 106
Chivers, J.E. 125
Cho, E.K. 156
Choi, M. 190
Chomitz, V.R. 130
Chong, W. 29
Chong, W.K. 12
Chotard, L. 179
Choudhury, B. 205
Christiansen, C. 149
Christman, M.F. 152
Chrysis, D. 53
Chung, P.P. 209
Cianfarani, S. 12
Ciccarelli, A. 6
Ciccarelli, E. 6
Cicognani, A. 166
Cirillo, G. 157
Clark, A.J. 90
Clark, V.J. 154
Clay, C.M. 13
Clayton, D.G. 112
Clement, K. 113
Clemente, M. 161
Clements, J. 205
Clifton, V.L. 49
Clodfelter, K.H. 40
Coakley, P. 145
Cocquet, J. 13
Cohn, R.D. 192
Cokus, S. 201
Colao, A. 6
Colditz, G. 152
Cole, J. 205
Cole, S.A. 155
Cole, T.J. 144
Collins, F. 150
Collins, J. 12
Collins, M.T. 8
Collins, S. 125

Colman, P.G. 104
Colombo, C. 112
Comuzzie, A.G. 155
Conneely, K.N. 150
Conrad, S.A. 180
Conway, G.S. 75
Cooke, N.E. 35
Cools, M. 84
Coop, G. 206
Cooper, J.D. 112
Cooper, R. 152
Cooper, S.F. 171
Cooper, T.K. 192
Coppens, S. 203
Coppola, A. 20
Corbeaux, T. 214
Corigliano, S. 28
Corrias, A. 30
Corsi, A.M. 154
Cortese, R. 158
Cossec, J.C. 26
Coste, A. 138
Coste, J. 77
Counts, D.R. 99
Courtney, R. 96
Coutifaris, C. 79
Cowell, C.T. 128
Cox, T.V. 158
Crabbe, R. 162
Crevillen, P. 202
Crock, P.A. 7
Cronin, M. 216
Crowe, B.J. 45
Crowley, W. 72
Cuccato, D. 62
Cudlip, S. 14
Cui, R. 204
Cummings, D.E. 119
Curro, F. 115
Curry, C.J. 34
Cuthbertson, D. 107
Cuzin, F. 201
Czernichow, P. 106, 157, 162

Darwin, C. 109
Dattani, M.T. 3, 12, 33, 75, 125
Davey-Smith, G. 148
Davies, H. 205
Davies, R. 158
Davis, E.A. 120
Davis, S. 199
Davis, S.I. 53
de Benoist, B. 28
de Cabo, R. 212
De Cristofaro, E. 166
De Herder, W. 6
De Menis, E. 6, 11
de Muinck Keizer-Schrama, S.M. 165
De Rosa, V. 125
de Sousa, G. 22, 141
de Vijlder, J.J. 168
Dean, C. 202
Dearth, R.K. 42
Debatin, K.M. 31
DeFazio, A. 205
DeFronzo, R.A. 155
Deghmoun, S. 157
Dehay, C. 203
Dekker-van der Sloot, M. 168
Del Maschio, A. 106
Delage, L. 89
Delalbre, A. 179
Delcroix, J.D. 209
deLeeuw, R.J. 156
Delemarre-van de Waal, H.A. 129
Delemer, B. 6
Delezoide, A.L. 27
Dellambra, E. 80
Delpech, M. 81
Demerath, E. 155
Deng, H.W. 187
Deng, H.Y. 187
Deng, L. 38
Denzer, C. 119
Deshaies, Y. 88
Desjardins, F. 213
Dewailly, D. 76
Dhallan, R. 216
di lorgi, N. 5
Di Rienzo, A. 154
Diamanti-Kandarakis, E. 76
Diamond, M.P. 79
Diano, S. 20
Dicks, E. 205
Dieguez, C. 9
Dierick, H.A. 175
Dietz, H.C. 192
Digilio, M.C. 34
Dijoud, F. 167
Dina, C. 147
Dinarello, C.A. 137

Kilpatrick, E.S. 103
Kilvington, F. 96
Kim, H.K. 56
Kim, S.H. 137
Kimber, W. 125
Kimm, L.R. 156
Kimura, N. 94
King, B. 203
Kirk, J.M. 12
Kleijer, W.J. 1
Klein, C. 33
Klein, E.C. 192
Klein, G. 213
Klein, R. 105
Klein, S. 127
Kleschevnikov, A.M. 209
Klibanski, A. 196
Kliewer, S.A. 190
Klingensmith, G.J. 110
Klinghammer, A. 31
Knaus, H. 99
Knerr, I. 31
Knight, B. 148, 154
Knight, B.A. 151
Knight, C.G. 181
Knight, D. 71
Knoepfelmacher, M. 4
Kobayashi, M. 136
Koberwitz, K. 152
Koelman, J.H. 168
Koenig, C. 158
Kohrle, J. 28
Kokko, A. 11
Koller, D. 48
Kollet, O. 63
Kollin, C. 164
Kolski-Andreaco, A. 99
Komura, D. 156
Kondo, T. 185
Kong, A. 149
Koopman, P. 71
Kopchick, J.J. 46
Korach, K.S. 84
Korner, A. 150, 152
Kostenuik, P. 56
Koster, J.C. 112
Kottler, M.L. 81
Kovacs, P. 150, 152
Koza, R.A. 177
Kozak, L.P. 177
Kramer, M.S. 105
Kratz, C.P. 33
Krause, J. 206
Krawiec, M. 164
Kretz, C. 81
Kreusch, A. 135
Kriauciunas, A. 57
Krischer, J. 107
Krishnamurthy, B. 104
Kroon, E. 101

Krude, H. 3, 17, 23
Kruit, J.K. 133
Kruithof, M.F. 48
Kudaravalli, S. 206
Kulkarni, N.H. 57
Kullberg, B.J. 137
Kulnane, L.S. 209
Kumar, T.R. 54, 55
Kumaran, K. 145
Kunde, J. 158
Kupelian, V. 73
Kuro-o, M. 68
Kurosu, H. 68
Kuznetsova, N. 65
Kwiterovich, P.O., Jr. 171
Kwon, Y.S. 176

Le Roux, C.W. 125
Leary, S.D. 145, 194
Lecointre, C. 167
Lecomte, P. 6
Lee, A.V. 42
Lee, B. 65
Lee, J.H. 73
Lee, K.K. 186
Lee, P.A. 76
Lee, S.K. 178
LeeHealey, C.J. 99
Leger, J. 77, 106, 162, 167
Legro, R.S. 76, 79
Lehtonen, R. 11
Leikin, S. 65
Leite, C.C. 4
Lemanske, R.F., Jr. 164
Lenburg, M.E. 152
Lenzi, A. 82
Leppert, P.C. 79
Lepri, F. 34
Lerin, C. 212
Lespinasse, J. 81
Lessan, N. 125
Leung, S.Y. 205
Levilliers, J. 81
Levin, A.A. 215
Levin, M. 121
Levy-Marchal, C. 133, 157
Lew, A.M. 104
Lewin, J. 158
Lewis, E. 137
Lewis, K. 212
Ley, R.E. 126, 127
Li, C. 29
Li, F. 134
Li, J. 29, 134
Li, J.L. 187
Li, M. 73
Li, T. 37
Li, W.P. 72
Li, Y. 29, 186
Liao, J. 24
Liao, L. 42
Liddle, J. 158
Liebhaber, S.A. 35
Lienhardt-Roussie, A. 81
Liese, A.D. 139, 140
Lin, J.Y. 204
Lin, L. 71, 75
Linder, B. 139, 141, 142
Lindgren, C.M. 148
Ling, J.Q. 37
Linne, Y. 144
Lipson, N. 84
Lipton, R.B. 212
Lister, C. 202
Little, B.M. 48
Littler, C. 189
Liu, A.H. 164

Liu, D. 176
Liu, G. 192
Liu, L.L. 139, 141
Liu, M. 57
Liu, S. 53
Liu, X.J. 111
Liu, Y.J. 187
Liu, Y.Z. 187
Liu, Z. 64
Liu, Z.W. 20
Liu, Z.X. 136
Lo Conte, R. 172
Loche, S. 1, 5, 30
Loeys, B.L. 192
Loh, K.L. 169
Lombardo, F. 115
Lomniczi, A. 183
London, S.E. 92
Long, J.R. 187
Lönn, M. 121
Looijenga, L. 205
Looijenga, L.H. 84
Loos, R.J. 148
Loots, B. 139
Lopez-Fernandez, J. 125
Lopez-Lluch, G. 212
Lord, J.M. 87
Lorenz-Depiereux, B. 54
Lorini, R. 5
Loris, C. 54
Louet, J.F. 138
Louey, S. 90
Louis, D.N. 205
Lovell-Badge, R. 12
Lu, Y. 53
Luca, G. 102
Lucas, A. 144
Luchtefeld, M. 213
Ludvigsson, J. 108
Ludwig, D.S. 130
Luo, Z.-J. 59
Luongo, C. 157
Lusis, A.J. 184
Luu-The, V. 91
Luzi, L. 106
Lyon, H. 152
Lystig, T.C. 121

M

Ma, Y.L. 57
Maahs, D.M. 110
MacAulay, C. 156
McCarthy, H.D. 143
McCarthy, M.I. 148, 151
MacCluer, J. 155
Maccoll, G. 72
McColl, J.H. 172
McCormack, A.L. 183
McCrimmon, R.J. 195

McCrindle, B.W. 114
McCrory, M.A. 134
MacDonald, J.R. 156
McFann, K. 107, 110
McGovern, P.G. 79
Machinis, K. 50
McIntosh, J.R. 208
Mackay, D.J. 151
McKenzie, M.D. 104
McKenzie, S. 125
McKinlay, J.B. 73
McMahon, R.P. 171
McNay, D.E. 3
McNay, E.C. 195
McNicol, A.M. 94
Maconochie, M. 198
McQueen, M.B. 152
Maes, C. 64
Maestroni, A. 106
Maghnie, M. 1, 5
Magrini, V. 126
Mahowald, M.A. 126
Maier, L.S. 73
Mak, P.A. 135
Makareeva, E. 65
Makinen, M.J. 11
Malagon, M.M. 9
Malecka-Tendera, E. 78
Malik, V.S. 130
Mamiya, S. 71
Mangelsdorf, D.J. 17, 190
Mannelli, M. 94
Mao, J. 29
Marchal, C.L. 106
Marchisotti, F.G. 49
Marcos, J. 91
Marcovina, S. 139, 140
Marcovina, S.M. 142
Mardis, E.R. 126
Marini, J.C. 65
Marinovic, D. 106
Marsh, B.J. 133
Marshall, C.R. 156
Martel, C. 91
Martin, J. 34
Martin, T.J. 57
Martinelli, S. 34
Martinez, F.D. 164
Martinez-Fuentes, A.J. 9
Martinovic, J. 27
Martyn, C.N. 44
Marui, S. 4
Maser-Gluth, C. 94
Masia, R. 112
Mason, J.I. 91
Mastronarde, D.N. 208
Masuyama, R. 64
Matarese, G. 125
Matchock, R.L. 190
Mathieu, M. 81

Mattocks, C. 194
Mauer, M. 105
Mauger, D.T. 164
Mauras, N. 45
Mayer-Davis, E.J. 141, 142
Mehta, S.D. 139
Mei, R. 156
Meier, J.J. 100
Meinecke, P. 1
Meitinger, T. 152
Melo, M.E. 4
Melzer, D. 148, 154
Mendonca, B.B. 4, 49
Mendoza, T. 177
Menon, R.K. 46
Menuelle, P. 39
Mertens, A.C. 197
Meschi, F. 106
Metcalf, B. 154
Metherell, L.A. 90
Meyer-Bahlburg, H.F. 93
Meyre, D. 147, 157
Michiels, S. 27
Miller, K.K. 196
Miller, W.L. 93
Miner, J.N. 58
Mirabeau, O. 3
Miraglia del Giudice, E. 157
Mitby, P. 197
Mitro, N. 135
Miyabayashi, K. 81
Miyamoto, K. 96
Miyoshi, M. 68
Mizutani, T. 96
Mobley, W.C. 209
Moe, O.W. 68
Moerman, A. 81
Mohammadi, M. 72
Mohan, S. 178
Mohlke, K.L. 150
Mohn, A. 115
Moldes, M. 113
Molinari, L. 28
Molini, V. 75
Molteni, V. 135
Monaghan, P. 211
Monden, T. 124
Monia, B.P. 136
Monks, D.A. 92
Montenegro, L.R. 49
Montgomery, C. 172
Montgomery, L. 156
Monting, J.S. 214
Montoye, T. 47
Montpetit, A. 147
Moonga, B.S. 54
Moorman, M.A. 101
Moosa, K. 28
Mora, S. 62
Moran, A. 100

Villar, A. 209
Vincent, D. 147
Vincent, S. 201
Visser, T.J. 19
von Puttkamer, J. 119
Voshol, P.J. 137
Voss, L.D. 154
Vottero, A. 78
Vu-Hong, T.A. 157
Vu, T.H. 37
Vulsma, T. 168

W

Wabitsch, M. 119, 122
Wada, Y. 81
Wade, J. 92
Wadwa, R.P. 110, 141
Wagenstaller, J. 54
Wagner, S. 73
Walenkamp, M.J.E. 48
Walker, M. 148, 151
Walker, N.M. 112
Walker, S.P. 191
Walsh, S. 186
Wan, X. 111
Wang, A. 136
Wang, D. 176
Wang, H. 184
Wang, J. 59
Wang, L. 153
Wang, M. 212
Wang, P.H. 99
Wang, S. 184
Wang, W. 29, 37
Wang, X. 38, 153
Wang, X.-F. 61
Wangensteen, T. 125
Ward, G.M. 128
Ward, L.M. 53
Ward, R.D. 10
Wareham, N.J. 144, 148
Warner, M. 74
Wasdell, M.B. 170
Wass, J.A. 14
Watanabe, R.M. 150
Watson, C.S. 39
Wauman, J. 47
Waxman, D.J. 40
Wayne, R.K. 199
Webb, T. 205
Weber, B.L. 205
Weedon, M.N. 148, 151, 154
Weetman, A.P. 23
Wehner, L.E. 33
Wei, E. 99
Wei, T. 57
Wei, Y. 28
Weikart-Yeckel, C. 195

Weis, M. 65
Weiss, B. 36
Weiss, M.D. 170
Weitzmann, M.N. 188
Wells, J. 194
Wells, J.C. 172
Wemeau, J.L. 6
West, B. 33
West , S. 205
West, T. 158
Westerhoff, H.V. 178
Westerlund, J. 24
Westerterp, K.R. 129
White, K.E. 53
White, S. 48
Whiteside-Mansell, L. 44
Wichmann, H.E. 152
Widaa, S. 205
Widlund, H.R. 204
Widmer, B. 112
Wielopolski, P.A. 165
Wiersinga, W.M. 23
Wiesel, T. 31
Wikstrom, A.M. 83
Wilensky, D.L. 204
Wilensky, R.L. 149
Wilhelm, D. 71
Wilkin, T.J. 154
Willer, C.J. 150
Williams, D.E. 139, 141
Williams, M.R. 110
Williamson, A. 172
Williamson, C.M. 198
Wilson, D.I. 91
Wilson, M.J. 71
Wilson, P.L. 65
Winkler, C. 95
Winzenberg, T. 171
Wit, J.M. 48
Witchel, S.F. 76
Withers, D.J. 125
Wolczynski, S. 81
Wolf, F. 73
Wolffenbuttel, K.P. 84
Wollmann, H. 161
Wong, C.H. 79
Wong, K.K. 156
Woo, S.B. 60
Wood, P.J. 91
Woodruff, T.K. 71
Woods, K.S. 3
Wooster, R. 205
Wright, S. 91
Wu, C. 209
Wu, J. 37
Wu, R.C. 138
Wudy, S.A. 87, 94
Wulff, H. 99
Wunsch, R. 141

X

Xia, W. 209
Xiao, P. 187
Xie, Y. 53
Xiong, D.H. 187
Xu, H.E. 190
Xu, J. 42
Xu, X. 153

Y

Yadav, K.K. 34
Yamada, G. 81
Yamada, K. 96
Yamada, M. 124
Yamaji, K. 136
Yamamoto, M. 68, 124
Yamashita, T. 188
Yamazaki, Y. 188
Yan, H. 59
Yang, F. 29
Yang, N. 38
Yang, R. 29
Yang, X. 17, 184
Yantha, J. 111
Yap, F. 128
Yaroslavskiy, B.B. 54
Yashiro, K. 71
Yasui, Y. 197
Yates, A. 205
Yazaki, J. 201
Yazawa, T. 96
Ye, Z. 176
Yee, S.-P. 39
Yokoya, S. 36
Yoshino, M. 96
Young, J. 8, 81
Yu, C. 59
Yu, H. 178
Yu, R.T. 17
Yu, X. 29, 53
Yu, Y. 29
Yuan, B. 53
Yuen, S.T. 205

Z

Zaidi, M. 54, 55
Zaidi, S. 54
Zallone, A. 54
Zampino, G. 34
Zeggini, E. 148
Zeiger, R.S. 164
Zelhof, A.C. 208
Zenaty, D. 167
Zeng, Q. 57
Zenker, M. 33
Zerbini, G. 106
Zhan, K. 209

Subject Index

insulin detemir versus NPH insulin study 108, 109

interferon-induced helicase-1 single nucleotide polymorphisms 112

intrahepatic islet transplantation and pulsatile insulin secretion 100, 101

islet antigen responses in nonobese diabetic mice and proinsulin tolerance 104

KCNJ11 mutation in developmental delay, epilepsy, and neonatal diabetes 112, 113

lipid abnormalities in youth 140

microcapsules for cell encapsulation 102

nocturnal hypoglycemia and awakening 195

potassium channel Kv1.3 therapeutic targeting in autoimmune disease 99, 100

renal function preceding microalbuminuria 106

statin therapy 110

steroid metabolism 84, 85

thyroxine therapy in autoimmune thyroiditis and type 1 diabetes 31

transient receptor potential vanilloid-1+ sensory neuron control of beta cell stress and islet inflammation 111

vitamin E supplementation study 115

Diabetes type 2

beta-cell ABCA1 modulation 133, 134

bile acid-binding resin prevention 136, 137

epidemiology 139, 140

genome-wide association studies 147–149

lipid abnormalities in youth 140

maturity-onset diabetes of the young and susceptibility 150, 151

screening in pediatric primary care 139

TCF7L2 gene variants 149, 150

transient neonatal diabetes mellitus genetic variation 151, 152

Dieting, sex hormone effects in boys 171, 172

Disorders of sex development, see Hypospadia

DMP1, see Dentin matrix protein 1

DNA methylation

Gnas cluster imprinted control region 198

human chromosome profiling 158, 159

Zac1 imprinted gene network regulation in embryonic growth 179, 180

DNA microarray

Arabidopsis transcription networks 186

ChIP-on-chip studies of estrogen receptor-α promoter-binding sites 176

whole genome microarray analysis of growth hormone-induced gene expression 178

Down syndrome

amyloid precursor protein effects on nerve growth factor transport in mouse model 209, 210

thyroxine therapy 168

ovarian wedge resection restoration of fertility in ERβ knockout mice 74, 75

European Youth Heart Study 193, 194

Evidence-based medicine

calcium supplementation and bone density 171

dieting and sex hormones in boys 171, 172

growth hormone therapy 161–163, 165, 166

inhaled corticosteroids in asthma 164, 165

insulin pumps in routine care 167, 168

orchidoplexy for undescended testes 164

oxandrolone and exercise for severe burns 169

oxytocin nasal spray for mothers of preterm infants 169, 170

physical activity determinants in adolescence 172

obesity prevention in children 172, 173

sleep hygiene and melatonin for attention deficit hyperactivity disorder 170

testosterone for bilateral anorchia in infancy 167

thyroxine treatment in Down syndrome 168

triptorelin for idiopathic early puberty 166

Exercise, see Physical activity

Notch, sustained signaling in pituitary development 12

Suppressors of cytokine signaling (SOCS), growth hormone modulation 47

Systems biology
adaptive point mutation 181
aggression studies in *Drosophila* 175, 176
Arabidopsis transcription networks 186
cancer research 178, 179
circadian clocks in peripheral tissues 180
diet-induced obesity, gene expression study in mice 177
estrogen receptor-α promoter-binding sites 176
glial glutamate metabolism in female puberty 183, 184
mate selection genetics 182, 183
natural selection on gene expression 181, 182
Sertoli cell bisphenol A injury genetic networks 185, 186
sexually dimorphic gene expression in mice 184, 185
whole genome microarray analysis of growth hormone-induced gene expression 178
Zac1 in embryonic growth 179, 180

T

T-box 1 (Tbx1), thyroid size and positioning 24, 25
T-box 3 (Tbx3), osteoblast proliferation regulation 178
Tbx1, *see* T-box 1
Tbx3, *see* T-box 3
TCF7L2, *see* Transcription factor 7-like 2
TDRD6, *see* Tudor domain containing protein 6
Telomerase, tumor activity 207
Testosterone
bilateral anorchia in infancy management 167
dieting effects in boys 171, 172
measurement 83, 84
population-level decline in American men 73, 74

therapy and cardiovascular risk markers in androgen-deficient women with hypopituitarism 196, 197

Thiazolidinediones, beta-cell ABCA1 modulation 133

Thymus, epithelium progenitor cells 214, 215

Thyroglobulin, dried blood spot thyroglobulin assessment of iodine status 28

Thyroid development
cervical arteries and developmental relocalization 23, 24
sodium/iodide symporter expression and fetal function onset 27, 28
Tbx1 in size and positioning 24, 25

Thyroid hormone
thyroxine therapy
autoimmune thyroiditis and type 1 diabetes 31
Down syndrome 168
timing effects in hypothyroidism 19, 20
triiodothyronine interactions with uncoupling protein-2 in feeding regulation 20, 21

Thyroid hormone receptors
circadian rhythm of expression 17, 18
phosphatidylinositol 3-kinase signaling 19

Thyroid-stimulating hormone (TSH)
congenital hypothyroidism diagnosis 25, 26
hyperthyrotropinemia in obesity 22, 23
upper limit in diagnostics 23

Thyrotropin, *see* Thyroid-stimulating hormone

Thyrotropin-releasing hormone (TRH), intracerebroventricular leptin stimulation 21, 22

Thyroxine, *see* Thyroid hormone

TNDM, *see* Transient neonatal diabetes mellitus

TNF-α, *see* Tumor necrosis factor-α

Transcription factor 7-like 2 (TCF7L2), gene variants in diabetes type 2 149, 150

Transient neonatal diabetes mellitus (TNDM), genetic variation 151, 152

Transient receptor potential vanilloid-1+ (TRPV1+), pancreatic sensory neuron control of beta cell stress and islet inflammation 111

TRH, *see* Thyrotropin-releasing hormone

Triiodothyronine, *see* Thyroid hormone

Triptorelin, idiopathic early puberty management 166

TRPV1+, *see* Transient receptor potential vanilloid-1+

TS, *see* Turner syndrome

TSH, *see* Thyroid-stimulating hormone

Tudor domain containing protein 6 (TDRD6), autoimmune polyendocrine syndrome type 1 autoantigen 7

Tumor necrosis factor-α (TNF-α), follicle-stimulating hormone response and bone function 55, 56

Turner syndrome (TS)
growth hormone therapy effects on aortic distensability and distension 165, 166
self-esteem and social adjustment in young women 77
Turner Syndrome Consensus Study Group guidelines 76, 77
X chromosome parental origin and clinical significance 78

U

UCP-2, *see* Uncoupling protein-2

Uncoupling protein-2 (UCP-2), triiodothyronine interactions in feeding regulation 20, 21